Functional Polymers as Innovative Tools in the Delivery of Antimicrobial Agents

Functional Polymers as Innovative Tools in the Delivery of Antimicrobial Agents

Editor

Umile Gianfranco Spizzirri

MDPI • Basel • Beijing • Wuhan • Barcelona • Belgrade • Manchester • Tokyo • Cluj • Tianjin

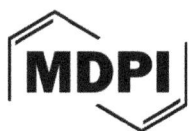

Editor
Umile Gianfranco Spizzirri
University of Calabria
Italy

Editorial Office
MDPI
St. Alban-Anlage 66
4052 Basel, Switzerland

This is a reprint of articles from the Special Issue published online in the open access journal *Pharmaceutics* (ISSN 1999-4923) (available at: https://www.mdpi.com/si/pharmaceutics/polymer_antimicrobial).

For citation purposes, cite each article independently as indicated on the article page online and as indicated below:

LastName, A.A.; LastName, B.B.; LastName, C.C. Article Title. *Journal Name* **Year**, *Volume Number*, Page Range.

ISBN 978-3-0365-3621-7 (Hbk)
ISBN 978-3-0365-3622-4 (PDF)

© 2022 by the authors. Articles in this book are Open Access and distributed under the Creative Commons Attribution (CC BY) license, which allows users to download, copy and build upon published articles, as long as the author and publisher are properly credited, which ensures maximum dissemination and a wider impact of our publications.

The book as a whole is distributed by MDPI under the terms and conditions of the Creative Commons license CC BY-NC-ND.

Contents

About the Editor vii

Umile Gianfranco Spizzirri
Functional Polymers as Innovative Tools in the Delivery of Antimicrobial Agents
Reprinted from: *Pharmaceutics* **2022**, *14*, 487, doi:10.3390/pharmaceutics14030487 1

Valentina Laverde-Rojas, Yamil Liscano, Sandra Patricia Rivera-Sánchez, Ivan Darío Ocampo-Ibáñez, Yeiston Betancourt, Maria José Alhajj, Cristhian J. Yarce, Constain H. Salamanca and Jose Oñate-Garzón
Antimicrobial Contribution of Chitosan Surface-Modified Nanoliposomes Combined with Colistin against Sensitive and Colistin-Resistant Clinical *Pseudomonas aeruginosa*
Reprinted from: *Pharmaceutics* **2021**, *13*, 41, doi:10.3390/pharmaceutics13010041 5

Joana Stokniene, Lydia C. Powell, Olav A. Aarstad, Finn L. Aachmann, Philip D. Rye, Katja E. Hill, David W. Thomas and Elaine L. Ferguson
Bi-Functional Alginate Oligosaccharide–Polymyxin Conjugates for Improved Treatment of Multidrug-Resistant Gram-Negative Bacterial Infections
Reprinted from: *Pharmaceutics* **2020**, *12*, 1080, doi:10.3390/pharmaceutics12111080 19

Maria Antonia Tănase, Adina Raducan, Petruţa Oancea, Lia Mara Diţu, Miruna Stan, Cristian Petcu, Cristina Scomoroşcenco, Claudia Mihaela Ninciuleanu, Cristina Lavinia Nistor and Ludmila Otilia Cinteza
Mixed Pluronic—Cremophor Polymeric Micelles as Nanocarriers for Poorly Soluble Antibiotics—The Influence on the Antibacterial Activity
Reprinted from: *Pharmaceutics* **2021**, *13*, 435, doi:10.3390/pharmaceutics13040435 41

Beatriz Ideriha Mathiazzi and Ana Maria Carmona-Ribeiro
Hybrid Nanoparticles of Poly (Methyl Methacrylate) and Antimicrobial Quaternary Ammonium Surfactants
Reprinted from: *Pharmaceutics* **2020**, *12*, 340, doi:10.3390/pharmaceutics12040340 63

Xiaojing Liu, Jingfu Jia, Shulei Duan, Xue Zhou, Anya Xiang, Ziling Lian and Fahuan Ge
Zein/MCM-41 Nanocomposite Film Incorporated with Cinnamon Essential Oil Loaded by Modified Supercritical CO_2 Impregnation for Long-Term Antibacterial Packaging
Reprinted from: *Pharmaceutics* **2020**, *12*, 169, doi:10.3390/pharmaceutics12020169 83

Gustavo Carreño, Adolfo Marican, Sekar Vijayakumar, Oscar Valdés, Gustavo Cabrera-Barjas, Johanna Castaño and Esteban F. Durán-Lara
Sustained Release of Linezolid from Prepared Hydrogels with Polyvinyl Alcohol and Aliphatic Dicarboxylic Acids of Variable Chain Lengths
Reprinted from: *Pharmaceutics* **2020**, *12*, 982, doi:10.3390/pharmaceutics12100982 95

Yin Wang and Hui Sun
Polymeric Nanomaterials for Efficient Delivery of Antimicrobial Agents
Reprinted from: *Pharmaceutics* **2021**, *13*, 2108, doi:10.3390/pharmaceutics13122108 113

Umile Gianfranco Spizzirri, Francesca Aiello, Gabriele Carullo, Anastasia Facente and Donatella Restuccia
Nanotechnologies: An Innovative Tool to Release Natural Extracts with Antimicrobial Properties
Reprinted from: *Pharmaceutics* **2021**, *13*, 230, doi:10.3390/pharmaceutics13020230 141

Urška Jančič and Selestina Gorgieva
Bromelain and Nisin: The Natural Antimicrobials with High Potential in Biomedicine
Reprinted from: *Pharmaceutics* **2022**, *14*, 76, doi:10.3390/pharmaceutics14010076 . . . . **173**

About the Editor

Umile Gianfranco Spizzirri received his degree in chemistry cum laude in 2001, and his PhD in 2005 from the University of Calabria. In 2004 he was a visiting researcher at the University of Texas at Austin (USA). He is currently a member of the Department of Pharmacy, Health and Nutrition Science at the University of Calabria. His research activities are mainly related to polymer chemistry for the preparation of stimuli-responsive drug delivery systems, polymers with tailored biological activity for biomedical applications, and functional polymers for the food industry. He is an author and co-author of 137 publications, including research and review articles as well as invited book chapters (more than 3500 total citations, and an H-index of 35).

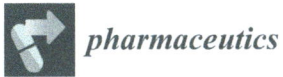

Editorial

Functional Polymers as Innovative Tools in the Delivery of Antimicrobial Agents

Umile Gianfranco Spizzirri

Department of Pharmacy, Health and Nutritional Sciences, University of Calabria, 87036 Rende, Italy; g.spizzirri@unical.it; Tel.: +39-0984-493298

Citation: Spizzirri, U.G. Functional Polymers as Innovative Tools in the Delivery of Antimicrobial Agents. *Pharmaceutics* **2022**, *14*, 487. https://doi.org/10.3390/pharmaceutics14030487

Received: 18 February 2022
Accepted: 21 February 2022
Published: 23 February 2022

Publisher's Note: MDPI stays neutral with regard to jurisdictional claims in published maps and institutional affiliations.

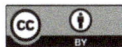

Copyright: © 2022 by the author. Licensee MDPI, Basel, Switzerland. This article is an open access article distributed under the terms and conditions of the Creative Commons Attribution (CC BY) license (https://creativecommons.org/licenses/by/4.0/).

Ubiquitous microorganisms such as bacteria, viruses, algae, and fungi induce several infectious diseases, representing crucial health challenges worldwide, due to increased antimicrobial resistance, high antimicrobial cost and adverse effects. The association between the growth of resistance mechanisms and the progress of new antimicrobial molecules is of great concern to public health. Therefore, it is important to consider innovative ways to face this resistance problem, such as the application of nanotechnologies, which are interesting alternatives to traditional antibiotic development approaches [1]. In the last decade, to overcome these issues and to successfully fight infections, new macromolecular carriers able to significantly improve the efficiency of antimicrobial species were proposed [2]. In this regard, antimicrobial delivery systems, properly entrapping these bioactive molecules, avoid their degradation by also decreasing the frequency of their administration [3]. This Special Issue explores different topics concerning recent progresses in the synthesis and characterization of suitable innovative macromolecular systems, proposed as carriers of specific antimicrobial molecules, to be employed in the biomedical and pharmaceutical fields.

Nowadays, the treatment of infections produced by multidrug-resistant bacteria expects as a last resort the employment of polymyxins, a potent class of peptide antibiotics. In order to overcome the limitations related to the nephro- and neurotoxicity of these compounds and to improve their antimicrobial activity and target specificity, several novel polymyxin derivatives are being developed, involving structural modifications of the peptides [4]. In this regard, conjugation to water-soluble polymers provides many advantages, such as sustained plasma half-life and reduced toxicity [5]. Nanoliposomes coated with highly deacetylated chitosan and colistin were prepared and characterized using dynamic light scattering and zeta potential measurements [6]. The antimicrobial activity of these formulations increased by four-fold against *P. aeruginosa*, but did not have any antimicrobial activity against multidrug-resistant bacteria. Alternatively, a low-molecular-weight alginate oligosaccharide, able to inhibit bacterial growth, adherence and biofilm development, and which potentiates the activity of antibiotics against Gram-negative multidrug-resistant pathogens, was proposed to create a bi-functional antibiotic polymer [7]. Hydroxyl and carboxyl functional groups in this oligosaccharide were successfully employed to prepare a colistin-based adduct that, combining the antimicrobial properties of both the antibiotics, was able to inhibit multidrug-resistant species, as well as Gram-negative *P. aeruginosa*, both in in vitro and in vivo experiments.

Alternatively, advanced micellar carriers were proposed for the encapsulation of norfloxacin, one of the most-used antibiotics from the class of fluoroquinolones, showing antibacterial activity against both Gram-positive and Gram-negative bacteria, and used to treat a large variety of urinary or respiratory tract infections [8]. Specifically, novel polymeric micelles based on Pluronic F127 and Cremophor EL were investigated as drug carriers for norfloxacin, exhibiting good activity against *S. aureus*, *E. faecalis*, and *E. coli*, while *P. aeruginosa* displayed low sensitivity to norfloxacin in all tested systems [9].

The involvement of nanoparticles in the preparation of new effective carriers to deliver antimicrobial agents was also deeply investigated [10]. This Special Issue explored the possibility of employing poly (methyl methacrylate) nanoparticles as carriers of microbicides, such as quaternary ammonium surfactants. In particular, antibacterial performances of the synthesized carriers, based on cetyl trimethyl ammonium bromide or dioctadecyl dimethyl ammonium bromide and poly (methyl methacrylate), were analyzed [11]. Antimicrobial properties were assessed by viability curves of *E. coli*, *S. aureus* and *C. albicans*. Significant inhibition against bacteria and yeast was observed only for cetyl trimethyl ammonium bromide, while dioctadecyl dimethyl ammonium bromide just displayed fungicidal activity against *C. albicans*.

Encapsulating antimicrobial species into nanoparticles and incorporating these nanoparticles with bio-based film to fabricate nanocomposite films represents an innovative and effective strategy to control the release of the active molecules. Specifically, a long-term antibacterial film nanocomposite composed by zein film and cinnamon essential oil-loaded MCM-41 silica nanoparticles was evaluated against *S. aureus* [12]. The results clearly highlighted that the addition of silica nanoparticles significantly improve the mechanical properties of zein films, prolonging, at the same time, the antibacterial effect of the cinnamon essential oil.

Alternatively, hydrogels appear to be excellent candidates as antibiotic delivery platforms slowing down the progression of bacterial resistance to antibiotics [13]. In this context, Carreno et al. (2020) proposed hydrophilic macromolecular systems synthesized by cross-linking polyvinyl alcohol and aliphatic dicarboxylic acids, such as glutaric acid, adipic acid or succinic acid to specific release linezolid, a chemotherapeutic agent able to treat bacterial resistance accepted for the treatment of complex skin infections [14]. The antibacterial tests against *E. faecium* bacterial strain confirmed that the sustained release of linezolid from a glutaric acid-based hydrogel showed the best antibacterial activity.

This Special Issue was completed by three reviews providing an overall view on the use of nanotechnology in the transport and release of antimicrobial molecules. In particular, Wang et al. (2021) analyzed the recent advances in the highly efficient delivery of antimicrobial agents by polymeric nanomaterials such as dendrimers, micelles, nanofibers, nanogels and vesicles [15]. The authors concluded that the versatility of the polymeric nanomaterials provided several benefits, showing significant potential in a wide variety of biomedical applications, such as fighting multidrug-resistant bacteria, wound healing and anti-biofilm. On the contrary, the other two reviews focused their attention on the delivery of specific antimicrobial agents. Spizzirri et al. (2021) discussed the most innovative strategies to synthesize nanodevices able to release antimicrobial natural extracts originating from herbs, plants, and agro-food waste by-products [16]. Finally, Jancic and Gorgieva highlighted the structure and properties of plant origin bromelain and antimicrobial peptide nisin, analyzing their mechanisms of action and the immobilization strategies involving macromolecular systems, in order to expand their application in the pharmaceutical and biomedical fields [17].

In conclusion, the challenges for the large-scale fabrication and translation from the bench to clinical trials of these polymeric systems to fight the multidrug resistance of several dangerous pathogens will represent a major focus in the coming decades. However, to overcome this issue, novelty from chemists and engineers, as well as regulatory policies able to simplify access to trials and patients are required.

Funding: This research received no external funding.

Conflicts of Interest: The author declares no conflict of interest.

References

1. Rubey, K.M.; Brenner, J.S. Nanomedicine to fight infectious disease. *Adv. Drug Deliv. Rev.* **2021**, *179*, 113996. [CrossRef] [PubMed]
2. Contera, S.; De La Serna, J.B.; Tetley, T.D. Biotechnology, nanotechnology and medicine. *Emerg. Top. Life Sci.* **2020**, *4*, 551–554. [PubMed]

3. Birk, S.E.; Boisen, A.; Nielsen, L.H. Polymeric nano- and microparticulate drug delivery systems for treatment of biofilms. *Adv. Drug Deliv. Rev.* **2021**, *174*, 30–52. [CrossRef] [PubMed]
4. Kanazawa, K.; Sato, Y.; Ohki, K.; Okimura, K.; Uchida, Y.; Shindo, M.; Sakura, N. Contribution of each amino acid residue in polymyxin B3 to antimicrobial and lipopolysaccharide binding activity. *Chem. Pharm. Bull.* **2009**, *57*, 240–244. [CrossRef] [PubMed]
5. Azzopardi, E.A.; Ferguson, E.L.; Thomas, D.W. The enhanced permeability retention effect: A new paradigm for drug targeting in infection. *J. Antimicrob. Chemother.* **2013**, *68*, 257–274. [CrossRef] [PubMed]
6. Laverde-Rojas, V.; Liscano, Y.; Rivera-Sánchez, S.P.; Ocampo-Ibáñez, I.D.; Betancourt, Y.; Alhajj, M.J.; Yarce, C.J.; Salamanca, C.H.; Oñate-Garzón, J. Antimicrobial contribution of chitosan surface-modified nanoliposomes combined with colistin against sensitive and colistin-resistant clinical *Pseudomonas aeruginosa*. *Pharmaceutics* **2021**, *13*, 41. [CrossRef] [PubMed]
7. Stokniene, J.; Powell, L.C.; Aarstad, O.A.; Aachmann, F.L.; Rye, P.D.; Hill, K.E.; David, T.W.; Ferguson, E.L. Bi-functional alginate oligosaccharide-polymyxin conjugates for improved treatment of multidrug-resistant gram-negative bacterial infections. *Pharmaceutics* **2020**, *12*, 1080. [CrossRef] [PubMed]
8. Faccendini, A.; Ruggeri, M.; Miele, D.; Rossi, S.; Bonferoni, M.C.; Aguzzi, C.; Grisoli, P.; Viseras, C.; Vigani, B.; Sandri, G.; et al. Norfloxacin-loaded electrospun scaffolds: Montmorillonite nanocomposite vs. free drug. *Pharmaceutics* **2020**, *12*, 325. [CrossRef] [PubMed]
9. Tanase, M.A.; Raducan, A.; Oancea, P.; Ditu, L.M.; Stan, M.; Petcu, C.; Scomoroscenco, C.; Ninciuleanu, C.M.; Nistor, C.L.; Cinteza, L.O. Mixed pluronic—Cremophor polymeric micelles as nanocarriers for poorly soluble antibiotics—The Influence on the antibacterial activity. *Pharmaceutics* **2021**, *13*, 435. [CrossRef] [PubMed]
10. Sanna, V.; Lubinu, G.; Madau, P.; Pala, N.; Nurra, S.; Mariani, A.; Sechi, M. Polymeric nanoparticles encapsulating white tea extract for nutraceutical application. *J. Agric. Food Chem.* **2015**, *63*, 2026–2032. [CrossRef] [PubMed]
11. Mathiazzi, B.I.; Carmona-Ribeiro, A.M. Hybrid nanoparticles of poly (methyl methacrylate) and antimicrobial quaternary ammonium surfactants. *Pharmaceutics* **2020**, *12*, 340. [CrossRef] [PubMed]
12. Liu, X.; Jia, J.; Duan, S.; Zhou, X.; Xiang, A.; Lian, Z.; Ge, F. Zein/MCM-41 nanocomposite film incorporated with cinnamon essential oil loaded by modified supercritical CO_2 impregnation for long-term antibacterial packaging. *Pharmaceutics* **2020**, *12*, 169. [CrossRef] [PubMed]
13. Forero-Doria, O.; Polo, E.; Marican, A.; Guzmán, L.; Venegas, B.; Vijayakumar, S.; Wehinger, S.; Guerrero, M.; Gallego, J.; Durán-Lara, E.F. Supramolecular hydrogels based on cellulose for sustained release of therapeutic substances with antimicrobial and wound healing properties. *Carbohydr. Polym.* **2020**, *242*, 116383. [CrossRef] [PubMed]
14. Carreño, G.; Marican, A.; Vijayakumar, S.; Valdés, O.; Cabrera-Barjas, G.; Castaño, J.; Durán-Lara, E.F. Sustained release of linezolid from prepared hydrogels with polyvinyl alcohol and aliphatic dicarboxylic acids of variable chain lengths. *Pharmaceutics* **2020**, *12*, 982. [CrossRef] [PubMed]
15. Wang, Y.; Sun, H. Polymeric nanomaterials for efficient delivery of antimicrobial agents. *Pharmaceutics* **2021**, *13*, 2108. [CrossRef] [PubMed]
16. Spizzirri, U.G.; Aiello, F.; Carullo, G.; Facente, A.; Restuccia, D. Nanotechnologies: An innovative tool to release natural extracts with antimicrobial properties. *Pharmaceutics* **2021**, *13*, 230. [CrossRef] [PubMed]
17. Jancic, U.; Gorgieva, S. Bromelain and nisin: The natural antimicrobials with high potential in biomedicine. *Pharmaceutics* **2022**, *14*, 76. [CrossRef] [PubMed]

Article

Antimicrobial Contribution of Chitosan Surface-Modified Nanoliposomes Combined with Colistin against Sensitive and Colistin-Resistant Clinical *Pseudomonas aeruginosa*

Valentina Laverde-Rojas [1], Yamil Liscano [2], Sandra Patricia Rivera-Sánchez [2,3], Ivan Darío Ocampo-Ibáñez [2], Yeiston Betancourt [2], Maria José Alhajj [4], Cristhian J. Yarce [4], Constain H. Salamanca [4,*] and Jose Oñate-Garzón [2,*]

1. Facultad de Salud, Programa de Medicina, Universidad Santiago de Cali, Calle 5 No. 62-00, Cali 760035, Colombia; valentina.laverde00@usc.edu.co
2. Facultad de Ciencias Básicas, Programa de Microbiología, Universidad Santiago de Cali, Calle 5 No. 62-00, Cali 760035, Colombia; yamil.liscano00@usc.edu.co (Y.L.); sandra.rivera04@usc.edu.co (S.P.-S.); ivan.ocampo00@usc.edu.co (I.D.O.-I.); yeiston.betancourt00@usc.edu.co (Y.B.)
3. Laboratorio de Salud Pública Departamental, Secretaria Departamental de Salud del Valle del Cauca, Gobernación del Valle del Cauca, Cali 760045, Colombia
4. Laboratorio de Diseño y Formulación de Productos Químicos y Derivados, Departamento de Ciencias Farmacéuticas, Facultad de Ciencias Naturales, Universidad Icesi, Cali 760035, Colombia; mariajoalhajj@hotmail.com (M.J.A.); cjyarce@icesi.edu.co (C.J.Y.)
* Correspondence: chsm70@gmail.com (C.H.S.); jose.onate00@usc.edu.co (J.O.-G.); Tel.: +57-2-5183900 (J.O.-G.)

Abstract: Colistin is a re-emergent antibiotic peptide used as a last resort in clinical practice to overcome multi-drug resistant (MDR) Gram-negative bacterial infections. Unfortunately, the dissemination of colistin-resistant strains has increased in recent years and is considered a public health problem worldwide. Strategies to reduce resistance to antibiotics such as nanotechnology have been applied successfully. In this work, colistin was characterized physicochemically by surface tension measurements. Subsequently, nanoliposomes coated with highly deacetylated chitosan were prepared with and without colistin. The nanoliposomes were characterized using dynamic light scattering and zeta potential measurements. Both physicochemical parameters fluctuated relatively to the addition of colistin and/or polymer. The antimicrobial activity of formulations increased by four-fold against clinical isolates of susceptible *Pseudomona aeruginosa* but did not have antimicrobial activity against multidrug-resistant (MDR) bacteria. Interestingly, the free coated nanoliposomes exhibited the same antibacterial activity in both sensitive and MDR strains. Finally, the interaction of colistin with phospholipids was characterized using molecular dynamics (MD) simulations and determined that colistin is weakly associated with micelles constituted by zwitterionic phospholipids.

Keywords: colistin; nanoliposomes; MDR-Bacteria; chitosan

1. Introduction

Colistin (CST) is an antimicrobial peptide that was reintroduced into clinical practice as a last resort for the treatment of infections caused by multi-drug resistant (MDR) Gram-negative bacteria [1]. CST is a cyclic heptapeptide consisting of a tripeptide side-chain acylated at the N terminus by a fatty acid tail and has a cationic charge at neutral pH [2]. This antibiotic has been used to control and prevent infectious diseases in animals for decades, but its excessive use has contributed to the emergence of CST-resistant Enterobacteriaceae [3,4], and possibly to the horizontal transmission of CST resistance from farm animals to humans [5]. The plasmid-mediated resistance to CST via carriage *mcr-1* was first described in 2016 [6], and has been propagated throughout several countries, becoming a serious public health problem, especially with the coexistence of other resistance genes such as Extended spectrum beta-lactamases (ESBL) and New Delhi metallo-beta-lactamase (NDM) [7]. Therefore, this situation poses a major challenge for the treatment of life-threatening Gram-negative bacterial infections.

Pseudomona aeruginosa is an opportunistic pathogen that causes life-threatening infections, such as sepsis and pneumonia [8]. It is frequently found in hospital settings and uses several mechanisms of natural resistance to multiple antibiotics. In this respect, infections caused by MDR clinical isolates of *P. aeruginosa* have increased patient mortality and morbidity in intensive care units [8]. Therefore, MDR strains of *P. aureginosa* resistant to CST is a serious risk to human health that must be urgently addressed. In fact, *P. aeruginosa* is categorized as priority 1 in the list of bacteria for which new antibiotics are urgently needed, according to the World Health Organization (WHO) [9].

The disproportionate relationship between the emergence and dissemination of resistance mechanisms and the development of new molecules with antimicrobial properties is of great concern to public health. Therefore, it is important to consider innovative ways to face this resistance problem, such as the application of nanotechnology, which is an interesting alternative to usual antibiotic development approaches [10–13]. In an in vitro study, the resistance of methicillin-resistant *Staphylococcus aureus* (MRSA) strains to ampicillin loaded inside Eudragit® polymer-coated nanoliposomes was markedly decreased [14], suggesting that the antimicrobial properties of the Eudragit® polymer contributed synergistically to the effect of the ampicillin. On the other hand, Chitosan is a biocompatible, biodegradable and non-toxic linear cationic biopolymer obtained from the deacetylation of chitin under alkaline conditions [15]. Chitosan is a polymer of interest for the development of nanoparticle-based drug delivery, which was approved as generally recognized as safe (GRAS) by the US Food and Drug Administration (US FDA) [16]. The degree of deacetylation and the molecular weight of chitosan affect its physicochemical properties and consequently its biological activity. For example, highly deacetylated chitosan is more biologically active than chitin and less deacetylated chitosan [17].

Molecular dynamics simulations provide valuable and reliable information about the interaction of peptides with membrane models [18,19], which is useful to understand the behavior of CST in relation to liposomal systems. An advantage of using micelles as opposed to lipid bilayers is the faster time scales of motion of dodecylphosphocholine (DPC) lipids [20]. The interaction of the peptide with the lipid macromolecular assembly induces a much faster response in micelles as opposed to bilayers and captures the essential features that modulate the peptide–membrane interaction [20].

Therefore, we evaluated the antimicrobial effect of the peptide CST in the presence of self-assembling nanosystems. The stages of the study were—(i) isolation of MDR clinical isolates of *P. aeruginosa* and their phenotypic characterization, (ii) characterization of CST in solution using in silico and experimental methods, (iii) development and characterization of liposomal nanosystems, and (iv) antimicrobial evaluation of the CST combined with highly deacetylated (>90%) chitosan-coated nanoliposomes against both susceptible and MDR clinical isolates of *P. aureginosa*.

2. Materials and Methods

2.1. Certified Bacterial Strains and Chemicals

P. aeruginosa ATCC® 27853 ™ was obtained from the American Type Culture Collection (ATCC; Rockville, MD, USA). Muller Hinton Cation-Adjusted Broth and Colistin Sulfate were purchased from Merck (Darmstadt, Germany). Cholesterol and dioleoyl phosphatidyl ethanolamine (DOPE) were obtained from Avanti Polar Lipids (Alabaster, AL, USA). Soy lecithin (Medick) was purchased from a local pharmacy (Cali-Colombia) and characterized in a recent study [21]. Chitosan with a deacetylation degree of >90% (MW = 477 KDa) was provided by the Laboratory of Design and Formulation of Chemicals and Derivatives of the Icesi University [22].

2.2. Isolation of Resistant P. aeruginosa and Phenotypic Characterization

Three MDR clinical isolates of *P. aureginosa* encoded as Pa01MDR, Pa02MDR, and Pa03MDR, and one antibiotic susceptible *P. aureginosa* clinical isolate (Pawt) were evaluated in this study. The antibiotic susceptibility, phenotypic characterization of the resistance of clinical isolates, and the minimal inhibitory concentration (MIC) for each antibiotic were confirmed using the VITEK® 2 Antimicrobial Susceptibility Testing card (VITEK® N272 -AST) in the VITEK® system 2 (Ref. 414164, Biomerieux), according to the clinical cut-off points defined by the Clinical Laboratory Standards Institute (CLSI) [23]. The antimicrobial agents used in the phenotypical characterization included piperacillin/tazobactam (TZP), ceftazidime (CAZ), Cefepim (FEP), Doripenem (DOR), Imipenem (IPM), Meropenem (MEM), Amikacin (AMK), Gentamicin (GEN), Ciprofloxacin (CIP), and Colistin (CST), were evaluated. The resistance to CST was confirmed by performing a broth macrodilution test in glass tubes and the in vitro MIC was determined according to the clinical breakpoints defined by the CLSI [24]. The *P. aeruginosa* ATCC® 27853 ™ strain was used as a reference strain.

2.3. Surface Tension Measurements

Measurement of CST surface tension was carried out using a surface tension meter (OCA15EC Dataphysics Instruments, Filderstadt, Germany) with the appropriate driver software (version 4.5.14 SCA22). The capture of the suspended droplet was recorded using an IDS video camera [25] and the solutions were prepared using dilutions from 5 mg/mL of reconstituted colistin with ultrapure water and phosphate-buffered saline at pH 7.2 (PBS, 138 mM NaCl, 3 mM KCl, 1.5 mM NaH_2PO_4, 8.1 mM Na_2HPO_4).

2.4. Chitosan-Coated Liposome Combined with CST

2.4.1. Preparation of the Chitosan-Coated Liposomes with CST

The liposomes were constructed using the ethanol injection method [25]. Briefly, the organic phase (ethanolic solutions of washed soy lecithin, cholesterol, and DOPE with a ratio of 3:3:1, respectively) was added to the aqueous phase (CST, 100 μg/mL in PBS). Equal volumes were used for the aqueous and organic phases. The resulting mixture was vortexed for one minute to form the liposomes. Then, the liposomal suspension was diluted in ultrapure water at a proportion of 1:4. Later, 1 mL of an aqueous solution of chitosan (1×10^{-4} M, pH = 7.0) with a degree of deacetylation >90% was added to 1 mL of the liposomal dispersion free and combined with CST at a rate of 50 μL/min. Finally, the mixture was left under constant magnetic stirring at 300 rpm for 8 h in a closed polypropylene beaker.

2.4.2. Physicochemical Characterization of Liposomal Systems

The particle size and zeta potential of the liposomes were determined using a Zetasizer Nano ZSP (Malvern Instrument, Cestershire, UK) with an He/Ne red laser (633 nm). The particle size was measured by dynamic light scattering (DLS) using a quartz flow cell (ZEN0023) and applying a light scattering angle from 173° to 25°. On the other hand, the zeta potential was measured using a disposable folded capillary cell (DTS1070). The instrument reports the particle size as the mean particle diameter (z-average), and the polydispersity index (PDI) ranges from 0 (monodisperse) to 1 (very wide distribution). All measurements were performed in triplicate after dilution of the freshly prepared liposome suspension in ultrapure water at a ratio of 5: 5000 *v/v*.

2.5. Molecular Dynamics of Colistin and Nanoliposomes

2.5.1. Construction of the Colistin 3D Structure

The SDF 2D structure of CST (Polymyxin E) was obtained from the Pubchem database (https://pubchem.ncbi.nlm.nih.gov/compound/5311054). The 3D structure of CST was constructed using Avogadro version 1.2 (https://avogadro.cc/) optimized with General Amber Force Field (GAFF) and steepest descent algorithm to obtain a PDB file for molecular dynamics (MD) [26,27].

2.5.2. CST in Aqueous Solution and Construction of CST inside of DPC Micelles

The CHARMM-GUI platform [28] was used to develop a micelle hydrated system consisting of 100 units of phospholipid DPC surrounding CST. DPC monolayers were constructed to visualize and understand the stability of one molecule of CST inside the micelle. GROMACS software version 2019.3 (University of Groningen, Groningen, The Netherlands) was used for molecular dynamics simulation [29]. The ion Monte Carlo method was used with 0.15 M NaCl, with a water thickness of 22.5 Å and CHARMM36m as a forcefield, which is suitable for describing the distribution of molecules within large systems such as micelles [30]. CST parametrization was performed with a CHARMM-GUI PDB reader [31] using par_all36_prot_lipid.prm. The behavior of CST in aqueous solution and inside of the micelle was compared.

2.5.3. Minimization Energy, Equilibration and MD

To ensure the absence of steric clashes between the CST and the micelle, the system was adjusted by heating to a temperature of 310 K at 1 fs (femtosecond)/step for 75 ps (picoseconds), relaxing the structure by energy minimization for 300 ps at a rate of 2 fs/step. The energy minimization of the system was obtained with the steepest descent algorithm (tolerance value of 1000 kJ·mol^{-1} nm^{-1}) in 5000 steps. The Berendsen algorithm was used to equilibrate the temperature and pressure of the system. After the system equilibration, the MD was run for data collection during 10 ns, using the Nose–Hoover and Parrinello–Rahman algorithms to adjust the temperature and pressure. The particle mesh Ewald summation was applied to handle the long-range electrostatic interactions [32].

2.5.4. MD and Interaction Analysis

The software VMD (Visual Molecular Dynamics, University of Illinois, Chicago, IL, USA) was used to visualize the simulation [33]. In order to determine the root mean square deviation (RMSD) and the hydrogen bond formation between colistin and the model system, a simulation analysis was performed using gromacs. Finally, the interactions were manually analyzed using Discovery Studio Visualizer version Client 2020 (https://discover.3ds.com/discovery-studio-visualizer-download) and Ligplot+ [34].

2.6. Antimicrobial Activity

The antimicrobial susceptibility was assessed through a broth macrodilution test in glass tubes following the suggestions proposed by the CLSI [23]. The clinical isolates of *P. aeruginosa* previously characterized as susceptible and resistant to CST were incubated at 37 °C for 18–24 h on Brain Heart Infusion (BHI) agar. One colony was initially resuspended in sterile water to reach a turbidity of 0.5 McFarland (approximately 1–4 × 10^8 colony forming units (CFU)/mL). The bacterial suspension was then diluted with Mueller–Hinton broth adjusted with cations to reach a concentration of approximately 2–7 × 10^5 CFU/mL. Subsequently, 1 mL of bacterial suspension and 1 mL of free CST were mixed in a glass tube using serial concentrations from 256 to 0.25 µg/mL and incubated at 37 °C for 18 h. For CST combined with nanoliposomes, the same volumes and the same incubation conditions were used, but the initial concentration of CST was adjusted to 64 µg/mL to be diluted in half to 0.25 µg/mL. PBS was used as a negative control and the ATCC strain was used as a reference to ensure reproducibility of the assays. After incubation, the MIC was determined by visual analysis. Assays were performed in triplicate.

3. Results and Discussion

3.1. Phenotypic Characterization of Clinical Isolates of MDR P. aeruginosa

The antibiotic susceptibility and resistance profiles of *P. aeruginosa* clinical isolates were constructed using six conventional antimicrobial categories (Table 1). The Pa*01MDR* strain was resistant to penicillin + β-lactamase inhibitor (TZP), to extended-spectrum cephalosporins (CAZ, FEP), to carbapenems (DOR, IPM, and MEM), and to polymyxins (CST), but it was susceptible to aminoglycosides (AMK, GEN) and fluoroquinolones (CIP).

Pa02MDR and Pa03MDR clinical isolates were resistant to all the antibiotics evaluated according to the clinical breakpoints defined by the CLSI guidelines [23].

Table 1. Bacterial resistance profile from phenotypic tests.

Scheme	MIC (µg/mL)									
	TZP	CAZ	FEP	DOR	IPM	MEM	AMK	GEN	CIP	CST
Pa ATCC	≤4/S	≤1/S	≤1/S	≤0.25/S	≤2/S	≤0.25/S	≤2/S	≤1/S	≤0.25/S	≤0.5/S
Pawt	8/S	4/S	2/S	0.5/S	1/S	≤0.25/S	≤2/S	≤1/S	≤0.25/S	≤0.5/S
Pa01MDR	≥128/R	≥64/R	≥64/R	≥8/R	≥16/R	≥16/R	8/S	4/S	0.5/S	≥8/R
Pa02MDR	≥128/R	≥64/R	≥64/R	≥8/R	≥16/R	≥16/R	≥64/R	≥16/R	≥4/R	≥8/R
Pa03MDR	≥128/R	≥64/R	≥64/R	≥8/R	≥16/R	≥16/R	≥64/R	≥16/R	≥4/R	≥8/R

S = Susceptibility strain, R = Resistant strain.

3.2. Surface Tension Measurements

The surface tension at different CST concentrations is shown in Figure 1.

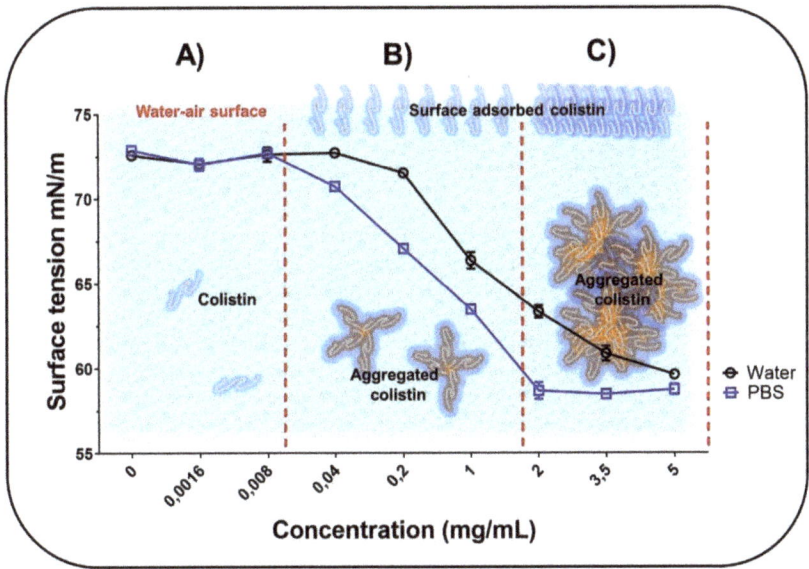

Figure 1. Characterization of the surface tension of Colistin (CST) in aqueous medium at different concentrations ranging from 0 to 0.008 mg/mL (A), from 0.008 to 2 mg/mL (B) and from 2 to 5 mg/mL (C).

The behavior of the surface tension against different concentrations of the CST follows a profile typical of amphiphilic molecules, which is consistent with the structural nature of CST. Besides, at low CST concentrations (<0.008 mg/mL in PBS and <0.04 mg/mL in water), the surface tension tends to remain constant at a typical value of $\sim 73 \times 10^{-3}$ mN/m at 25 °C (Figure 1A). This suggests that at these concentrations, the CST is mainly solubilized within the solution bulk with very few chains in the surface area. However, increasing the peptide concentration from 0.04 to 5 mg/mL in water and from 0.008 to 2 mg/mL in PBS leads to a decrease in surface tension from ~73 to ~60 mN/m and from ~73 to ~59 mN/m, respectively (Figure 1B). Therefore, at such concentrations, CST may begin to localize at the air–water surface, as well as in the solution bulk, where other association effects between the different peptide chains also start to take place, forming CST–CST aggregates. In this form, the peptide acts as a surfactant in an aqueous medium, decreasing the cohesive forces between water molecules located at the interface [35]. Finally, the CST–CST aggregates prevailed at the higher peptide concentrations in water (5 mg/mL) and PBS (2 mg/mL) (Figure 1C). Notably, the CST–CST aggregates were formed at a lower concentration in PBS than in ultrapure water. This may be due to the charge shielding effect generated when the phosphate anions of PBS are attracted to the cationic groups of CST until the peptide is electrically neutralized. Thus, the low polarization of the peptide interface promotes rapid and easy aggregation of CST–CST [36]. Therefore, depending on whether the CST is free or added, it is possible to obtain a greater or lesser antimicrobial effect. However, this mechanism is not fully elucidated, even though the few studies focused on evaluating this type of effect found that free forms have more antimicrobial activity than added forms [37,38].

3.3. Physicochemical Characterization of Liposomal Systems

The characteristics of the uncoated and chitosan-coated liposomal systems in the presence and absence of CST are shown in Figure 2. For the uncoated liposomes, the particle size was 208.7 ± 1.6 nm, which increased considerably to 1610.7 ± 537.0 nm when combined with CST. On the contrary, the free chitosan-coated liposomes had a particle size of 178.3 ± 1.6 nm, while combined with CST they reached 485.0 ± 9.8 nm, showing a compaction effect compared to uncoated liposomes (Figure 2A). Likewise, the PDI of these systems strongly depends on the coating with chitosan and its combination with CST (Figure 2B). The PDI for the uncoated liposomes was 0.217 ± 0.012, but an abrupt increase was observed when they were combined with CST (Figure 2B). In the case of chitosan-coated liposomes, the combination with CST also caused an increase of the PDI from 0.007 ± 0.005 to 0.468 ± 0.017 (Figure 2B). As shown in Figure 2C, the zeta potential was -48.8 ± 3.7 mV for the uncoated liposomes, and it increased to -23.2 ± 1.7 mV when they were combined with CST. This suggests that the positively charged CST locates on the liposomal surface, but the positive charge density is not sufficient to reverse the negative charge contributed by the phosphate groups of the phospholipids. Oppositely, the free chitosan-coated liposomes had a zeta potential of $+13.1 \pm 0.4$ mV, which decreased slightly to $+5.3 \pm 0.3$ mV when they were combined with CST.

All these results can be explained considering that under the methodology used, the liposomes based on lecithin, DOPE, and cholesterol are nanometric, very uniform in size, and with a negative surface potential, as previously described for such systems [14]. However, when these liposomes are coated with highly deacetylated chitosan, a slight size contraction, a greater homogenization of the size populations (to a point of high uniformity), and an inversion of the surface charge occur, indicating that the chitosan is completely deposited on the liposomal surface. These results suggest that the chitosan coating process occurs in a highly organized manner and forms a very well-defined system. Interestingly, there is not an additive effect between the positive charges of chitosan and CST on the zeta potential (Figure 2C), suggesting that there is a competition between both molecules for binding to the liposomal surface. Thus, when chitosan-coated liposomes are combined with CST, the latter would be displaced by chitosan forming a slightly more organized and less polydisperse system (Figure 2D). On the other hand, CST could mediate contacts between liposomes [39] or interacts differently with liposomes leading to increased size and subsequent changes in the aggregation indices of liposomes and to more polydisperse systems, which is consistent with the high dynamism of this peptide, which can form a balance between its chains and aggregates.

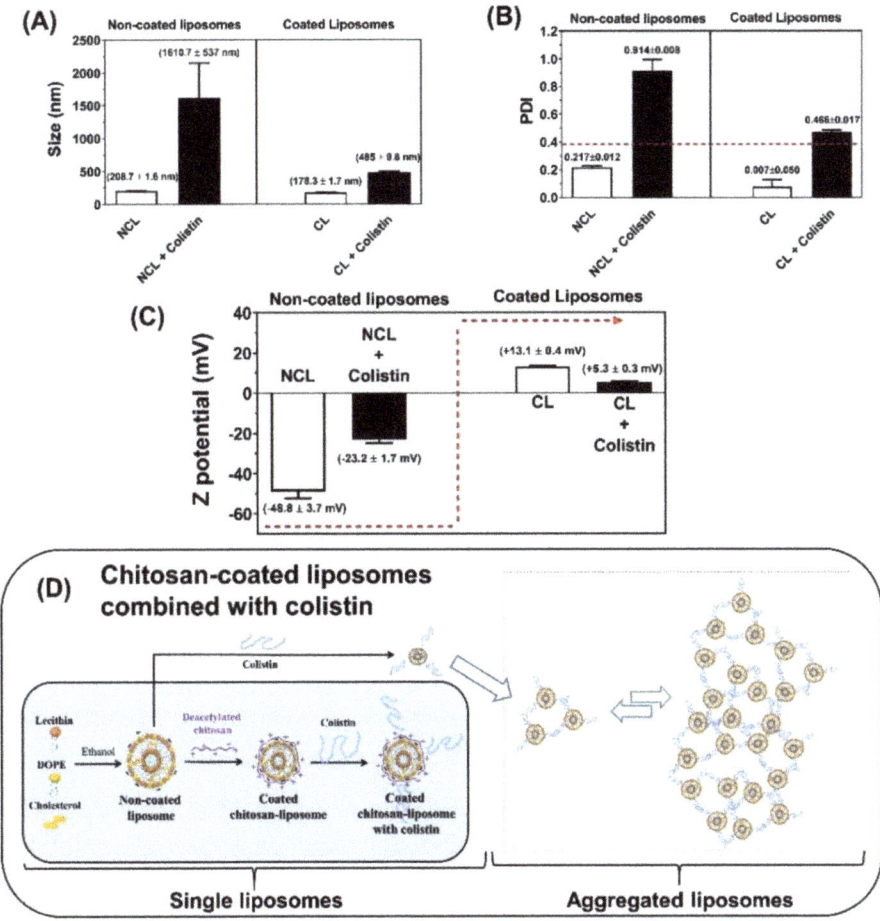

Figure 2. Physicochemical characterization of uncoated and chitosan-coated liposomes in the presence and absence of CST. (**A**) Particle size, (**B**) Polydispersity index-PDI, (**C**) Zeta potential, (**D**) Schematic representation of the liposomal coating process and its interaction with CST. NCL—Non-coated liposomes; CL—coated liposomes.

3.4. Molecular Dynamics of CST Combined with Nanoliposomes

To complement the results obtained in the Section 3.3 and understand how CST interacts with uncoated nanoliposomes, micelle-type aggregation systems were built with DPC phospholipids (which is zwitterionic, like those that constitute nanoliposomal formulations) and the CST was initially placed inside the system. Although the nanosystems built above (Section 2.4.1) are lamellar liposomes, we simulated DPC micelles to elucidate the initial motion of the peptide upon insertion into the membrane because micelles are commonly used as bilayer membrane mimetics to study the interaction protein–membrane [40] and the data obtained from these two systems, bilayers and micelles, can be used in a complementary fashion [41].

After 7 ns, most of the CST comes out of the DPC micelle due to its strong hydrogen bond interaction with the water molecules surrounding the micelle. CST appears at 2 ns (Figure 3B) and is even more visible at 7 ns (Figure 3C). This is consistent with the results shown in Figure 2A,B since it reveals that CST is positioned on the external surface of nanoliposomes, thereby increasing the size and the Z potential value. Although the DPC headgroup carries a highly electronegative phosphate center comprised of four strong hydrogen-bond acceptor oxygen atoms [20], the binding between CST and DPC micelles is reduced.

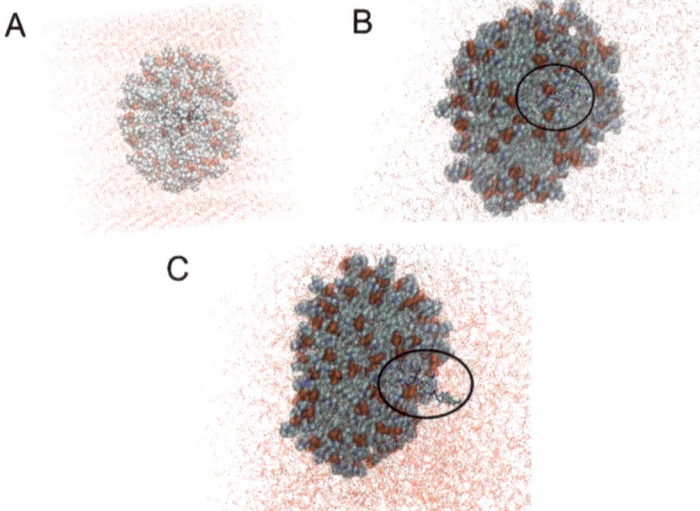

Figure 3. CST interaction with dodecylphosphocholine (DPC) micelle through 10 ns (**A**) DPC Micelle with CST at 0 ns. (**B**) DPC micelle with CST at 2 ns (**C**) DPC micelle with CST at 7 ns. Black circle highlights the CST.

Figure 4A shows the RMSD between CST and the hydrated DPC micelle, and of CST immersed in water only. In the latter, the RMSD varies little, apparently because of the constant formation of hydrogen bonds between CST and water which remains at an average of 33 hydrogen bonds during the 10 ns (Figure 4B). Contrarily, the RMSD of the CST placed inside the micelle shows that it stays in the micelle for 7 ns, and the RMSD increases to approximately 3 nm, suggesting that CST migrates from the micelle core toward the water surrounding the DPC in agreement with what was shown in Figure 3. The number of hydrogen bonds with water molecules increases progressively until it reaches 20 at 7 ns. CST has six L-diaminobutyric acid residues, and five of these can form hydrogen bonds. Also, two threonine residues provide donor and acceptor atoms for the formation of relatively weaker hydrogen bonds.

Interactions between CST and hydrated micelle by hydrogen bonds are shown in Figure 5. At 0 ns, no hydrogen bonds exist between CST and DPC (Figure 5A). The few hydrogen bonds formed are intramolecular for CST as seen in Supplement 1, where a minimal hydrophobic interaction with DPC is observed. The number of hydrogen bonds between CST and DPC remains almost constant, ranging between 7 and 10 interactions from 1 to 7 ns. Conversely, there are no interactions between CST and the water molecules surrounding the micelles at 0 ns, but they increase considerably as time passes (Figure 5B). There were also few hydrophobic interactions between CST and DPC, going from two interactions at 0 ns to one at 7 ns (Table S1), suggesting that the hydrophobic interactions between the acyl chain of CST and the hydrophobic region of the micelle is not enough to compensate the polar interactions between side chains and backbone polar groups of CST with water molecules.

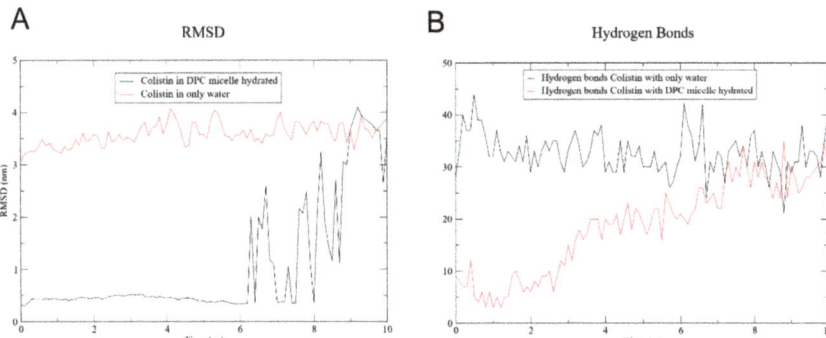

Figure 4. CST molecular dynamics (MD) analysis. (**A**) Root mean square deviation (RMSD) of the DPC micelle with CST and CST in water only. (**B**) Hydrogen bonds of DPC micelle with CST and CST in water only.

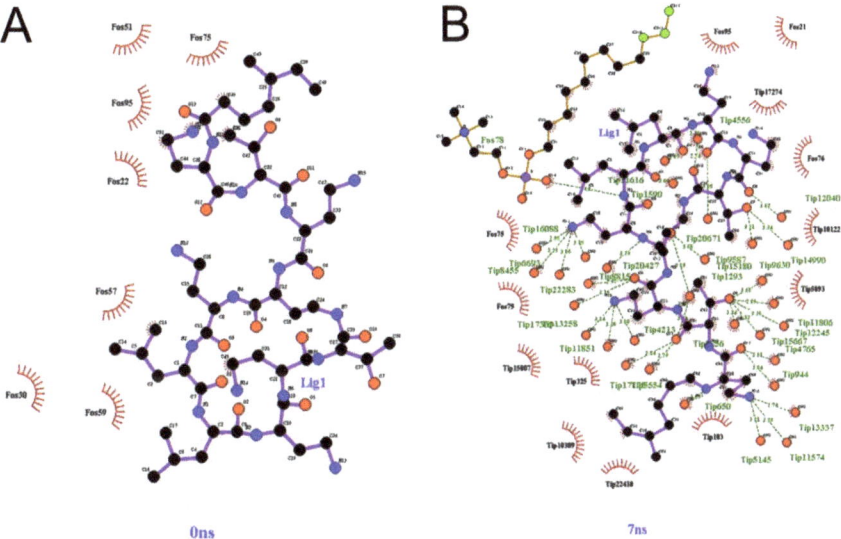

Figure 5. Interaction between CST and DPC micelle hydrated atoms (**A**) at 0 ns. (**B**) At 7ns. Fos: DPC molecule. Lig: CST. Tip: water molecule.

3.5. Antimicrobial Activity

The antibacterial activities of free CST (CST), coated nanoliposome without CST (CL), and coated nanoliposome combined with CST (CL + CST) were evaluated against different susceptible and MDR *P. aeruginosa* clinical isolates (Table 2). CST exhibited a MIC of 2 µg/mL for both Pa ATCC 27853 and Pa*wt*. CST was initially attracted to the bacterial surface because of the electrostatic interaction between the positively charged αγ-diaminobutyric acid residues and the negatively charged phosphate groups of lipid A of lipopolysaccharide (LPS) [42]. There, CST displaces the divalent cations (Ca^{2+} and Mg^{2+}) from the LPS layer, therefore increasing the fluidity and permeability of the membrane, leading to the release of cytoplasmic content and finally cell death [2]. On the other hand, MIC values for MDR clinical isolates ranged between 8 to 16 µg/mL. Resistance to CST is closely related to the loss of its affinity for LPS because of the neutralization of the negative charge of the phosphate groups of LPS by the addition of aminoarabinose and ethanolamine residues [43]. However, even though the surface membrane charge has been reduced, CST still exhibits antimicrobial activity against MDR strains at moderately higher concentrations (Table 2). This is because the membrane of CST-resistant bacteria is still negatively charged [44] due to anionic phospholipids that are exposed on the surface, which could interact electrostatically with cationic CST.

Table 2. Antimicrobial activity (MIC) of CST, CST-free coated nanoliposomes (CL) and CST-coated nanoliposomes (CL + CST) against sensitive and multidrug resistant (MDR) strains of *P. aeruginosa*.

Strain	MIC (µg/mL)		
	CST	CL + CST	CL *
Pa ATCC 27853	2	0.5	5.96
Pa*wt*	2	0.5	5.96
Pa01MDR	8	8	5.96
Pa02MDR	16	16	5.96
Pa03MDR	8	8	5.96

* Final chitosan concentration coating the nanoliposomes.

CL + CST reduced the MIC in susceptible strains by four-fold (Table 2). This antimicrobial contribution against *P. aeruginosa* is provided by highly deacetylated chitosan as reported in previous studies [22,45]. To explain these results, two hypotheses could be proposed—(i) cationic chitosan and CST may interact with the membrane simultaneously since both can be attracted by the anionic charge of the membrane [42,45,46]. This way, the destabilizing effect that chitosan adds to the effect of CST on the membrane could explain the decrease in MIC; (ii) while CST acts on the membrane, chitosan could penetrate the cell wall and membrane and travel to the nucleus where it could interfere with mRNA synthesis, causing a decrease in MIC [47].

However, CL + CST did not increase the antimicrobial effect of CST on MDR strains (Table 2). This can be explained according to the results obtained by the physicochemical characterization of the nanoliposomes and by the MD simulations (Figures 2 and 3) where the localization of chitosan and colistin outside of the nanosystem was revealed. In this way, several cationic CST molecules remain in solution because they would not be attracted by the neutralized LPS of MDR strains [43], and thus, the cationic charge of CST would not be neutralized by the phosphate groups of LPS, unlike with susceptible strains. Therefore, in the CL + CST system, both cationic molecules CST and chitosan compete with each other as seen in Figure 2C, preventing the latter from encountering the bacteria because of electrostatic repulsion with CST and avoiding an additive antimicrobial effect, in contrast to that observed in sensitive strains.

Interestingly, the nanoliposome coated with high degree deacetylated chitosan without CST (CL) showed antimicrobial activity in the third dilution equivalent to 1.25×10^{-5} M (5.96 µg/mL) (Table 2). A previous study reported an approximate MIC of chitosan with a degree of deacetylation of >90% against *P. aeruginosa* [45]. Our results suggests that chitosan has a similar antimicrobial effect in all strains regardless of the resistance level to CST and therefore, the decrease in the anionic charge magnitude of the bacterial surface by LPS modification in CST-resistant strains does not affect the antibacterial function of this polymer. In addition, the antibacterial effect of highly deacetylated chitosan is not altered by the presence of β-lactamases, carbapenemases, or by structural changes in prokaryotic ribosome and DNA gyrase. Studies have reported that chitosan exhibits a membranolytic effect against MDR bacteria [48,49], a consistent approach considering that the cell membrane remains anionic despite resistance to colistin [44], therefore, both sensitive and MDR strains could electrostatically attract chitosan to the surface. However, recent evidence revealed that chitosan penetrates the cell membrane of *P. aeruginosa*, releasing the cell contents and aggregating the residue cytoplasmic material into a mass. It was presumed that the cytoplasmic material was agglomerated by flocculation of chitosan after entering the cell [50], an effect that would overcome the resistance mechanisms mentioned above. Finally, so far, this finding could mean highly deacetylated chitosan is a potential antimicrobial agent to use against CST-resistant MDR strains.

4. Conclusions

CST behaves differently in water or PBS buffer, depending on its concentration. At low concentrations, it is solubilized in the bulk while at higher concentrations it behaves in two specific ways. First, it decreases the surface tension due to its adsorption at the air–aqueous medium interface. Second, it aggregates within the solution, establishing a condition of high dynamism between the aggregated and non-aggregated forms.

The liposomes have a homogeneous nanometric size and with negative zeta potentials, and when they are combined with the coating polymers (chitosan), they form more compact and homogeneous systems, but with positive zeta potential. Conversely, the combination of liposomal systems with CST leads to the formation of larger and more polydisperse systems, suggesting a random interaction between the liposomal surface (coated and uncoated) and the peptide. This result agrees with those obtained with in silico studies, which show that CST has a greater tropism towards the external aqueous medium than towards phospholipids. Based on this, we assume that CST amounts are in equilibrium between the internal and external environment of the nanoliposome. We will confirm this hypothesis in later studies using in silico lamellar systems.

Finally, combining CST with coated nanoliposomes increased its antimicrobial activity by four-fold against sensitive *P. aeruginosa* but did not make any contribution against MDR strains. Interestingly, coated nanoliposomes without CST exhibited the same antimicrobial activity in susceptible and MDR strains. Thus, this polymer is considered a potential antibiotic that should be further explored against MDR *P. aeruginosa*.

Supplementary Materials: The following are available online at https://www.mdpi.com/1999-4923/13/1/41/s1, Table S1: Interactions between colistin and micelle hydrated system at 0 ns and 7 ns. LIG: colistin; H: hydrogen; O: oxygen; TIP: water; C: carbon.

Author Contributions: V.L.-R. performed the pendant drop methodology, built and characterizes liposomal systems and performed antimicrobial activity against sensitive bacteria. Y.L. performed the modeling of the interaction between colistin and micelles. Y.B., I.D.O.-I. and S.P.R.-S. collected the MDR strains and determined the antibacterial activity of the nanoformulations. M.J.A. and C.J.Y. contributed to the development, characterization and analysis of results of liposomal systems. C.H.S. and J.O.-G. designed the study, analyzed the results and wrote the manuscript. All authors have read and agreed to the published version of the manuscript.

Funding: This research was funded by the Universidad Santiago de Cali, grant number DGI-COCEIN No 512-621120-1529, and the APC of the open access journal was funded by the Universidad Santiago de Cali.

Institutional Review Board Statement: Not applicable.

Informed Consent Statement: Not applicable.

Data Availability Statement: There are not limitations in the Data Availability Statement.

Acknowledgments: The authors thank the Universidad Santiago de Cali, Universidad Icesi and Secretaría de Salud Pública del Valle del Cauca.

Conflicts of Interest: The authors declare no conflict of interests.

References

1. Van der Weide, H.; Vermeulen-de Jongh, D.M.C.; van der Meijden, A.; Boers, S.A.; Kreft, D.; ten Kate, M.T.; Falciani, C.; Pini, A.; Strandh, M.; Bakker-Woudenberg, I.A.J.M.; et al. Antimicrobial activity of two novel antimicrobial peptides AA139 and SET-M33 against clinically and genotypically diverse Klebsiella pneumoniae isolates with differing antibiotic resistance profiles. *Int. J. Antimicrob. Agents* **2019**, *54*, 159–166. [CrossRef]
2. Poirel, L.; Jayol, A.; Nordmanna, P. Polymyxins: Antibacterial activity, susceptibility testing, and resistance mechanisms encoded by plasmids or chromosomes. *Clin. Microbiol. Rev.* **2017**, *30*, 557–596. [CrossRef]
3. Boyen, F.; Vangroenweghe, F.; Butaye, P.; De Graef, E.; Castryck, F.; Heylen, P.; Vanrobaeys, M.; Haesebrouck, F. Disk prediffusion is a reliable method for testing colistin susceptibility in porcine *E. coli* strains. *Vet. Microbiol.* **2010**, *144*, 359–362. [CrossRef]

4. Kieffer, N.; Poirel, L.; Nordmann, P.; Madec, J.Y.; Haenni, M. Emergence of colistin resistance in Klebsiella pneumoniae from veterinary medicine. *J. Antimicrob. Chemother.* **2014**, *70*, 1265–1267. [CrossRef]
5. Olaitan, A.O.L.; Thongmalayvong, B.; Akkhavong, K.; Somphavong, S.; Paboriboune, P.; Khounsy, S.; Morand, S.; Rolain, J.M. Clonal transmission of a colistin-resistant *Escherichia coli* from a domesticated pig to a human in Laos. *J. Antimicrob. Chemother.* **2015**, *70*, 3402–3404.
6. Liu, Y.Y.; Wang, Y.; Walsh, T.R.; Yi, L.X.; Zhang, R.; Spencer, J.; Doi, Y.; Tian, G.; Dong, B.; Huang, X.; et al. Emergence of plasmid-mediated colistin resistance mechanism MCR-1 in animals and human beings in China: A microbiological and molecular biological study. *Lancet Infect. Dis.* **2016**, *16*, 161–168. [CrossRef]
7. Baron, S.; Hadjadj, L.; Rolain, J.M.; Olaitan, A.O. Molecular mechanisms of polymyxin resistance: Knowns and unknowns. *Int. J. Antimicrob. Agents* **2016**, *48*, 583–591. [CrossRef]
8. Abd El-Baky, R.M.; Masoud, S.M.; Mohamed, D.S.; Waly, N.G.F.M.; Shafik, E.A.; Mohareb, D.A.; Elkady, A.; Elbadr, M.M.; Hetta, H.F. Prevalence and some possible mechanisms of colistin resistance among multidrug-resistant and extensively drug-resistant pseudomonas aeruginosa. *Infect. Drug Resist.* **2020**, *13*, 323–332. [CrossRef]
9. WHO Publishes List of Bacteria for Which New Antibiotics are Urgently Needed. Available online: https://www.who.int/news-room/detail/27-02-2017-who-publishes-list-of-bacteria-for-which-new-antibiotics-are-urgently-needed (accessed on 16 August 2020).
10. Fernando, S.; Gunasekara, T.; Holton, J. Antimicrobial Nanoparticles: Applications and mechanisms of action. *Sri Lankan J. Infect. Dis.* **2018**, *8*, 2–11. [CrossRef]
11. Wang, L.; Hu, C.; Shao, L. The antimicrobial activity of nanoparticles: Present situation and prospects for the future. *Int. J. Nanomed.* **2017**, *12*, 1227–1249. [CrossRef]
12. Kumar, M.; Curtis, A.; Hoskins, C. Application of Nanoparticle Technologies in the Combat against Anti-Microbial Resistance. *Pharmaceutics* **2018**, *10*, 11. [CrossRef]
13. Salamanca, C.H.; Yarce, C.J.; Roman, Y.; Davalos, A.F.; Rivera, G.R. Application of nanoparticle technology to reduce the anti-microbial resistance through β-lactam antibiotic-polymer inclusion nano-complex. *Pharmaceuticals* **2018**, *11*, 19. [CrossRef]
14. Arévalo, L.M.; Yarce, C.J.; Oñate-Garzón, J.; Salamanca, C.H. Decrease of antimicrobial resistance through polyelectrolyte-coated nanoliposomes loaded with β-lactam drug. *Pharmaceuticals* **2019**, *12*, 1. [CrossRef]
15. Kean, T.; Thanou, M. Biodegradation, biodistribution and toxicity of chitosan. *Adv. Drug Deliv. Rev.* **2010**, *62*, 3–11. [CrossRef]
16. Garg, U.; Chauhan, S.; Nagaich, U.; Jain, N. Current advances in chitosan nanoparticles based drug delivery and targeting. *Adv. Pharm. Bull.* **2019**, *9*, 195–204. [CrossRef]
17. Kumirska, J.; Weinhold, M.X.; Czerwicka, M.; Kaczyski, Z.; Bychowska, A.; Brzozowski, K.; Thming, J.; Stepnowski, P. Influence of the Chemical Structure and Physicochemical Properties of Chitin- and Chitosan-Based Materials on Their Biomedical Activity. In *Biomedical Engineering, Trends in Materials Science*; Laskovski, A., Ed.; InTech: London, UK, 2011; pp. 25–64. ISBN 978-953-307-513-6.
18. Aragón-Muriel, A.; Ausili, A.; Sánchez, K.; Rojasa, O.E.; Mosquera, J.L.; Polo-Cerón, D.; Oñate-Garzón, J. Studies on the interaction of alyteserin 1c peptideand its cationic analogue with model membranes imitating mammalian and bacterial membranes. *Biomolecules* **2019**, *9*, 527. [CrossRef]
19. Liscano, Y.; Salamanca, C.H.; Vargas, L.; Cantor, S.; Laverde-Rojas, V.; Oñate-Garzón, J. Increases in hydrophilicity and charge on the polar face of alyteserin 1c helix change its selectivity towards gram-positive bacteria. *Antibiotics* **2019**, *8*, 238. [CrossRef] [PubMed]
20. Khandelia, H.; Kaznessis, Y.N. Molecular dynamics simulations of the helical antimicrobial peptide ovispirin-1 in a zwitterionic dodecylphosphocholine micelle: Insights into host-cell toxicity. *J. Phys. Chem. B* **2005**, *109*, 12990–12996. [CrossRef] [PubMed]
21. Yarce, C.J.; Alhajj, M.J.; Sanchez, J.D.; Oñate-Garzón, J.; Salamanca, C.H. Development of Antioxidant-Loaded Nanoliposomes Employing Lecithins with Different Purity Grades. *Molecules* **2020**, *25*, 5344. [CrossRef] [PubMed]
22. Ciro, Y.; Rojas, J.; Oñate-Garzon, J.; Salamanca, C.H. Synthesis, characterisation and biological evaluation of ampicillin-chitosan-polyanion nanoparticles produced by ionic gelation and polyelectrolyte complexation assisted by high-intensity sonication. *Polymers* **2019**, *11*, 1758. [CrossRef] [PubMed]
23. CLSI. *Performance Standards for Antimicrobial Susceptibility Testing*, 29th ed.; CLSI Supplement M100; Clinical and Laboratory Standars Institute: Wayne, PA, USA, 2019.
24. Turlej-Rogacka, A.; Xavier, B.B.; Janssens, L.; Lammens, C.; Zarkotou, O.; Pournaras, S.; Goossens, H.; Malhotra-Kumar, S. Evaluation of colistin stability in agar and comparison of four methods for MIC testing of colistin. *Eur. J. Clin. Microbiol. Infect. Dis.* **2018**, *37*, 345–353. [CrossRef] [PubMed]
25. Yarce, C.; Vargas, L.; Salamanca, C.; Cantor, S.; Rojas, A.O.; Oñate-Garzón, J. Evaluation of the Antimicrobial Activity of Cationic Peptides Loaded in Surface-Modified Nanoliposomes against Foodborne Bacteria. *Int. J. Mol. Sci.* **2019**, *20*, 680.
26. Wang, J.; Wolf, R.M.; Caldwell, J.W.; Kollman, P.A.; Case, D.A. Development and testing of a general Amber force field. *J. Comput. Chem.* **2004**, *25*, 1157–1174. [CrossRef] [PubMed]
27. Hanwell, M.D.; Curtis, D.E.; Lonie, D.C.; Vandermeerschd, T.; Zurek, E.; Hutchison, G.R. Avogadro: An advanced semantic chemical editor, visualization, and analysis platform. *J. Cheminform.* **2012**, *4*, 17. [CrossRef] [PubMed]
28. Jo, S.; Kim, T.; Iyer, V.G.; Im, W. CHARMM-GUI: A web-based graphical user interface for CHARMM. *J. Comput. Chem.* **2008**, *29*, 1859–1865. [CrossRef]

29. Abraham, M.J.; Murtola, T.; Schulz, R.; Páll, S.; Smith, J.C.; Hess, B.; Lindah, E. Gromacs: High performance molecular simulations through multi-level parallelism from laptops to supercomputers. *SoftwareX* **2015**, *1–2*, 19–25. [CrossRef]
30. Huang, J.; Mackerell, A.D. CHARMM36 all-atom additive protein force field: Validation based on comparison to NMR data. *J. Comput. Chem.* **2013**, *34*, 2135–2145. [CrossRef]
31. Jo, S.; Cheng, X.; Islam, S.M.; Huang, L.; Rui, H.; Zhu, A.; Lee, H.S.; Qi, Y.; Han, W.; Vanommeslaeghe, K.; et al. CHARMM-GUI PDB manipulator for advanced modeling and simulations of proteins containing nonstandard residues. *Adv. Protein Chem. Struct. Biol.* **2014**, *96*, 235–265.
32. Petersen, H.G. Accuracy and efficiency of the particle mesh Ewald method. *J. Chem. Phys.* **1995**, *103*, 3668–3679. [CrossRef]
33. Humphrey, W.; Dalke, A.; Schulten, K. VMD: Visual molecular dynamics. *J. Mol. Graph.* **1996**, *14*, 33–38. [CrossRef]
34. Laskowski, R.A.; Swindells, M.B. LigPlot+: Multiple ligand-protein interaction diagrams for drug discovery. *J. Chem. Inf. Model.* **2011**, *51*, 2778–2786. [CrossRef] [PubMed]
35. Shchukin, E.D.; Amelina, E.A. Surface modification and contact interaction of particles. *J. Dispers. Sci. Technol.* **2003**, *24*, 377–395. [CrossRef]
36. Sudhölter, E.J.R.; Engberts, J.B.F.N. Salt effects on the critical micellar concentration, iodide counterion binding, and surface micropolarity of 1-methyl-4-dodecylpyridinium iodide micelles. *J. Phys. Chem.* **1979**, *83*, 1854–1859. [CrossRef]
37. Lee, D.L.; Mant, C.T.; Hodges, R.S. A novel method to measure self-association of small amphipathic molecules: Temperature profiling in reversed-phase chromatography. *J. Biol. Chem.* **2003**, *278*, 22918–22927. [CrossRef] [PubMed]
38. Chen, Y.; Mant, C.T.; Farmer, S.W.; Hancock, R.E.; Vasil, M.L.; Hodges, R.S. Rational design of alpha-helical antimicrobial peptides with enhanced activities and specificity/therapeutic index. *J. Biol. Chem.* **2005**, *280*, 12316–12329. [CrossRef] [PubMed]
39. Cajal, Y.; Rogers, J.; Berg, O.G.; Jain, M.K. Intermembrane molecular contacts by polymyxin B mediate exchange of phospholipids. *Biochemistry* **1996**, *35*, 299–308. [CrossRef]
40. Cheng, X.; Kim, J.K.; Kim, Y.; Bowie, J.U.; Im, W. Molecular dynamics simulation strategies for protein-micelle complexes. *Biochim. Biophys. Acta Biomembr.* **2016**, *1858*, 1566–1572. [CrossRef]
41. Franzin, C.M.; Teriete, P.; Marassi, F.M. Structural similarity of a membrane protein in micelles and membranes. *J. Am. Chem. Soc.* **2007**, *129*, 8078–8079. [CrossRef]
42. Morrison, D.C.; Jacobs, D.M. Binding of polymyxin B to the lipid A portion of bacterial lipopolysaccharides. *Immunochemistry* **1976**, *13*, 813–818. [CrossRef]
43. Olaitan, A.O.; Morand, S.; Rolain, J.M. Mechanisms of polymyxin resistance: Acquired and intrinsic resistance in bacteria. *Front. Microbiol.* **2014**, *5*, 1–18. [CrossRef]
44. Soon, R.L.; Nation, R.L.; Cockram, S.; Moffatt, J.H.; Harper, M.; Adler, B.; Boyce, J.D.; Larson, I.; Li, J. Different surface charge of colistin-susceptible and -resistant Acinetobacter baumannii cells measured with zeta potential as a function of growth phase and colistin treatment. *J. Antimicrob. Chemother.* **2011**, *66*, 126–133. [CrossRef] [PubMed]
45. Je, J.Y.; Kim, S.K. Chitosan derivatives killed bacteria by disrupting the outer and inner membrane. *J. Agric. Food Chem.* **2006**, *54*, 6629–6633. [CrossRef] [PubMed]
46. Sahariah, P.; Másson, M. Antimicrobial Chitosan and Chitosan Derivatives: A Review of the Structure-Activity Relationship. *Biomacromolecules* **2017**, *18*, 3846–3868. [CrossRef] [PubMed]
47. Rabea, E.I.; Badawy, M.E.T.; Stevens, C.V.; Smagghe, G.; Steurbaut, W. Chitosan as antimicrobial agent: Applications and mode of action. *Biomacromolecules* **2003**, *4*, 1457–1465. [CrossRef] [PubMed]
48. Park, S.C.; Nam, J.P.; Kim, J.H.; Kim, Y.M.; Nah, J.W.; Jang, M.K. Antimicrobial action of water-soluble β-chitosan against clinical multi-drug resistant bacteria. *Int. J. Mol. Sci.* **2015**, *16*, 7995–8007. [CrossRef] [PubMed]
49. Hoque, J.; Adhikary, U.; Yadav, V.; Samaddar, S.; Konai, M.M.; Prakash, R.G.; Paramanandham, K.; Shome, B.R.; Sanyal, K.; Haldar, J. Chitosan Derivatives Active against Multidrug-Resistant Bacteria and Pathogenic Fungi: In Vivo Evaluation as Topical Antimicrobials. *Mol. Pharm.* **2016**, *13*, 3578–3589. [CrossRef]
50. Ju, X.; Chen, J.; Zhou, M.; Zhu, M.; Li, Z.; Gao, S.; Ou, J.; Xu, D.; Wu, M.; Jiang, S.; et al. Combating Pseudomonas aeruginosa Biofilms by a Chitosan-PEG-Peptide Conjugate via Changes in Assembled Structure. *ACS Appl. Mater. Interfaces* **2020**, *12*, 13731–13738. [CrossRef]

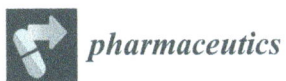

Article

Bi-Functional Alginate Oligosaccharide–Polymyxin Conjugates for Improved Treatment of Multidrug-Resistant Gram-Negative Bacterial Infections

Joana Stokniene [1,*], Lydia C. Powell [1], Olav A. Aarstad [2], Finn L. Aachmann [2], Philip D. Rye [3], Katja E. Hill [1], David W. Thomas [1] and Elaine L. Ferguson [1]

1. Advanced Therapies Group, School of Dentistry, College of Biomedical and Life Sciences, Cardiff University, Heath Park, Cardiff CF14 4XY, UK; l.c.powell@swansea.ac.uk (L.C.P.); hillke1@cardiff.ac.uk (K.E.H.); thomasdw2@cardiff.ac.uk (D.W.T.); fergusonel@cardiff.ac.uk (E.L.F.)
2. Norwegian Biopolymer Laboratory (NOBIPOL), Department of Biotechnology and Food Sciences, NTNU Norwegian University of Science and Technology, 7491 Trondheim, Norway; olav.a.aarstad@ntnu.no (O.A.A.); finn.l.aachmann@ntnu.no (F.L.A.)
3. AlgiPharma AS, 1337 Sandvika, Norway; phil.rye@algipharma.com
* Correspondence: stoknienej@cardiff.ac.uk; Tel.: +44-(0)2922-510663

Received: 19 October 2020; Accepted: 9 November 2020; Published: 11 November 2020

Abstract: The recent emergence of resistance to colistin, an antibiotic of last resort with dose-limiting toxicity, has highlighted the need for alternative approaches to combat infection. This study aimed to generate and characterise alginate oligosaccharide ("OligoG")–polymyxin (polymyxin B and E (colistin)) conjugates to improve the effectiveness of these antibiotics. OligoG–polymyxin conjugates (amide- or ester-linked), with molecular weights of 5200–12,800 g/mol and antibiotic loading of 6.1–12.9% w/w, were reproducibly synthesised. In vitro inflammatory cytokine production (tumour necrosis factor alpha (TNFα) ELISA) and cytotoxicity (3-(4,5-dimethylthiazol-2-yl)-2,5-diphenyltetrazolium bromide (MTT) of colistin (2.2–9.3-fold) and polymyxin B (2.9–27.2-fold) were significantly decreased by OligoG conjugation. Antimicrobial susceptibility tests (minimum inhibitory concentration (MIC), growth curves) demonstrated similar antimicrobial efficacy of ester- and amide-linked conjugates to that of the parent antibiotic but with more sustained inhibition of bacterial growth. OligoG–polymyxin conjugates exhibited improved selectivity for Gram-negative bacteria in comparison to mammalian cells (approximately 2–4-fold). Both OligoG–colistin conjugates caused significant disruption of *Pseudomonas aeruginosa* biofilm formation and induced bacterial death (confocal laser scanning microscopy). When conjugates were tested in an in vitro "time-to-kill" (TTK) model using *Acinetobacter baumannii*, only ester-linked conjugates reduced viable bacterial counts (~2-fold) after 4 h. Bi-functional OligoG–polymyxin conjugates have potential therapeutic benefits in the treatment of multidrug-resistant (MDR) Gram-negative bacterial infections, directly reducing toxicity whilst retaining antimicrobial and antibiofilm activities.

Keywords: gram-negative bacteria; multidrug resistance; polymer therapeutics; colistin; polymyxin B

1. Introduction

Antimicrobial resistance (AMR) is a significantly growing global challenge that is associated with elevated morbidity and mortality rates, high healthcare costs and >700,000 deaths annually [1,2]. Excessive use of antibiotics in animal husbandry, agriculture, and human and veterinary medicine has contributed to a dramatic increase in life-threatening multi- and pan-drug resistant bacterial infections [3]. This environmental exposure has been compounded by decreases in the development of novel antimicrobials and it has been predicted that AMR could result in 10 million annual deaths by 2050 [4]. According to the World Health Organisation (WHO), Gram-negative bacteria such as carbapenem-resistant *Pseudomonas aeruginosa* and *Acinetobacter baumannii*, extended spectrum β-lactamase-producing and carbapenem-resistant *Klebsiella pneumoniae* and *Escherichia coli* represent a major clinical threat and burden to public health [5]. It has been estimated that Gram-negative bacterial resistance resulted in 960,000 hospital admission days in Europe in 2017 [6].

Polymyxins (Scheme 1), such as polymyxin B and colistin (polymyxin E), are a potent class of polypeptide antibiotics. Despite the clinical efficacy of colistin against Gram-negative bacteria, it is recommended for employment as an antibiotic of last resort, both to avoid resistance and, importantly, due to dose-limiting nephro- and neurotoxicity [7]. To reduce this toxicity and optimise antimicrobial activity, drug absorption and target specificity, several novel derivatives of polymyxin antibiotics are being developed [8–11]. Structural modifications have involved the N-terminal fatty acyl moiety or Dab side chains and demonstrated the importance of Dab at residue five in antimicrobial activity [12]. Progression to clinical trials of these polymyxin derivatives has, however, been limited due to their narrow spectrum of antimicrobial activity, and their cytotoxicity/poor tolerability in animal studies [13].

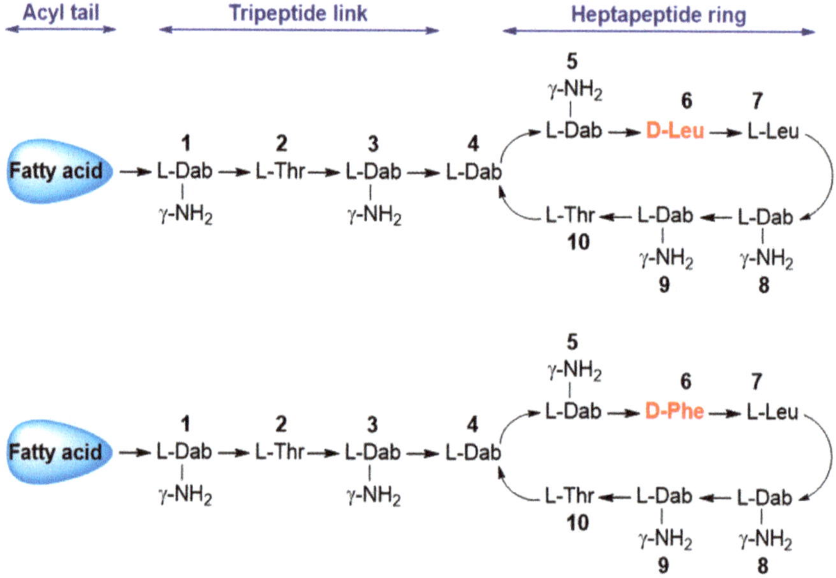

Scheme 1. Graphic structure of (**a**) colistin and (**b**) polymyxin B. The hydrophilic heptapeptide ring is linked to a hydrophobic acyl tail through a tripeptide fragment. The only structural difference between both molecules is an amino acid residue at position 6: D-leucine in colistin is replaced by D-phenylalanine in polymyxin B. Composition of the fatty acyl tail: 6-methyloctanoic acid for polymyxin B1/E1 and 6-methylheptanoic acid for polymyxin B2/E2.

Polymer therapeutics have emerged as a promising strategy to combat antimicrobial resistance, particularly when used to reinstate "old" antibiotics [14]. Conjugation of an antibiotic to a water-soluble polymer offers many advantages compared to small molecule drugs, including reduced toxicity/immunogenicity, prolonged plasma half-life and improved pharmacodynamic targeting through the enhanced permeability and retention (EPR) effect [15]. Colistin has previously been conjugated to both, dextrin [16] and poly(ethylene glycol) (PEG) [17], however, complete restoration of antibiotic activity was not achieved after amylase-unmasking of dextrin–colistin conjugates, presumably due to the presence of oligosaccharides attached to the colistin amine groups [18]. The use of alternative conjugation chemistry may offer the opportunity to optimise reinstatement of antibiotic activity at sites of infection/inflammation [19]. Moreover, conjugation of the antibiotic to bioactive polysaccharides affords the opportunity to deliver anti-infective bi-functional polymer therapeutics.

Although alginates, like dextrin, are recognised as non-toxic by the Food and Drug Administration (FDA), their large molecular weight and lack of mammalian, alginate-degrading enzymes has limited their use in protein/peptide conjugation. More recently, a low molecular weight alginate oligosaccharide (OligoG, Mn 3200 g/mol), was extracted as a sodium salt from marine algae (*Laminaria hyperborea*) with >85% of residues being composed of α-L-guluronic acid. Although OligoG has no (MIC) value, it inhibits bacterial growth, adherence and biofilm development, and potentiates the activity of antibiotics against Gram-negative MDR pathogens [20–24]. This low molecular weight alginate also possesses hydroxyl and carboxyl functional groups that can be used for drug conjugation.

We hypothesised that conjugation of guluronic-rich, low molecular weight alginates to antibiotics, such as polymyxins, could create a bi-functional antibiotic polymer therapeutic [25]; combining the antimicrobial properties of both the antibiotic and the alginate, while simultaneously reducing systemic toxicity of the antibiotic, and facilitating size-dependent targeting by the EPR effect at the site of infection. Polymyxins were chosen as a model drug because previous studies have demonstrated that OligoG can enhance the antimicrobial efficacy of colistin against MDR, Gram-negative *P. aeruginosa* both in vitro and in vivo [26].

The aim of the study was to generate and characterise a bi-functional polymyxin conjugate using OligoG to optimise the antimicrobial function of these last resort antibiotics. A range of OligoG-polymyxin conjugates were synthesised and their physicochemical properties, in vitro cytotoxicity and biological activity characterised. Antimicrobial activity was assessed using MIC assays, growth curves, confocal laser scanning microscopy (CLSM) imaging and "time-to-kill" (TTK) studies.

2. Materials and Methods

2.1. Materials

OligoG CF-5/20 and the high molecular weight alginate PRONOVA UP MVG (>60% guluronic acid and Mw of 200,000 g/mol) were provided by AlgiPharma AS (Sandvika, Norway). The LIVE/DEAD® Baclight™ Bacterial Viability kit was from Invitrogen Molecular Probes (Paisley, UK). Pullulan gel filtration standards were from Polymer Laboratories (Church Stretton, UK). All chemicals were obtained from either Fisher Scientific (Loughborough, UK) or Sigma-Aldrich (Poole, UK) unless otherwise stated and were of analytical grade.

2.2. Cell Lines and Cell Culture

Human kidney proximal tubule cells (HK-2) were obtained from the American Type Culture Collection (ATCC) (Manassas, VA, USA) and screened to be free of mycoplasma contamination before use. Keratinocyte serum-free (K-SFM) medium (with L-glutamine), bovine pituitary extract (BPE, 0.05 mg/mL), human recombinant epidermal growth factor (EGF, 5 ng/mL), 0.05% *w/v* trypsin-0.53 mM ethylenediaminetetraacetic acid (EDTA) were from Invitrogen Life Technologies (Paisley, UK).

2.3. Bacterial Isolates and Growth Media

The bacterial strains (Table S1) used have been previously described [20,27]. Bacteria were grown on either tryptone soy agar (TSA) or blood agar (BA) plates supplemented with 5% *v/v* defibrinated horse blood. Bacterial overnight cultures were grown in tryptone soy (TS) broth and Mueller–Hinton (MH) broth was used for susceptibility testing. All media were from LabM (Bury, UK). Artificial sputum (AS) medium was prepared as previously described by Pritchard et al. [24].

2.4. Synthesis of OligoG–Polymyxin Conjugates

To synthesise amide (A)-linked conjugates (Scheme 2a), OligoG (1000 mg, 0.3 mmol), 1-ethyl-3-(3-dimethylaminopropyl) carbodiimide hydrochloride (EDC; 96.8 mg, 0.5 mmol) and

N-hydroxysulfosuccinimide (sulfo-NHS; 109.6 mg, 0.5 mmol) were dissolved under stirring (15 min at 21 °C) in distilled water (dH$_2$O; 10 mL). To this, colistin sulphate (146.7 mg, 0.1 mmol) or polymyxin B (144.4 mg, 0.1 mmol) was added followed by drop-wise addition of NaOH (0.5 M) until pH 8 was reached. The reaction mixture was stirred for 2 h at 21 °C, then stored at −20 °C prior to purification.

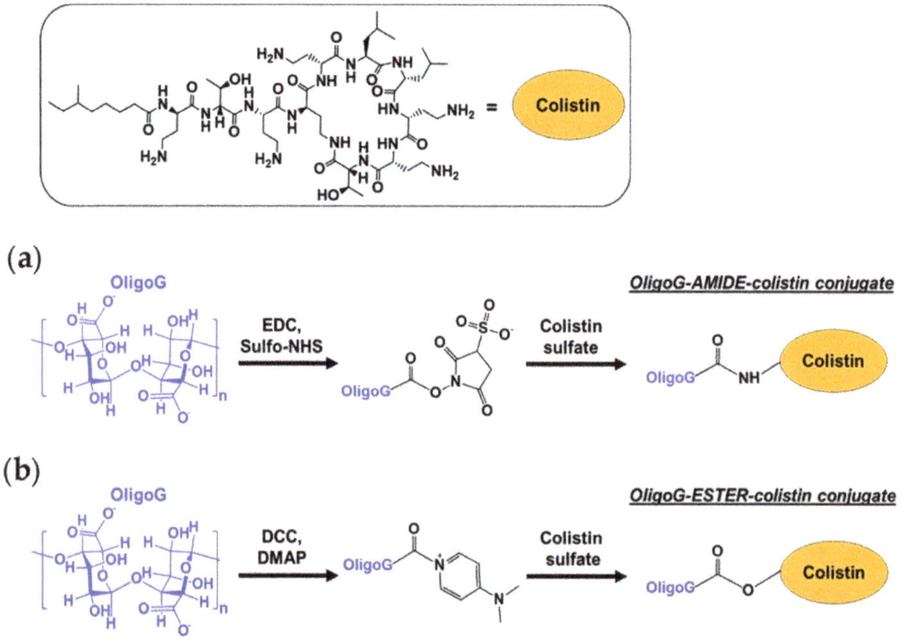

Scheme 2. Schematic showing steps in the synthesis of the OligoG–colistin conjugate. (**a**) Using an amide linker (OligoG–A–colistin conjugate). (**b**) Using an ester linker (OligoG–E–colistin conjugate).

To synthesise ester (E)-linked conjugates (Scheme 2b), OligoG (1000 mg, 0.3 mmol), N,N′-dicyclohexyl carbodiimide (DCC; 64.5 mg, 0.3 mmol), 4-dimethylaminopyridine (DMAP; 6.4 mg, 0.05 mmol) and colistin sulphate (146.7 mg, 0.1 mmol) or polymyxin B (144.4 mg, 0.1 mmol) were dissolved while stirring overnight at 21 °C in anhydrous DMSO (10 mL). The reaction was stopped by pouring the mixture into excess chloroform (~100 mL). Formed precipitates were collected by filtration and dissolved in dH$_2$O (10 mL), then stored at −20 °C prior to purification.

2.5. Purification of OligoG–Polymyxin Conjugates

OligoG–polymyxin conjugates were purified from the reaction mixture by fast protein liquid chromatography (FPLC) using an AKTA Purifier system (GE Healthcare; Amersham, UK) connected to a prepacked Superdex 75 16/600 GL column with a UV detector and a fraction collector (Frac-950). Data analysis was performed using Unicorn 5.31 software (2011; GE Healthcare; Amersham, UK). Samples (2 mL) were injected into a 2 mL loop using phosphate buffered saline (PBS) buffer (pH 7.4) as a mobile phase at 1 mL/min. Fractions were collected, pooled and lyophilised. Then, conjugates were re-dissolved in a minimal volume of dH$_2$O and dialysed (1000 g/mol cut-off) against 5 × 1 L dH$_2$O to remove PBS salts. The final conjugates were lyophilised and stored at −20 °C.

2.6. Characterisation of OligoG–Polymyxin Conjugates

Size exclusion chromatography with multi-angle light scattering detection (SEC-MALS) or refractive index detection (SEC-RI), were used to measure the approximate molecular weight and polydispersity of the conjugates. SEC-MALS was performed at ambient temperature on an HPLC system consisting of a solvent reservoir, on-line degasser, automatic sample injector, HPLC isocratic pump, pre-column and serially connected columns (TSKgel 4000 and 2500 PWXL). The column outlet was connected to a Dawn HELEOS-II multi-angle laser light scattering photometer (Wyatt, MO, USA) ($\lambda 0$ = 663.8 nm) followed by a Shodex RI-501 RI detector. The eluent was 0.15 M NaNO3 with 0.01 M EDTA, pH 6.0 and the flow rate was 0.5 mL/min. Samples (10 mg/mL) were filtered (pore size 0.45 µm) before injection and analysed twice with injection volumes of 25 and 50 µL. A weighted specific refractive index increment (dn/dc) value was calculated from the % w/w colistin using dn/dc = 0.150 and 0.185 for alginate and colistin, respectively. Data were collected and processed using the Astra software (version 7.3.0; Wyatt, USA).

The SEC-RI system consisted of two TSK gel columns (G5000PWXL and G3000PWXL) (Tosoh, Germany) in series connected to a Gilson 133 differential refractometer (Middleton, WI, USA). Samples were prepared in PBS (3 mg/mL) and eluted using PBS (pH 7.4) as the mobile phase at a flow rate of 1 mL/min. Cirrus GPC software (version 3.2, 2006) from Polymer Laboratories (Church Stretton, UK,) was used for data analysis. Molecular weight was determined relative to pullulan molecular weight standards.

The FPLC system described above, connected to a Superdex 75 (10/300 GL) column, was also used to assess conjugate purity. Samples (3 mg/mL in PBS) were injected into a 100 µL loop at 0.5 mL/min. The area under the curve was used to estimate the percentage of free and conjugated antibiotic. The total polymyxin content of conjugates was determined by bicinchoninic acid (BCA) assay using colistin sulphate or polymyxin B standards.

Before and after OligoG conjugation, the number of available primary amine groups on colistin and polymyxin B was determined using the ninhydrin assay. First, a lithium acetate buffer (4 M) was prepared by dissolving lithium acetate dihydrate 40.81% w/v in dH$_2$O. Acetic acid (glacial) was added to reach pH 5.2 before adjusting the final volume. Next, ninhydrin reagent was prepared by dissolving ninhydrin 2% w/v and hydrindantin 0.3% w/v in 7.5 mL of DMSO and 2.5 mL of lithium acetate buffer. Test compounds (86 µL) were diluted with ninhydrin reagent (1:1) and heated in a water bath (100 °C) for 15 min. Samples were subsequently cooled to room temperature and mixed with 50% v/v ethanol solution (130 µL). Then, aliquots (100 µL) were transferred into the wells of a 96-well microtitre plate and analysed spectrophotometrically at 570 nm. Calibration of the assay was achieved using ethanolamine (0–0.1158 mM).

NMR spectroscopy was used to confirm OligoG–polymyxin conjugation (Supplementary Materials).

2.7. Drug Release of OligoG–Polymyxin Conjugates

To compare the rate of degradation of OligoG–polymyxin conjugates, solutions were prepared (3 mg/mL) in either (i) PBS at pH 5, (ii) PBS at pH 7, or (iii) PBS at pH 7 containing alginate lyase from *Sphingobacterium multivorum* (1 U/mL) and incubated at 37 °C for 0, 2, 4, 6, 24 and 48 h. Upon collection, samples were immediately snap-frozen in liquid nitrogen and stored at −20 °C. Time-dependent changes in molecular weight and free polymyxin content were determined by SEC-RI and FPLC, respectively.

2.8. Characterisation of In Vitro Toxicity

A 3-(4,5-dimethylthiazol-2-yl)-2,5-diphenyltetrazolium bromide (MTT) assay was used to measure cell viability and proliferation of HK-2 cells. Cells were seeded into sterile 96-well microtitre plates at 1×10^5 cells/mL (100 µL/well) and allowed to adhere for 24 h at 37 °C. The following day, the old medium was replaced with test compounds (0–1 mg/mL polymyxin base) dissolved in filter-sterilised K-SFM. After 67 h incubation at 37 °C, filter-sterilised MTT solution (20 µL of a 5 mg/mL solution in PBS) was added to each well and incubated for a further 5 h at 37 °C. Finally, the medium was carefully removed, and the formazan crystals were solubilised in DMSO (100 µL) for 30 min. Absorbance was measured at 550 nm using a Fluostar Omega microplate reader. The results are stated as percentage cell viability compared with the untreated control cells. Data are expressed as mean ± SEM (n = 18).

Release of the cytokine, tumour necrosis factor alpha (TNFα), by HK-2 cells (1×10^5 cells/mL) after exposure to free- and OligoG-conjugated antibiotic (0–1 mg/mL polymyxin base) was assessed using an enzyme-linked immunosorbent assay (ELISA) kit. After 72 h incubation, the 96-well microtitre plates were centrifuged (226× g, 3 min), the supernatant was collected, diluted with reagent diluent (1:1) and analysed with the TNFα ELISA kit according to the manufacturer's instructions (Fisher Scientific; Loughborough, UK). Plates were analysed spectrophotometrically at 450 nm. In parallel, 100 µL of K-SFM was added to the wells of the centrifuged plates containing cells and MTT assays were performed. A standard curve was used to calculate TNFα concentrations in the test samples, which were then multiplied by the dilution factor (×2) and divided by cell viability for each drug concentration (from the MTT assay). Two outliers were identified and removed using robust regression and the outlier removal (ROUT) method (Q coefficient = 0.2%). Data are expressed as mean ± SEM ($n = 6$).

2.9. Antimicrobial Activity of OligoG–Polymyxin Conjugates

The minimum inhibitory concentration (MIC) of colistin (as sulphate salt) and polymyxin B and their conjugates was determined using the broth microdilution method in MH broth in accordance with standard guidelines [28]. Test organisms were suspended in MH broth (100 µL, 5×10^5 colony forming units (CFU)/mL) and incubated in 96-well microtitre plates in serial two-fold dilutions of the test compounds. The MIC was defined as the lowest concentration of test compound that produced no visible growth after 16–20 h. Results were expressed as mode ($n = 3$). For the purpose of calculating selectivity index (SI), MIC values lower than 0.008 were taken as the lowest concentration tested. Selective activities of the polymyxins and OligoG–polymyxin conjugates were calculated as follows:

$$\text{Selectivity index (SI)} = IC_{50} \text{ (µg/mL)}/\text{MIC (µg/mL)}.$$

To investigate whether alginate oligomer degradation is required for antimicrobial activity, MIC assays were also conducted in the presence of alginate lyase (1 and 10 U/mL), whereby alginate lyase was added to the MH broth during microtitre plate set up. In addition, alginate oligomer–colistin conjugates (3 mg/mL) were incubated in PBS at pH 7 containing bacterial alginate lyase (1 and 10 U/mL) at 37 °C for 24 h, before preparing microtitre plates as described above.

To more closely mimic in vivo environmental conditions, the antimicrobial activity of test compounds was studied in the presence of mucin, by supplementing MH broth with porcine stomach (type II) mucin (0.2 and 2% w/v) and used to set up the 96-well plates according to the standard MIC protocol. To account for turbidity caused by mucin, resazurin dye solution (30 µL, 0.01% w/v in dH$_2$O) was added to each well and incubated for a further 3 h at 37 °C. Colour changes were observed and recorded.

To study the antimicrobial efficacy of test compounds under more clinically relevant conditions, the MIC protocol was performed using AS medium instead of MH broth. The plates were incubated with resazurin as described above.

A checkerboard assay was used to assess synergy of test compounds with azithromycin dihydrate. Here, stock solutions of test compounds (8 × MIC) and serial two-fold dilutions of azithromycin dihydrate (16–1/16 × MIC) were freshly prepared in MH broth. Test compound solutions (100 µL) were placed in the wells of row 1, then serially diluted along the ordinate with MH broth. Serially diluted azithromycin dihydrate solutions (50 µL) were then added to the wells in decreasing concentration along the abscissa. Each microtitre well was inoculated with the test organism (5×10^5 CFU/mL) and incubated at 37 °C for 20 h. The fractional inhibitory concentration index (FICI) was calculated by comparing the MIC values of the individual agents with the MIC value of the combined treatments [29]. Drug combinations were considered synergistic when the mean FICI was ≤0.5, additive when the FICI was between 0.5 and 2, indifferent when the FICI was between 2 and 4, and antagonistic when the FICI was ≥4 [30]. Results were expressed as median values ($n = 3$).

To study the effect of test compounds on bacterial pharmacokinetic profiles, 96-well microtitre plates were set up according to the standard MIC protocol, then placed in a Fluostar Omega Microplate Reader at 37 °C, and absorbance at 600 nm was measured hourly for 48 h. Results were expressed as mean values ($n = 3$). Unconjugated colistin plus OligoG, OligoG and the high molecular weight, biologically inactive alginate, PRONOVA, at equivalent concentrations used in amide-linked or ester-linked conjugates, were used as controls.

2.10. Anti-Biofilm Activity of OligoG–Polymyxin Conjugates

To analyse the effect of test compounds on biofilm formation, solutions of test compounds in MH broth were inoculated (1:10) with *P. aeruginosa* R22 (standardised to 10^7 CFU/mL) in a Greiner glass-bottomed optical 96-well plate. The plate was then wrapped in parafilm and incubated (37 °C, 20 rpm) for 24 h. The supernatant was carefully removed and replaced with 10% *v/v* LIVE/DEAD stain in PBS prior to imaging. CLSM of Syto 9 ($\lambda_{ex}/\lambda_{em}$ maximum, 480/500 nm) and propidium iodide ($\lambda_{ex}/\lambda_{em}$ maximum, 490/635 nm) was performed using a Leica SP5 confocal microscope with ×63 lens (under oil) and a step size of 0.79 µm. Z-stack CLSM images were analysed using COMSTAT image analysis software [31] and results were expressed as mean ± SEM ($n = 15$).

2.11. Pharmacokinetic–Pharmacodynamic (PK–PD) Model

A two-compartment static dialysis bag model (adapted from Azzopardi et al. [32]) was used to study the PK–PD profile of OligoG–colistin conjugates. First, the ability of the dialysis membrane to control diffusion of test compounds was assessed. The inner compartment (IC) contained OligoG–colistin or colistin sulphate (10 mg/mL colistin base; 5 mL) in PBS and the outer compartment (OC) contained sterile PBS (15 mL). The aseptically sealed beaker was incubated (37 °C, 70 rpm) for 48 h. Samples were collected at various time points from each compartment and stored at −20 °C prior to analysis of colistin content by BCA assay.

A modified experimental set-up was used to investigate the concentration- and time-dependent antimicrobial activity of test compounds using a TTK assay (48 h). Here, the total volume in the system was considered, with the IC containing test compounds at MIC (colistin sulphate 0.25 µg/mL; OligoG–A–colistin 0.125 µg/mL colistin base; OligoG–E–colistin 0.125 µg/mL colistin base) or 2 × MIC (OligoG–A–colistin 0.25 µg/mL colistin base; OligoG–E–colistin 0.25 µg/mL colistin base) in PBS. The OC contained MH broth inoculated with *A. baumannii* 7789 (5×10^5 CFU/mL). Samples were collected from the OC (0, 2, 4, 6, 24 and 48 h) and colony counts (CFU/mL) determined using drop counts. Treatments were considered bactericidal if the reduction in viable bacterial counts was ≥3 $\log_{10}$ CFU/mL (equivalent to 99.9% of the initial inoculum) and bacteriostatic if the decrease was <3 $\log_{10}$ CFU/mL [33,34]. Growth (no test compounds) and sterility (no bacteria) controls were also performed.

2.12. Statistical Analysis

GraphPad Prism (version 6.01, 2012; San Diego, CA, USA) was used for statistical analysis. Statistical significance was indicated by *, where * $p < 0.05$, ** $p < 0.01$, *** $p < 0.001$ and **** $p < 0.0001$. Analysis of variance (ANOVA) was used to evaluate multiple group comparisons ($n \geq 3$) followed by Dunnett's post hoc test to account for multiple comparisons.

3. Results

3.1. Synthesis and Characterisation of OligoG–Polymyxin Conjugates

The characteristics of the OligoG–antibiotic conjugates synthesised in this study are summarised in Table 1 and Table S2. Polymyxin B conjugates typically showed less drug loading (6.1–8% *w/w*) than the colistin conjugates (8.1–12.9% *w/w*). SEC-MALS, SEC-RI and FPLC analysis confirmed the presence of high molecular weight conjugates with <6% unbound drug (Figures S1 and S2, Table S3).

The mean molecular weight of amide- and ester-linked conjugates (measured by SEC-MALS) was 8200–12,800 g/mol and 5200–6200 g/mol, respectively. The ninhydrin assay indicated that 2–4 amine groups were used for binding to OligoG via amide conjugation. Diffusion-ordered spectroscopy (DOSY) NMR confirmed covalent coupling of OligoG to colistin. Signals corresponding to OligoG and colistin in the samples had the same diffusion coefficient (1.26×10^{-10} m^2/s), indicative of covalent coupling (Figure S3). OligoG–A–colistin conjugate samples appeared to contain some free OligoG while the DOSY spectrum for OligoG–E–colistin conjugate showed the presence of both, free OligoG and colistin in the sample.

Table 1. Summary of the properties of the OligoG-polymyxin conjugates synthesised in this study.

Tested Compound	Mw (g/mol) (PDI) by SEC-MALS	Polymyxin Content (% w/w)	Molar Ratio (per Colistin)	Conjugated NH$_2$ per Molecule	Free Polymyxin (%)
OligoG–A–colistin					
Mean	9220 (1.3)	9.4	4.3	3.4	3.2
Range	8200–12,300 (1.2–1.4)	8.1–12.5	3.1–5.0	2.7–4.6	1.5–5.7
OligoG–E–colistin					
Mean	5550 (1.3)	10.9	3.8	N/A	2.7
Range	5200–5900 (1.2–1.3)	8.3–12.9	3.0–4.9	N/A	2.0–3.5
OligoG–A–polymyxin B					
Mean	10,950 (1.4)	7.1	6.0	2.0	1.6
Range	9100–12,800 (1.3–1.5)	6.1–8.0	5.1–6.8	1.9–2.0	1.6
OligoG–E–polymyxin B	6200 (1.2)	7.0	5.9	N/A	2.7

Abbreviations: A, amide; E, ester; PDI, polydispersity index (given in brackets); SEC-MALS, size exclusion chromatography with multi-angle light scattering detection; N/A, not applicable.

3.2. Stability of OligoG–Polymyxin Conjugates

Both ester- and amide-linked conjugates of OligoG–colistin and OligoG–polymyxin B incubated in PBS at either pH 5 or pH 7 showed no significant decrease in molecular weight (Figure S4). Conjugates were slightly less stable at pH 7, compared to pH 5. Conversely, alginate lyase effectively triggered ~30% of colistin and ~90% of polymyxin B release (increase in % free drug) within 24 h from these conjugates at 1 U/mL. There was little difference in total drug release between amide- and ester-linked conjugates.

3.3. Cytotoxicity of OligoG–Polymyxin Conjugates

The concentration-dependent cytotoxicity of unmodified antibiotics, OligoG and OligoG-polymyxin conjugates in HK-2 cells is shown in Figure 1. OligoG was not cytotoxic at <10 mg/mL. Cytotoxicity was greatest for the free drugs (colistin sulphate half maximal inhibitory concentration (IC$_{50}$ = 0.026 mg/mL), polymyxin B (0.011 mg/mL)); slightly reduced by ester conjugation (OligoG–E–colistin (IC$_{50}$ = 0.057 mg/mL), OligoG–E–polymyxin B (0.032 mg/mL)); and significantly reduced for the amide-linked conjugates (OligoG–A–colistin (IC$_{50}$ = 0.242 mg/mL), OligoG–A–polymyxin B (0.299 mg/mL)). ELISA showed that the unmodified antibiotics induced greater TNFα release than the conjugates (Figure 1c). OligoG–E–polymyxin B caused the highest release of TNFα, compared to the other conjugates, but this was still lower than the unmodified drug.

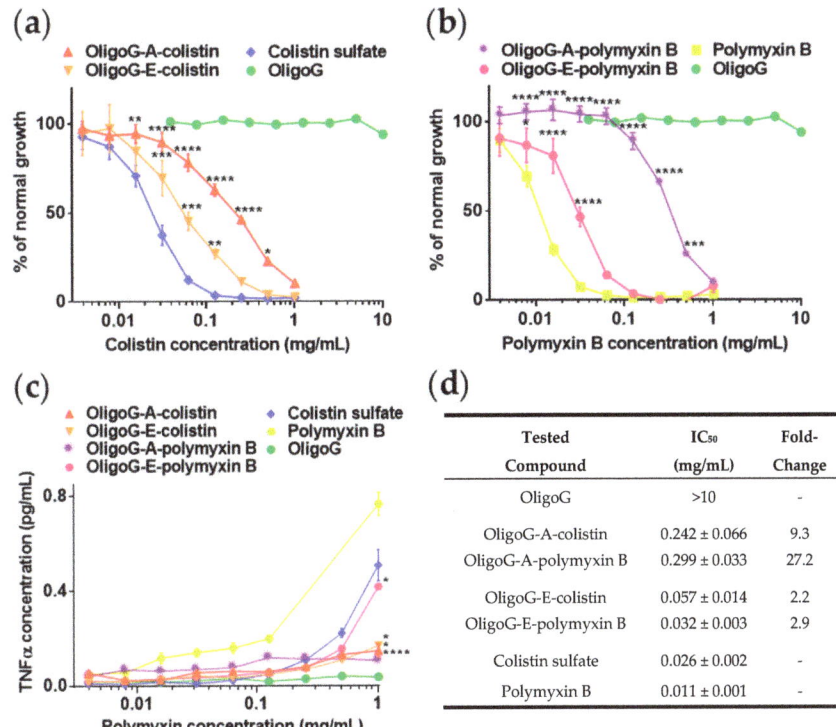

Figure 1. In vitro cytotoxicity of OligoG–polymyxin conjugates in human kidney proximal tubule cells (HK-2) cells. Cell viability determined by 3-(4,5-dimethylthiazol-2-yl)-2,5-diphenyltetrazolium bromide (MTT) assay after 72 h incubation. (**a**) Colistin sulphate. (**b**) Polymyxin B. Data are presented as mean % of untreated control ± SEM ($n = 18$). (**c**) Tumour necrosis factor alpha (TNFα) release in HK-2 cells after incubation with OligoG–polymyxin conjugates for 72 h (±SEM; $n = 6$). (**d**) Half maximal inhibitory concentration (IC$_{50}$) values (±SEM) and fold-change (MTT assay) of tested compounds in HK-2 cells. Significance is indicated by *, where * $p < 0.05$, ** $p < 0.01$, *** $p < 0.001$, **** $p < 0.0001$ compared to colistin sulphate or polymyxin B controls. Abbreviations: A, amide; E, ester.

3.4. Antimicrobial Activity of OligoG–Polymyxin Conjugates

The effects of conjugation on antimicrobial efficacy against a range of Gram-negative pathogens varied between the conjugates and antibiotic (Table 2). Whilst ester-conjugation resulted in similar (≤2-fold differences) or decreased MIC values for OligoG–colistin and –polymyxin B conjugates, the amide-linked conjugates demonstrated increased MIC values. This effect was particularly evident for the polymyxin B conjugates, where MICs were increased by 4- to 32-fold. OligoG conjugation did not improve the bactericidal efficacy of colistin in colistin-resistant strains (Table 2). Both OligoG–polymyxin conjugates exhibited substantially improved selectivity for Gram-negative bacteria in comparison to mammalian cells, compared to unmodified colistin sulphate (1.7–4.7-fold) and polymyxin B (2.3–4.1-fold) (Table S4).

The antimicrobial activity of the conjugates was also assessed in the presence of alginate lyase or following pre-incubation with alginate lyase (Table S5), where no significant change was observed for either amide- or ester-bonded conjugates.

In contrast, when mucin was added to the broth, antimicrobial activity of OligoG–polymyxin conjugates decreased in a dose-dependent manner (Table S6). The presence of unconjugated OligoG with colistin sulphate or polymyxin B did not alter the antimicrobial activity of the free antibiotic.

Table 2. Minimum inhibitory concentration (MIC) determinations of OligoG–polymyxin conjugates against a range of Gram-negative bacterial pathogens.

Isolate	Tested Compound MIC (µg/mL Drug Base)					
	Colistin Sulphate	Polymyxin B	OligoG–E–Colistin	OligoG–E–Polymyxin B	OligoG–A–Colistin	OligoG–A–Polymyxin B
P. aeruginosa R22	0.5	0.25	1	0.25	2	4
P. aeruginosa MDR 301	0.5	0.5	0.5	0.5	1	2
P. aeruginosa NH57388A	0.25	0.25	0.25	0.25	0.5	1
P. aeruginosa NCTC 10662	0.125	0.063	0.25	0.25	1	4
K. pneumoniae KP05 506	0.125	0.125	0.125	0.25	0.125	0.5
K. pneumoniae IR25	0.063	0.125	0.125	0.125	1	4
A. baumannii MDR ACB	0.5	0.125	**0.25**	**0.063**	1	2
A. baumannii 7789	0.25	0.125	**0.125**	0.5	**0.125**	0.5
E. coli AIM-1	<0.008	<0.004	0.008	0.016	0.008	0.063
E. coli IR57	0.125	0.5	0.25	0.5	0.125	2
E. coli 5702	0.031	0.063	0.031	0.063	0.063	0.25
E. coli NCTC 10418	0.125	0.25	0.5	0.25	0.25	4
E. coli PN21	8	8	16	8	32	32
E. coli PN25	8	4	8	4	32	32
E. coli PN26	0.125	0.125	0.25	0.25	0.5	0.5
E. coli ATCC 25922	0.25	0.5	1	0.5	1	16

Increased antimicrobial activity of conjugated polymyxin (MIC ≥ 1-fold lower compared to colistin sulphate or polymyxin B controls) is shown in bold. Abbreviations: A, amide; E, ester.

Differences in antimicrobial activity of both, free- and OligoG-bound antibiotics were observed in AS medium compared to MH broth (Table S7). In most cases, using the checkerboard assay, an indifferent or additive effect was observed when azithromycin dihydrate was combined with OligoG–colistin or colistin sulphate (Table S8). Generally, OligoG conjugation did not alter the efficacy of the antibiotic combination, except for *A. baumannii* 7789, where the additive effect of colistin sulphate + azithromycin dihydrate (FICI = 1.14) became indifferent when azithromycin dihydrate was combined with OligoG–colistin conjugates (FICI >2.5). However, the combination of azithromycin dihydrate with OligoG–E–colistin resulted in a synergistic effect for the *E. coli* National Collection of Type Culture (NCTC) 10418 isolate (FICI = 0.46).

Bacterial growth curves of *P. aeruginosa* MDR 301 (Figure 2) showed that the OligoG–colistin conjugates delayed bacterial growth in a concentration-dependent manner (indicated by the longer lag-phase), and exponential growth was similarly slower compared to the untreated control. Growth inhibition (up to >48 h) was noted for the OligoG–colistin conjugates at $\geq 2 \times$ MIC, while higher equivalent concentrations of colistin sulphate were required ($\geq 8 \times$ MIC) to achieve comparable efficacy. Neither amide- nor ester-linked conjugates had an effect on time to onset of bacterial growth. Both, OligoG–A–colistin and OligoG–E–colistin conjugates, at their MIC (1 and 0.5 µg/mL colistin base, respectively), demonstrated a delayed lag phase of >24 h and >18 h, respectively. Typically, colistin covalently conjugated to OligoG showed similar activity to the combined mixture of unconjugated colistin and OligoG at equivalent concentrations. Furthermore, neither OligoG nor Pronova alone had any significant effect in reducing bacterial growth, when an equivalent concentration to that contained in OligoG–colistin conjugates was used.

3.5. Anti-Biofilm Activity of OligoG–Polymyxin Conjugates

CLSM of biofilms grown in the presence of free and OligoG-bound colistin ($\geq$MIC) showed a marked effect on biofilm formation (Figure 3). For example, the OligoG–E–colistin conjugate, at its MIC (1 µg/mL colistin base), caused obvious bacterial clumping, disruption of biofilm structure, and cell death (as noted by increased numbers of red cells). COMSTAT analysis revealed a significant reduction in biofilm thickness for all treatments ($\geq$MIC) ($p < 0.05$) and biofilm roughness was significantly increased by OligoG–colistin conjugates ($\geq$MIC) and colistin sulphate (MIC) treatments ($p < 0.05$). Both OligoG–colistin conjugates ($2 \times$ MIC) significantly reduced biofilm biomass compared to untreated control ($p < 0.05$), whereas no significant change was observed with colistin sulphate (up to $2 \times$ MIC).

3.6. Pharmacokinetic–Pharmacodynamic (PK–PD) Model

In the PK-PD model (Figure 4), when antibiotic was placed in the IC, colistin diffused more rapidly than the OligoG–colistin conjugates (1 mg/mL in the OC was reached at 2.83 h (colistin) < 10.47 h (OligoG–E–colistin) < 17.35 h (OligoG–A–colistin)). Colistin sulphate, at MIC (0.25 µg/mL) and the OligoG–E–colistin conjugate at $2 \times$ MIC (0.25 µg/mL colistin base) caused substantial bacterial killing after 4 h (<3 $\log_{10}$ CFU/mL) (Figure 4b). Both treatments caused a reduction in viable bacterial counts compared to the control (~5-fold lower) and the initial starting bacterial concentration (~2-fold lower). However, no antimicrobial effect was observed with the OligoG–A–colistin conjugate up to $2 \times$ MIC.

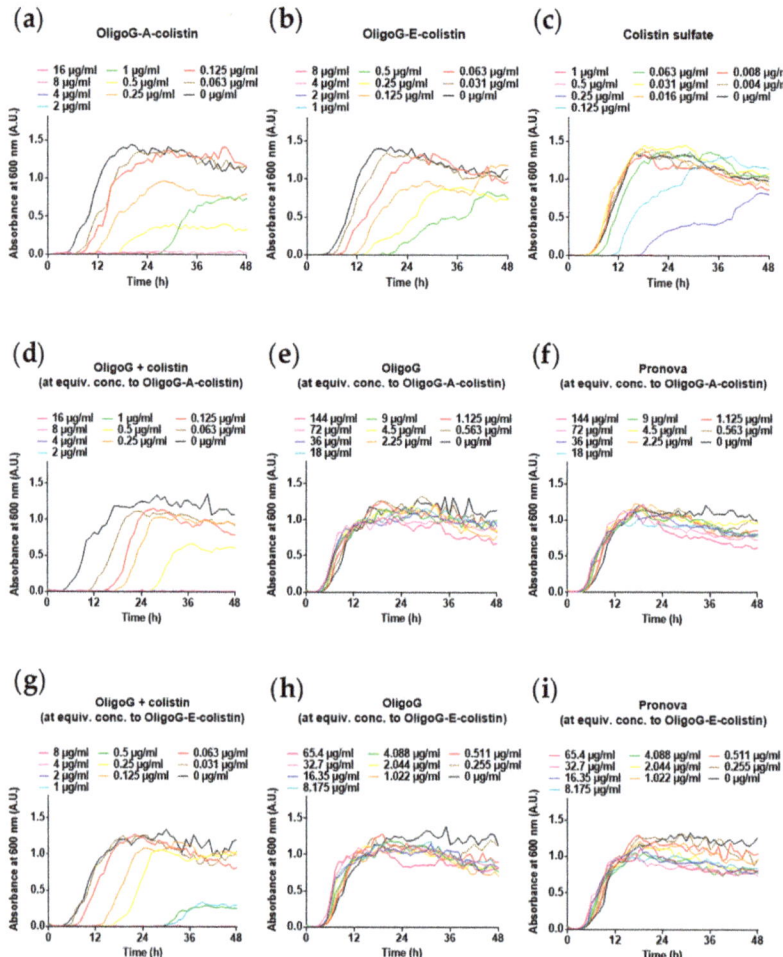

Figure 2. Bacterial growth curves for *P. aeruginosa* MDR 301 (48 h) in the presence of the following antimicrobials. (**a**) OligoG–A–colistin conjugate. (**b**) OligoG–E–colistin conjugate. (**c**) Colistin sulphate. (**d**) Colistin sulphate plus OligoG control for amide-linked conjugate. (**e**) OligoG control for amide-linked conjugate. (**f**) PRONOVA control for amide-linked conjugate. (**g**) Colistin sulphate plus OligoG control for ester-linked conjugate. (**h**) OligoG control for ester-linked conjugate. (**i**) PRONOVA control for ester-linked conjugate. Controls were used at the equivalent concentrations used in the corresponding amide- or ester-linked conjugates ($n = 3$). Abbreviations: A, amide; E, ester.

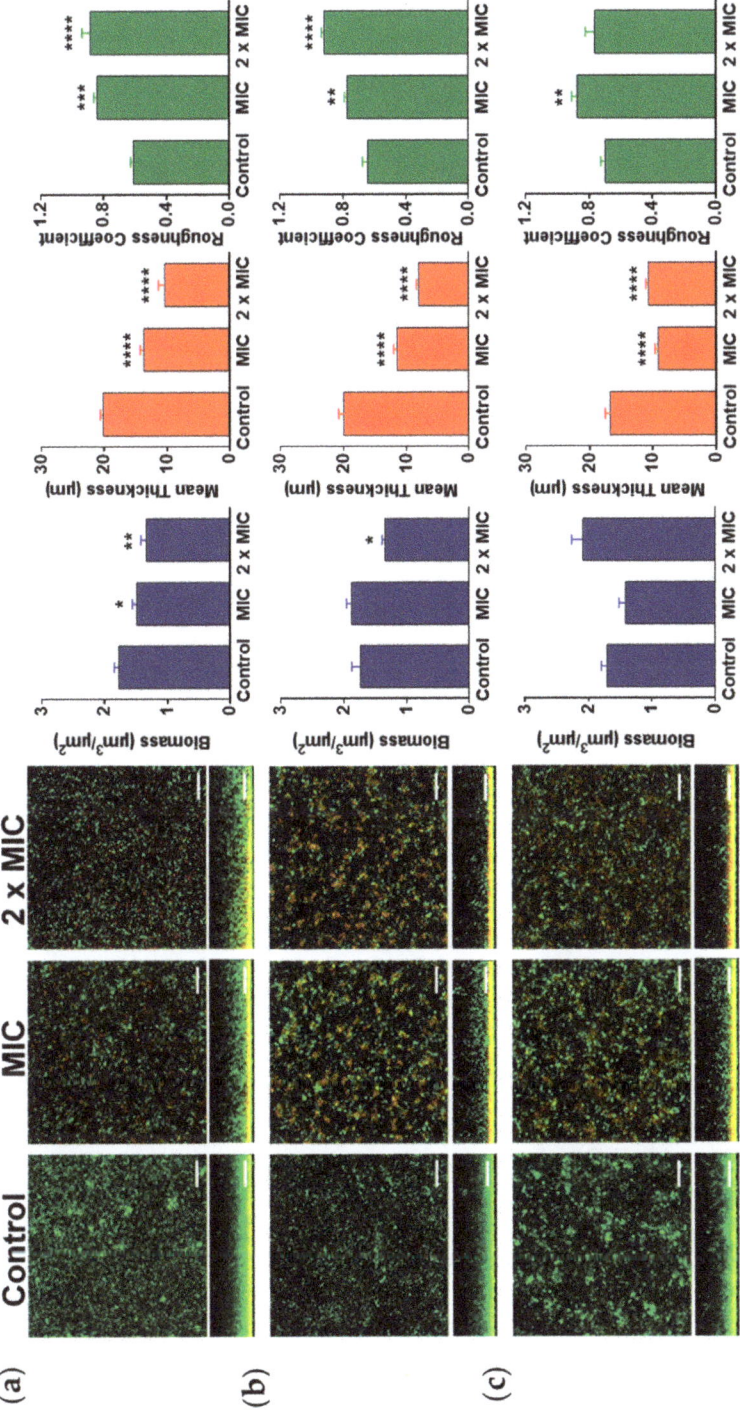

Figure 3. Biofilm formation assay showing LIVE/DEAD (green/red, respectively) stained confocal laser scanning microscopy (CLSM) images (aerial and cross-sectional views, scale bar, 35 μm) of *P. aeruginosa* R22 biofilms grown for 24 h in the presence of (**a**) OligoG–A–colistin (MIC, 2 μg/mL colistin base), (**b**) OligoG–E–colistin (MIC, 1 μg/mL colistin base) and (**c**) colistin sulphate (MIC, 0.5 μg/mL colistin base). Corresponding COMSTAT analysis of the CLSM images is also shown (±SEM; $n = 15$). Significance is indicated by *, where * $p < 0.05$, ** $p < 0.01$, *** $p < 0.001$, **** $p < 0.0001$ compared to an untreated control.

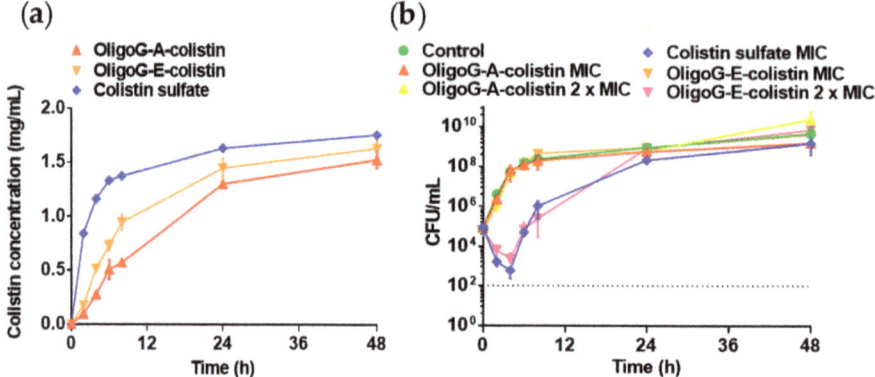

Figure 4. Pharmacokinetic–pharmacodynamic (PK–PD) model to compare diffusion of free- and OligoG-conjugated colistin. (**a**) Change in colistin concentration in the outer compartment over 48 h (measured by BCA assay). Data are expressed as mean ± SD ($n = 3$). (**b**) Viability count of *A. baumannii* 7789 in a "time-to-kill" (TTK) model. Data represent mean colony forming units (CFU) ± SD ($n = 3$). Dotted line, lower limit of detection (10^2 CFU/mL). Abbreviations: A, amide; E, ester.

4. Discussion

4.1. Rationale for Development of OligoG–Polymyxin Conjugates

In recent years, interest in developing polymyxin derivatives to improve the therapeutic index or provide activity towards bacterial strains that are not currently susceptible to polymyxins has grown considerably [35]. Structural modifications, such as removal or substitution of the N-terminal acyl chain, reduction in the number of positive charges, polymer conjugation and the introduction of hydrophobic residues, have all been explored in an attempt to improve activity, reduce adverse side effects and elucidate structure–activity relationships [36,37]. These studies have demonstrated the critical importance of the amphipathicity of polymyxin molecules for their antimicrobial activity, which stems from the charged Dab residues and hydrophobic tail. This study compared the activity and toxicity of OligoG–polymyxin conjugates containing reversible or irreversible linking chemistries, to improve the therapeutic index of the polymyxins.

To form an amide bond between OligoG and polymyxin antibiotics, the carboxyl groups of the polymer were first activated by EDC in the presence of sulfo-NHS to create a stable amine-reactive intermediate [38]. The resultant amine-reactive sulfo-NHS ester was then bound to primary amines on the polymyxins. We hypothesised that amide-linked conjugates would rely on degradation of the OligoG backbone by alginate lyase. There are no known mammalian enzymes capable of degrading alginate, but bacterial alginate lyase from *K. pneumoniae* and *P. aeruginosa* has been found in cystic fibrosis patients' lungs [39] and could provide an opportunity for site-specific release of a therapeutic payload from an alginate conjugated drug. Although alginate lyases from these bacteria are generally considered to be mannuronate-specific, it has been shown that they may also demonstrate moderate to low activity towards guluronate [40]. Non-biodegradable polymers whose molecular weight is below the renal threshold (<40,000 g/mol) are expected to be readily excreted from the body [41], so the conjugates synthesised in the present study should be readily excreted by the kidney. Furthermore, sugar residues and/or linker groups that remain attached to the antibiotic Dab residues after polymer degradation, may result in reduced antimicrobial activity, as observed with amide-linked dextrin–colistin conjugates [18]. In parallel, ester-linked OligoG–polymyxin conjugates were formed using Steglich esterification. Here, the polymer carboxyl groups were activated by DCC, with DMAP as a catalyst [42]. The resultant O-acylisourea intermediate was then bound to hydroxyl groups on the polymyxins. Addition of DMAP as a catalyst compensates for hydroxyls being poorer nucleophiles than amines (which can cause spontaneous rearrangement of the *O*-acylisourea intermediate into undesirable *N*-acylurea) by reacting with *O*-acylisourea to form an acyl pyridinium species. Reaction of DMAP with *O*-acylisourea forms an acyl pyridinium intermediate that is unable to form intramolecular by-products but can react with a hydroxyl group to form an ester bond [43]. Ester-linkage permits complete release of the native antibiotic at low or high pH, and by enzymatic activity and reactive oxygen species at sites of infection [44]. Moreover, release of intact OligoG at the target site would restore intrinsic antimicrobial activity of the polymer, which would further enhance its antibiotic efficacy in vivo.

4.2. Physicochemical Characterisation of OligoG–Polymyxin Conjugates

Covalent attachment of OligoG to colistin was confirmed using several methods. DOSY is an indirect method that can detect if the polymer and peptide are chemically linked as they will have the same diffusion coefficient if bound together in solution [45] while SEC detects an increase in size caused by an increase in molecular weight. In a control experiment using SEC-MALS, OligoG with 10% *w/w* added colistin yielded almost identical RI chromatograms as pure OligoG, confirming that the observed shift in elution profile for the OligoG–colistin conjugates was not simply due to electrostatic interactions between OligoG and free colistin. DOSY confirmed successful conjugation using both amide and ester linkers. Nevertheless, DOSY also detected unbound colistin in the OligoG–E–colistin sample and SEC-MALS analysis did not show an increased molecular weight compared to free OligoG. This may be caused by hydrolysis of the ester linkage during measurement (in D_2O at 25 °C), rather than insufficient removal of unreacted material, highlighting the importance of using multiple analytical methods to characterise these complex molecules.

4.3. Biological Characterisation of OligoG–Polymyxin Conjugates

Polymyxin antibiotics have been reported to cause severe nephrotoxicity in up to 53.5% of patients [46] due to extensive reabsorption of the drug by renal tubular cells [47]. OligoG–polymyxin conjugates in the present study exhibited a marked decrease in in vitro cytotoxicity in kidney cells when compared to unmodified antibiotics. As expected, ester-linked polymyxin conjugates were considerably more cytotoxic towards HK-2 cells compared to amide-linked conjugates. Since the positively charged Dab residues are known to mediate polymyxin toxicity, and 2–4 of these primary amines were used for irreversible (amide-linked) conjugation with OligoG, this result was unsurprising.

Antimicrobial efficacy of all OligoG–polymyxin conjugates was comparable to that of the parent antibiotic. However, attachment of OligoG in the bi-functional molecule was unable to overcome colistin resistance. For colistin-sensitive strains, conjugate MIC values were below the Clinical and Laboratory Standards Institute [48] and European Committee on Antimicrobial Susceptibility Testing [49] susceptibility breakpoints (≤2 µg/mL) for polymyxins. Importantly, ester-linked conjugates showed full retention of the antimicrobial activity of the free drug, while the antimicrobial activity of the amide-linked conjugates was reduced by more than two-fold, presumably because of residual sugars and/or linker groups on the antibiotic amine groups. Although these studies did not test the stability of the conjugates in bacterial growth medium, it is likely that hydrolysis of the ester bond would occur during the MIC assay incubation. This may explain the smaller decrease in antimicrobial activity seen with ester-linked conjugates compared to amide-linked ones. Greater selectivity of OligoG–A–polymyxin conjugates for Gram-negative bacteria in comparison to mammalian cells suggests better tolerability and reduced side effects in vivo and substantially improved efficacy at clinically relevant concentrations compared to the free antibiotic. In addition, studies with alginate lyase suggested that either OligoG degradation is not necessary for antibiotic activity, or that alginate oligomers are broken down by bacterial enzymes. Nevertheless, compared to dextrin–colistin conjugates described in previous studies [16], alginate oligomer–conjugates were significantly more potent (more than five-fold change). This may be due to the larger molecular weight of dextrin causing steric hindrance or the charge difference between the two polymers, but more likely, it can be attributed to the inherent biological activity of OligoG itself [20].

Sustained antibiotic release was demonstrated by slower bacterial growth in the presence of OligoG–colistin conjugates, which was dose-dependent. In this study, lower concentrations of OligoG–colistin conjugates, compared to free colistin, were required to inhibit bacterial growth which was sustained for up to 48 h. OligoG–E–colistin delayed the onset of bacterial growth for much longer than amide-linked conjugates, suggesting that, after systemic administration, OligoG–E–colistin conjugates might achieve better therapeutic activity in vivo. Similarly, when PEG was attached to colistin via a labile ester bond, sustained drug release led to equivalent or better antimicrobial activity against *A. baumannii* and *P. aeruginosa* isolates [17].

In a clinical setting, binding of colistin to sputum biomolecules (e.g., mucin) in the airways could negatively impact antibiotic effectiveness and availability. Indeed, Huang et al. [50] demonstrated >100-fold increase in MIC values of both, colistin and polymyxin B, when mucin was added to the bacterial culture medium. A four-fold increase in the MIC of colistin was also reported when the assay was conducted in AS medium instead of MH broth, thought to be caused by bacterial growth disruption, structural modifications of lipopolysaccharides or direct colistin–mucin interactions [24]. Although recent studies have demonstrated the ability of OligoG to bind mucin [51], conjugation of OligoG to colistin and polymyxin B did not affect the ability of the antibiotic to bind mucin or alter the effect of nutrient-deficient medium.

In practice, patients with severe infections of MDR pathogens are usually treated with combinations of two or more antibiotics to overcome or prevent drug resistance. When we combined OligoG–colistin conjugates with azithromycin dihydrate, an antibiotic that has previously shown enhanced efficacy in combination with OligoG [20], antimicrobial activity of the drug was enhanced, but only additively. Similarly, He et al. [52] reported additive effects in *P. aeruginosa* when they combined a low molecular weight alginate oligosaccharide (Mw < 10 kDa) with azithromycin, suggesting that the alginate oligosaccharide component of OligoG–colistin conjugates may be responsible for the additive effects observed in our study.

Chronic airway infections by *P. aeruginosa* affect more than 80% of CF patients and contribute to a progressive decline in lung function [53]. Marked disruption of *P. aeruginosa* biofilm formation was observed when they were grown in the presence of both OligoG–colistin conjugates, although only the ester-linked conjugate induced bacterial clumping (≥MIC) which might be associated with the higher cationic charge of colistin. This is in keeping with the findings of Powell et al. [23] who showed that OligoG, at concentrations ≥0.5%, caused *P. aeruginosa* aggregation, while higher concentrations (≥2%) caused significant disruption of bacterial biofilm formation and growth.

4.4. PK–PD Modelling

Drug TTK profiles and colistin release rate from amide- or ester-linked OligoG–colistin conjugates were investigated using an in vitro two-compartment PK–PD model. Predictably, diffusion of colistin, which was mirrored by a time-dependent increase in drug concentration in the OC, was substantially faster than the OligoG conjugates. When the ester-linked OligoG–colistin conjugate was contained in the IC, diffusion of colistin was more pronounced than when the amide-linked conjugate was tested, presumably due to the unstable nature of the ester bond. *A. baumannii* is an opportunistic pathogen that can causes serious infections often associated with multidrug resistant strains and has an 8.4–36.5% mortality rate [54]. In the present TTK study, although colistin sulphate at MIC (0.25 µg/mL colistin base) and the OligoG–E–colistin conjugate at 2 × MIC (0.25 µg/mL colistin base) exhibited rapid initial antimicrobial efficacy, marked bacterial re-growth was observed at 24 h. Previous studies have reported the impact of hetero-resistance of *A. baumannii* clinical isolates to colistin that allowed significant bacterial re-growth at 24 h at 32 × MIC [55] and 64 × MIC [56]. The reduction of viable bacterial counts by <3 $\log_{10}$ CFU/mL compared to the initial inoculum was indicative of bacteriostatic activity only. Similarly, bacteriostatic activity of colistin, at its MIC, towards *A. baumannii* clinical isolates has been demonstrated, indicating a 2-fold decrease in CFU/mL at 4–6 h post-dose [57]. Importantly, previous studies saw significant bactericidal activity of colistin when carbapenem-resistant *A. baumannii* isolates were treated with higher concentrations of the antibiotic (≥4 × MIC) [58]. Observations in the present study support the clinical limitations of conventional colistin therapy, due to concentration-dependent nephrotoxicity, which may limit the optimal dosing and efficacy of the antibiotic.

The findings of this study indicate that the ester-linked OligoG–colistin conjugate could be a suitable alternative to conventional colistin, as it demonstrated equivalent antimicrobial effectiveness (0.25 µg/mL colistin base) but exhibited significantly lower cytotoxicity in human kidney cells. Following systemic administration of colistimethate sodium (Colomycin®; prodrug of colistin), the plasma colistin concentration at steady-state is 0.5–4 µg/mL [59]. Clinically, nephrotoxicity is an important limiting factor to colistin dosing, therefore, a plasma concentration of 2 µg/mL is desirable to target bacterial pathogens with MIC values ≤1 µg/mL [60]. To avoid acute kidney injury, a maximum plasma concentration of 2.42 µg/mL is recommended [61]. Yet, the clinical susceptibility breakpoint for colistin against *Acinetobacter* spp. is 2 µg/mL [48,49], which gives it a narrow therapeutic index in vivo. Due to the EPR effect, OligoG–E–colistin conjugates are expected to accumulate within infected tissues, so higher antibiotic concentrations (>0.25 µg/mL colistin base, equivalent to >2 × MIC) could theoretically be achieved much quicker than with the unmodified antibiotic. Sustained release over 48 h and concentration-dependent antibacterial efficacy of colistin has been achieved using dextrin–colistin conjugates [32]. In that study, colistin was covalently linked to dextrin through an amide bond, so "unmasking" of antibiotic relied on α-amylase-mediated degradation of the polymer. The fact that the OligoG–A–colistin conjugate did not show any antimicrobial effect in the PK–PD model in this study could be attributed to the absence of alginate lyase in the culture medium or the presence of residual saccharides attached to colistin which would not be present on antibiotic released from the ester-linked conjugates. Recently, it has been demonstrated that, even after complete amylase degradation of dextrin in amide-linked dextrin-colistin conjugates, the colistin molecule was still attached to at least one linker with varying lengths of glucose units [18]. These findings suggest that complete "unmasking" or release of colistin is a pre-requisite for reinstatement of antibiotic activity.

Importantly, the therapeutic benefits of OligoG–colistin conjugates might have been underestimated by the in vitro assays. Passive accumulation of conjugates at sites of in vivo bacterial infection due to the EPR effect, alongside the local reduced pH, reactive oxygen species and esterase activity as well as alginate lyase could all promote the controlled release of the drug from the polymer, and might further enhance the efficacy of the drug in vivo and thus, reduce the doses required to eradicate infection.

5. Conclusions

This study has established, for the first time, the potential therapeutic benefits of using OligoG conjugation to reduce antibiotic toxicity, while maintaining antimicrobial activity against MDR Gram-negative bacterial pathogens. These studies also demonstrate that complete detachment of the polymer from the bioactive compound is required to restore its full biological efficacy, with residual sugars shown to impede complete regeneration of activity. As OligoG has been shown to enhance the antimicrobial activity of macrolides, tetracyclines and β-lactams antibiotics, against a range of MDR Gram-negative bacteria [20], OligoG conjugation might also improve the pharmacokinetics of other toxic, water-insoluble or otherwise undeliverable drugs. Polymer conjugates like the OligoG–polymyxins offer a novel approach to repurpose "old" antibiotics into safer, less toxic bi-functional compounds to meet the increasingly urgent need for new antimicrobial therapies.

Supplementary Materials: The following are available online at http://www.mdpi.com/1999-4923/12/11/1080/s1, Figure S1: Size exclusion chromatography with multi-angle light scattering detection (SEC-MALS) analysis of OligoG-conjugates (three different batches of OligoG–A–colistin (OAC) and one batch of OligoG–E–colistin (OEC)), showing overlaid refractive index chromatograms and corresponding Mw-time calibration lines. The injected mass was 250 µg for all samples. Abbreviations: A, amide; E, ester, Figure S2: SEC-MALS analysis of OligoG in the absence and presence of 10% *w/w* colistin, showing that they do not form strong complexes since the elution profile is identical, Figure S3: Diffusion-ordered spectroscopy (DOSY) of (a–c) three different batches of OligoG–A–colistin conjugates and (d) one batch of OligoG–E–colistin conjugate. The assignment of the unique signals for OligoG and colistin is indicated at the top of each panel and the red lines indicate the average diffusion coefficients of the molecules, Figure S4: Drug release of OligoG–polymyxin conjugates in phosphate buffered saline (PBS) at pH 5, pH 7 or pH 7 containing alginate lyase (AlgL). (a) Content of free polymyxin and (b) change in molecular weight were determined by fast protein liquid chromatography (FPLC) and size exclusion chromatography with refractive index detection (SEC-RI), respectively, over 48 h incubation. Abbreviations: A, amide; E, ester, Table S1: Gram-negative bacterial isolates used for characterisation of OligoG–polymyxin conjugates, Table S2: Physicochemical characteristics and batch details of OligoG–polymyxin conjugates used in this study, Table S3: Weight and number average molecular weights of OligoG and OligoG–colistin conjugates, Table S4: Selectivity index (SI) values of OligoG–polymyxin conjugates against a range of Gram-negative bacterial pathogens, Table S5: Microbiological efficacy (MICs) of OligoG–colistin conjugates in the presence of alginate lyase in Mueller–Hinton (MH) broth or after pre-incubation with alginate lyase against Gram-negative bacterial pathogens, Table S6: Microbiological efficacy (MICs) of polymyxins and antibiotic conjugates in the absence and presence of mucin against Gram-negative bacterial pathogens, Table S7: Comparison of the effect of growth medium (AS medium and MH broth) on antimicrobial activity (MIC determinations) of polymyxins and antibiotic conjugates, Table S8: Fractional inhibitory concentration index (FICI) values of OligoG–colistin conjugates or colistin in combination with azithromycin dihydrate, Methods: NMR spectroscopy.

Author Contributions: Conceptualization, J.S., E.L.F., D.W.T. and K.E.H.; Investigation, J.S., L.C.P. (participated in the confocal imaging experiments and analysis), O.A.A. and F.L.A. (SEC-MALS and DOSY experiments and analysis); Formal analysis, J.S., E.L.F., D.W.T., K.E.H.; Writing—Review and Editing, J.S., E.L.F., D.W.T., K.E.H. and P.D.R. All authors read and approved the final manuscript.

Funding: This work was supported by funding from the Research Council of Norway (228542/O30, 281920 and 226244), AlgiPharma AS, Sandvika, Norway and UK Medical Research Council (MR/N023633/1).

Acknowledgments: We thank Timothy Walsh (Department of Medical Microbiology and Infectious Disease, Cardiff University, UK) for the colistin resistant bacterial isolates. We thank Anne Tøndervik and Håvard Sletta for intellectual discussions about the research and Alexander Åstrand (AlgiPharma AS) for helpful comments on the manuscript.

Conflicts of Interest: This work was partly supported by funding from AlgiPharma AS, Sandvika, Norway who also provided the alginates used in the study. The authors (D.W.T. and K.E.H.) declare previous research funding from AlgiPharma AS. P.D.R. is CSO at AlgiPharma AS.

References

1. O'Neill, J. Tackling Drug-Resistant Infections Globally: Final Report and Recommendations. 2016. Available online: https://amr-review.org/Publications.html (accessed on 6 November 2020).
2. Zaman, S.B.; Hussain, M.A.; Nye, R.; Mehta, V.; Mamun, K.T.; Hossain, N. A review on antibiotic resistance: Alarm bells are ringing. *Cureus* **2017**, *9*, e1403. [CrossRef]
3. Schäberle, T.F.; Hack, I.M. Overcoming the current deadlock in antibiotic research. *Trends Microbiol.* **2014**, *22*, 165–167. [CrossRef] [PubMed]
4. O'Neill, J. Antimicrobial Resistance: Tackling a Crisis for the Health and Wealth of Nations. 2014. Available online: https://amr-review.org/Publications.html (accessed on 6 November 2020).
5. World Health Organization (WHO). Antibacterial Agents in Clinical Development. 2017. Available online: https://www.who.int/medicines/areas/rational_use/antibacterial_agents_clinical_development/en/ (accessed on 6 November 2020).
6. Nouvellet, P.; Robotham, J.V.; Naylor, N.R.; Woodford, N.; Ferguson, N.M. Potential impact of novel diagnostics and treatments on the burden of antibiotic resistant in *Escherichia coli*. *BioRxiv* **2016**, 052944.
7. Falagas, M.E.; Kasiakou, S.K.; Saravolatz, L.D. Colistin: The revival of polymyxins for the management of multidrug-resistant Gram-negative bacterial infections. *Clin. Infect. Dis.* **2005**, *40*, 1333–1341. [CrossRef] [PubMed]
8. Brown, P.; Abbott, E.; Abdulle, O.; Boakes, S.; Coleman, S.; Divall, N.; Duperchy, E.; Moss, S.; Rivers, D.; Simonovic, M.; et al. Design of next generation polymyxins with lower toxicity: The discovery of SPR206. *ACS Infect. Dis.* **2019**, *5*, 1645–1656. [CrossRef] [PubMed]
9. Su, M.; Wang, M.; Hong, Y.; Nimmagadda, A.; Shen, N.; Shi, Y.; Gao, R.; Zhang, E.; Cao, C.; Cai, J. Polymyxin derivatives as broad-spectrum antibiotic agents. *Chem. Commun.* **2019**, *55*, 13104–13107. [CrossRef]

10. Vaara, M. Polymyxin derivatives that sensitize Gram-negative bacteria to other antibiotics. *Molecules* **2019**, *24*, 249. [CrossRef]
11. Vaara, M. New polymyxin derivatives that display improved efficacy in animal infection models as compared to polymyxin B and colistin. *Med. Res. Rev.* **2018**, *38*, 1661–1673. [CrossRef]
12. Kanazawa, K.; Sato, Y.; Ohki, K.; Okimura, K.; Uchida, Y.; Shindo, M.; Sakura, N. Contribution of each amino acid residue in polymyxin B_3 to antimicrobial and lipopolysaccharide binding activity. *Chem. Pharm. Bull.* **2009**, *57*, 240–244. [CrossRef]
13. Velkov, T.; Roberts, K.D.; Thompson, P.E.; Li, J. Polymyxins: A new hope in combating Gram-negative superbugs? *Future Med. Chem.* **2016**, *8*, 1017–1025. [CrossRef]
14. Cal, P.M.; Matos, M.J.; Bernardes, G.J. Trends in therapeutic drug conjugates for bacterial diseases: A patent review. *Expert. Opin. Ther. Pat.* **2017**, *27*, 179–189. [CrossRef] [PubMed]
15. Azzopardi, E.A.; Ferguson, E.L.; Thomas, D.W. The enhanced permeability retention effect: A new paradigm for drug targeting in infection. *J. Antimicrob. Chemother.* **2013**, *68*, 257–274. [CrossRef] [PubMed]
16. Ferguson, E.L.; Azzopardi, E.; Roberts, J.L.; Walsh, T.R.; Thomas, D.W. Dextrin-colistin conjugates as a model bioresponsive treatment for multidrug resistant bacterial infections. *Mol. Pharm.* **2014**, *11*, 4437–4447. [CrossRef]
17. Zhu, C.; Schneider, E.K.; Wang, J.; Kempe, K.; Wilson, P.; Velkov, T.; Li, J.; Davis, T.P.; Whittaker, M.R.; Haddleton, D.M. A traceless reversible polymeric colistin prodrug to combat multidrug-resistant (MDR) Gram-negative bacteria. *J. Control. Release* **2017**, *259*, 83–91. [CrossRef]
18. Varache, M.; Powell, L.C.; Aarstad, O.A.; Williams, T.L.; Wenzel, M.N.; Thomas, D.W.; Ferguson, E.L. Polymer masked-unmasked protein therapy: Identification of the active species after amylase activation of dextrin-colistin conjugates. *Mol. Pharm.* **2019**, *16*, 3199–3207. [CrossRef]
19. Yang, J.S.; Xie, Y.J.; He, W. Research progress on chemical modification of alginate: A review. *Carbohydr. Polym.* **2011**, *84*, 33–39. [CrossRef]
20. Khan, S.; Tøndervik, A.; Sletta, H.; Klinkenberg, G.; Emanuel, C.; Onsøyen, E.; Myrvold, R.; Howe, R.A.; Walsh, T.R.; Hill, K.E.; et al. Overcoming drug resistance with alginate oligosaccharides able to potentiate the action of selected antibiotics. *Antimicrob. Agents Chemother.* **2012**, *56*, 5134–5141. [CrossRef]
21. Powell, L.C.; Sowedan, A.; Khan, S.; Wright, C.J.; Hawkins, K.; Onsøyen, E.; Myrvold, R.; Hill, K.E.; Thomas, D.W. The effect of alginate oligosaccharides on the mechanical properties of Gram-negative biofilms. *Biofouling* **2013**, *29*, 413–421. [CrossRef]
22. Powell, L.C.; Pritchard, M.F.; Emanuel, C.; Onsøyen, E.; Rye, P.D.; Wright, C.J.; Hill, K.E.; Thomas, D.W. A nanoscale characterization of the interaction of a novel alginate oligomer with the cell surface and motility of *Pseudomonas aeruginosa*. *Am. J. Respir. Cell Mol. Biol.* **2014**, *50*, 483–492. [CrossRef]
23. Powell, L.C.; Pritchard, M.F.; Ferguson, E.L.; Powell, K.A.; Patel, S.U.; Rye, P.D.; Sakellakou, S.M.; Buurma, N.J.; Brilliant, C.D.; Copping, J.M.; et al. Targeted disruption of the extracellular polymeric network of *Pseudomonas aeruginosa* biofilms by alginate oligosaccharides. *NPJ Biofilms Microbiomes* **2018**, *4*, 13. [CrossRef]
24. Pritchard, M.F.; Powell, L.C.; Jack, A.A.; Powell, K.; Beck, K.; Florance, H.; Forton, J.; Rye, P.D.; Dessen, A.; Hill, K.E.; et al. A low-molecular-weight alginate oligosaccharide disrupts pseudomonal microcolony formation and enhances antibiotic effectiveness. *Antimicrob. Agents Chemother.* **2017**, *61*, e00762-17. [CrossRef] [PubMed]
25. Duncan, R. The dawning era of polymer therapeutics. *Nat. Rev. Drug. Discov.* **2003**, *2*, 347–360. [CrossRef] [PubMed]
26. Hengzhuang, W.; Song, Z.; Ciofu, O.; Onsøyen, E.; Rye, P.D.; Høiby, N. OligoG CF-5/20 disruption of mucoid *Pseudomonas aeruginosa* biofilm in a murine lung infection model. *Antimicrob. Agents Chemother.* **2016**, *60*, 2620–2626. [CrossRef] [PubMed]
27. Yang, Q.; Li, M.; Spiller, O.B.; Andrey, D.O.; Hinchliffe, P.; Li, H.; Maclean, C.; Niumsup, P.; Powell, L.C.; Pritchard, M.F.; et al. Balancing mcr-1 expression and bacterial survival is a delicate equilibrium between essential cellular defence mechanisms. *Nat. Commun.* **2017**, *8*, 2054. [CrossRef] [PubMed]
28. Jorgensen, J.H.; Turnidge, J.D. Chapter 71—Susceptibility test methods: Dilution and disk diffusion methods. In *Manual of Clinical Microbiology*, 11th ed.; Jorgensen, J.H., Pfaller, M., Carroll, K., Funke, G., Landry, M., Richter, S., Warnock, D., Eds.; ASM Press: Washington, DC, USA, 2015; pp. 1253–1273.
29. Hsieh, M.H.; Yu, C.M.; Yu, V.L.; Chow, J.W. Synergy assessed by checkerboard: A critical analysis. *Diagn. Microbiol. Infect. Dis.* **1993**, *16*, 343–349. [CrossRef]

30. Bonapace, C.R.; Bosso, J.A.; Friedrich, L.V.; White, R.L. Comparison of methods of interpretation of checkerboard synergy testing. *Diagn. Microbiol. Infect. Dis.* **2002**, *44*, 363–366. [CrossRef]
31. Heydorn, A.; Nielsen, A.T.; Hentzer, M.; Sternberg, C.; Givskov, M.; Ersbøll, B.K.; Molin, S. Quantification of biofilm structures by the novel computer program comstat. *Microbiology* **2000**, *146*, 2395–2407. [CrossRef]
32. Azzopardi, E.A.; Ferguson, E.L.; Thomas, D.W. Development and validation of an in vitro pharmacokinetic/pharmacodynamic model to test the antibacterial efficacy of antibiotic polymer conjugates. *Antimicrob. Agents. Chemother.* **2015**, *59*, 1837–1843. [CrossRef]
33. Clinical and Laboratory Standards Institute (CLSI). Methods for Determining Bactericidal Activity of Antimicrobial Agents; Approved Guideline (M26-A). 1999. Available online: https://clsi.org/standards/products/microbiology/documents/m26/ (accessed on 6 November 2020).
34. Levison, M.E.; Levison, J.H. Pharmacokinetics and pharmacodynamics of antibacterial agents. *Infect. Dis. Clin. N. Am.* **2009**, *23*, 791–815. [CrossRef]
35. Vaara, M. Polymyxins and their potential next generation as therapeutic antibiotics. *Front. Microbiol.* **2019**, *10*, 1689. [CrossRef]
36. Rabanal, F.; Cajal, Y. Recent advances and perspectives in the design and development of polymyxins. *Nat. Prod. Rep.* **2017**, *34*, 886–908. [CrossRef] [PubMed]
37. Brown, P.; Dawson, M.J. Development of new polymyxin derivatives for multi-drug resistant Gram-negative infections. *J. Antibiot.* **2017**, *70*, 386–394. [CrossRef] [PubMed]
38. Hermanson, G.T. Zero-length crosslinkers. In *Bioconjugate Techniques*, 3rd ed.; Academic Press: Boston, MA, USA, 2013; Chapter 4, pp. 259–273.
39. Simpson, J.A.; Smith, S.E.; Dean, R.T. Alginate may accumulate in cystic fibrosis lung because the enzymatic and free radical capacities of phagocytic cells are inadequate for its degradation. *Biochem. Mol. Biol. Int.* **1993**, *30*, 1021–1034. [PubMed]
40. Wong, T.Y.; Preston, L.A.; Schiller, N.L. Alginate lyase: Review of major sources and enzyme characteristics, structure-function analysis, biological roles, and applications. *Annu. Rev. Microbiol.* **2000**, *54*, 289–340. [CrossRef]
41. Greco, F.; Vicent, M. Polymer-drug conjugates: Current status and future trends. *Front. Biosci.* **2008**, *13*, 2744–2756. [CrossRef]
42. Li, C.; Yu, D.F.; Newman, R.A.; Cabral, F.; Stephens, L.C.; Hunter, N.; Milas, L.; Wallace, S. Complete regression of well-established tumors using a novel water-soluble poly(l-glutamic acid)-paclitaxel conjugate. *Cancer Res.* **1998**, *58*, 2404–2409.
43. Tsakos, M.; Schaffert, E.S.; Clement, L.L.; Villadsen, N.L.; Poulsen, T.B. Ester coupling reactions-an enduring challenge in the chemical synthesis of bioactive natural products. *Nat. Prod. Rep.* **2015**, *32*, 605–632. [CrossRef]
44. Wong, P.T.; Choi, S.K. Mechanisms of drug release in nanotherapeutic delivery systems. *Chem. Rev.* **2015**, *115*, 3388–3432. [CrossRef]
45. Dalheim, M.Ø.; Vanacker, J.; Najmi, M.A.; Aachmann, F.L.; Strand, B.L.; Christensen, B.E. Efficient functionalization of alginate biomaterials. *Biomaterials* **2016**, *80*, 146–156. [CrossRef]
46. Spapen, H.; Jacobs, R.; Gorp, V.V.; Troubleyn, J.; Honoré, P.M. Renal and neurological side effects of colistin in critically ill patients. *Ann. Intensive Care* **2011**, *1*, 14. [CrossRef]
47. Sandri, A.M.; Landersdorfer, C.B.; Jacob, J.; Boniatti, M.M.; Dalarosa, M.G.; Falci, D.R.; Behle, T.F.; Bordinhão, R.C.; Wang, J.; Forrest, A.; et al. Population pharmacokinetics of intravenous polymyxin B in critically ill patients: Implications for selection of dosage regimens. *Clin. Infect. Dis.* **2013**, *57*, 524–531. [CrossRef] [PubMed]
48. Clinical and Laboratory Standards Institute (CLSI). Performance Standards for Antimicrobial Susceptibility Testing (M100). 2020. Available online: https://clsi.org/standards/products/microbiology/documents/m100/ (accessed on 6 November 2020).
49. European Committee on Antimicrobial Susceptibility Testing (ECAST). Breakpoint Tables for Interpretation of MICs and Zone Diameters. 2019. Available online: http://www.eucast.org/clinical_breakpoints/ (accessed on 6 November 2020).
50. Huang, J.X.; Blaskovich, M.A.T.; Pelingon, R.; Ramu, S.; Kavanagh, A.; Elliott, A.G.; Butler, M.S.; Montgomery, A.B.; Cooper, M.A. Mucin binding reduces colistin antimicrobial activity. *Antimicrob. Agents Chemother.* **2015**, *59*, 5925–5931. [CrossRef] [PubMed]

51. Pritchard, M.F.; Oakley, J.L.; Brilliant, C.D.; Rye, P.D.; Forton, J.; Doull, I.J.M.; Ketchell, I.; Hill, K.E.; Thomas, D.W.; Lewis, P.D. Mucin structural interactions with an alginate oligomer mucolytic in cystic fibrosis sputum. *Vib. Spectrosc.* **2019**, *103*, 102932. [CrossRef]
52. He, X.; Hwang, H.M.; Aker, W.G.; Wang, P.; Lin, Y.; Jiang, X.; He, X. Synergistic combination of marine oligosaccharides and azithromycin against *Pseudomonas aeruginosa*. *Microbiol. Res.* **2014**, *169*, 759–767. [CrossRef] [PubMed]
53. Gaspar, M.C.; Couet, W.; Olivier, J.C.; Pais, A.A.C.C.; Sousa, J.J.S. *Pseudomonas aeruginosa* infection in cystic fibrosis lung disease and new perspectives of treatment: A review. *Eur. J. Clin. Microbiol. Infect. Dis.* **2013**, *32*, 1231–1252. [CrossRef] [PubMed]
54. Falagas, M.E.; Rafailidis, P.I. Attributable mortality of *Acinetobacter baumannii*: No longer a controversial issue. *Crit. Care* **2007**, *11*, 134. [CrossRef] [PubMed]
55. Li, J.; Rayner, C.R.; Nation, R.L.; Owen, R.J.; Spelman, D.; Tan, K.E.; Liolios, L. Heteroresistance to colistin in multidrug-resistant *Acinetobacter baumannii*. *Antimicrob. Agents Chemother.* **2006**, *50*, 2946–2950. [CrossRef]
56. Owen, R.J.; Li, J.; Nation, R.L.; Spelman, D. In vitro pharmacodynamics of colistin against *Acinetobacter baumannii* clinical isolates. *J. Antimicrob. Chemother.* **2007**, *59*, 473–477. [CrossRef]
57. Tan, T.Y.; Ng, L.S.; Tan, E.; Huang, G. In vitro effect of minocycline and colistin combinations on imipenem-resistant *Acinetobacter baumannii* clinical isolates. *J. Antimicrob. Chemother.* **2007**, *60*, 421–423. [CrossRef]
58. Song, J.Y.; Kee, S.Y.; Hwang, I.S.; Seo, Y.B.; Jeong, H.W.; Kim, W.J.; Cheong, H.J. In vitro activities of carbapenem/sulbactam combination, colistin, colistin/rifampicin combination and tigecycline against carbapenem-resistant *Acinetobacter baumannii*. *J. Antimicrob. Chemother.* **2007**, *60*, 317–322. [CrossRef]
59. Nation, R.L.; Garonzik, S.M.; Li, J.; Thamlikitkul, V.; Giamarellos-Bourboulis, E.J.; Paterson, D.L.; Turnidge, J.D.; Forrest, A.; Silveira, F.P. Updated US and European dose recommendations for intravenous colistin: How do they perform? *Clin. Infect. Dis.* **2016**, *62*, 552–558. [CrossRef] [PubMed]
60. Landersdorfer, C.B.; Nation, R.L. Colistin: How should it be dosed for the critically ill? *Semin. Respir. Crit. Care Med.* **2015**, *36*, 126–135. [CrossRef] [PubMed]
61. Sorlí, L.; Luque, S.; Grau, S.; Berenguer, N.; Segura, C.; Montero, M.M.; Álvarez-Lerma, F.; Knobel, H.; Benito, N.; Horcajada, J.P. Trough colistin plasma level is an independent risk factor for nephrotoxicity: A prospective observational cohort study. *BMC Infect. Dis.* **2013**, *13*, 380. [CrossRef] [PubMed]

Publisher's Note: MDPI stays neutral with regard to jurisdictional claims in published maps and institutional affiliations.

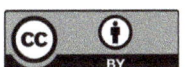

© 2020 by the authors. Licensee MDPI, Basel, Switzerland. This article is an open access article distributed under the terms and conditions of the Creative Commons Attribution (CC BY) license (http://creativecommons.org/licenses/by/4.0/).

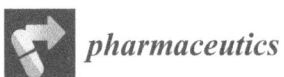

Article

Mixed Pluronic—Cremophor Polymeric Micelles as Nanocarriers for Poorly Soluble Antibiotics—The Influence on the Antibacterial Activity

Maria Antonia Tănase [1], Adina Raducan [1], Petruța Oancea [1], Lia Mara Dițu [2], Miruna Stan [3], Cristian Petcu [4,*], Cristina Scomoroșcenco [4], Claudia Mihaela Ninciuleanu [4], Cristina Lavinia Nistor [4] and Ludmila Otilia Cinteza [1,*]

[1] Physical Chemistry Department, University of Bucharest, 030018 Bucharest, Romania; maria.a.tanase@gmail.com (M.A.T.); adina.raducan@g.unibuc.ro (A.R.); petruta.oancea@unibuc.ro (P.O.)
[2] Microbiology Department, Faculty of Biology, University of Bucharest, 60101 Bucharest, Romania; lia-mara.ditu@bio.unibuc.ro
[3] Department of Biochemistry and Molecular Biology, Faculty of Biology, ICUB-Research Institute of the University of Bucharest, University of Bucharest, 050095 Bucharest, Romania; miruna.stan@bio.unibuc.ro
[4] National Institute for Research and Development in Chemistry and Petrochemistry-ICECHIM, Polymer Department, 202 Spl. Independentei, 060021 Bucharest, Romania; cristina.scomoroscenco@icechim-pd.ro (C.S.); claudia.ninciuleanu@icechim-pd.ro (C.M.N.); cristina.nistor@icechim-pd.ro (C.L.N.)
* Correspondence: cpetcu@icf.ro (C.P.); ocinteza@gw-chimie.math.unibuc.ro (L.O.C.)

Abstract: In this work, novel polymeric mixed micelles from Pluronic F127 and Cremophor EL were investigated as drug delivery systems for Norfloxacin as model antibiotic drug. The optimal molar ratio of surfactants was determined, in order to decrease critical micellar concentration (CMC) and prepare carriers with minimal surfactant concentrations. The particle size, zeta potential, and encapsulation efficiency were determined for both pure and mixed micelles with selected composition. In vitro release kinetics of Norfloxacin from micelles show that the composition of surfactant mixture generates tunable extended release. The mixed micelles exhibit good biocompatibility against normal fibroblasts MRC-5 cells, while some cytotoxicity was found in all micellar systems at high concentrations. The influence of the surfactant components in the carrier on the antibacterial properties of Norfloxacin was investigated. The drug loaded mixed micellar formulation exhibit good activity against clinical isolated strains, compared with the CLSI recommended standard strains (*Staphylococcus aureus* ATCC 25923, *Enterococcus faecalis* ATCC 29213, *Pseudomonas aeruginosa* ATCC 27853, *Escherichia coli* ATCC 25922). *P. aeruginosa* 5399 clinical strain shows low sensitivity to Norfloxacin in all tested micelle systems. The results suggest that Cremophor EL-Pluronic F127 mixed micelles can be considered as novel controlled release delivery systems for hydrophobic antimicrobial drugs.

Keywords: mixed polymeric micelles; drug delivery; antibiotics; Pluronic F127

1. Introduction

Infectious disease treatments continue to impose the extensive use of antibiotics. Despite the remarkable advances made in the last century in the synthesis of new drugs with antimicrobial activity, there are many deficiencies, such as high toxicity, low solubility, reduced bioavailability, and inadequate release profile for both new and old antibiotics successfully used in the present therapies. The main issue, however, remains the multidrug resistance, which produce a huge burden on the global health system.

To overcome these drawbacks, in the last decades, nanosized drug delivery systems have been generate increasing interest of the scientific community, due to their unique physicochemical properties. The advantages of these nanoparticulate carriers in antimicrobial formulations include targeted delivery to the infection site, improved cellular internalization and drug stability, higher solubility, and sustained drug release [1]. The quinolone and their derivatives fluoroquinolone antibiotics are the most efficient class of topoisomerase inhibitors, used to treat bacterial infections caused by both Gram-positive and Gram-negative bacteria [2]. Their mechanism of action consists in the inhibition of topoisomerase enzymes (DNA gyrase implicated in genome replication and transcription), which inhibits the relaxation of supercoiled DNA and promotes the breakage of double stranded DNA [3]. Their broad antimicrobial spectrum is due to their ability to cross bacterial cell wall and cytoplasmic membranes via passive diffusion mechanism, being is strongly dependent on the lipid composition [4]. Consequently, the antibacterial activity of fluoroquinolones appears to result from the combination of efficient cellular membrane penetration and DNA gyrase inhibiting activity. Norfloxacin (1-ethyl-6-fluoro-l,4-dihydro-4-oxo-7-(1-piperazinyl)-3-quinoline carboxylic acid) is one of the most used antibiotics from the class of fluoroquinolones [5]. Due to its complex structure, it shows superior antibacterial activity against both gram positive and gram-negative bacteria, and is used to treat a large variety of respiratory or urinary tract infections.

Norfloxacin is considered as a poorly soluble drug, despite of the experimental partition coefficient log P that is reported in literature ranging from -0.43 to -1.52, quite different from the value obtained from theoretical calculation (-0.92 to 1.44) [6]. However, the large value of negative thermodynamic potential of solvation in the apolar solvent explains the poor bioavailability (less than 40%) and short half-time (3–4 h) in serum [7]. Various drug delivery systems were proposed to prolong the release, and good results have been obtained. Encapsulation in polymeric material guar gum, sodium carboxymethyl cellulose, and hydroxypropyl cellulose lead to an extended the Norfloxacin release over a period of 7–12 h [8]. A sustained release of the drug was also reported using Norfloxacin loaded proniosomes and lipid polymer hybrid nanoparticles [9].

Taking into account the advantages of different nanostructured vectors, various drug delivery systems for Norfloxacin (NFLX) have been proposed to increase its solubility, stability to chemical and photodegradation, and to improve the therapeutic benefits. For example, Ahmad et al. [10] are proposing a series of liposomal preparations of Norfloxacin with variable concentrations of phosphatidylcholine, based on the charge transfer complex between drug and phosphatidylcholine molecules. In another study, Norfloxacin-loaded nanosponges based on cyclodextrin to maximize oral absorption were proposed [11]. Norfloxacin-stearic acid solid-lipid nanoparticles were also successfully used as an oral delivery formulation [12]. Another hybrid drug delivery system containing Norfloxacin loaded into TiO_2 nanoparticles followed by encapsulation onto poly lactic acid was found to be a suitable carrier with high antibacterial activity [13].

Nanocarriers as delivery systems for antibiotics enhance drug solubility, modulate drug release characteristics, and are also valuable tools in fighting antibiotic resistance [14]. Advanced drug delivery systems are studied for the encapsulation of norfloxacin [15] and other quinolones [16], but very rare micellar systems are investigated [17].

Micelles dispersions, from classic surfactants or polymeric surfactants, are currently used in many pharmaceutical products with various applications, from infusible solutions with chemotherapeutics or antibiotics to ocular formulations. Most of the pharmaceutical products contains as solubilizers nonionic surfactants, such as Tweens or Cremophors. Cremophor EL is FDA-approved nonionic emulsifier, used as a solubilizing agent for many years [18], produced by reacting castor oil with ethylene oxide. Therefore, it contains a mixture of unmodified castor oil and a large variety of polyethylene glycols, polyethoxylated glycerols, polyethoxylated fatty acids, and mono-, di-, and tri-esters of glycerol that are polyethoxylated to different degrees [19]. Due to its excellent emulsifying capacity, Cremophor is used for solubilization, protection, and delivery of different lipophilic active pharmaceutical ingredients (API). Numerous studies highlight Cremophor toxicity, namely anaphylactic hypersensitivity reactions, allergic shock, lipoprotein patterns and hyperlipidemia, neurotoxicity and hypotension, also at low concentration [20]. Also, some papers indicate that Cremophor can modify the toxicity profile of some active pharmaceutical ingredients [20].

Polymeric surfactants are considered a safer and more convenient alternative to classic surfactants, due to their low CMC values, good biocompatibility profile, and high drug entrapment efficiency since they possess large hydrophobic inner core. Among them, the most investigated class are polyethylene oxide-polypropylene oxide block copolymers (Pluronics or Poloxamers). These group of surfactants are FDA approved and used in various nanocarriers, in micelles, gels, and polymer stabilized nanoemulsions, to solubilize and improve the bioavailability of the poorly water-soluble active pharmaceutical ingredients. Their specific tri-block copolymer structure offers advantage regarding the modification of the release and are widely used as a carrier for controlled drug delivery [21]. Another significant advantage is that aqueous solutions of Pluronics in the presence of acids, alkalis, and metal ions are very stable [22]. Also, these polymeric micelles are more investigated because they do not show demicellization (micellar aggregate breaking) upon dilution in the presence of biological fluids such as blood and tearing.

Micellar carriers that contain Pluronic polymers exhibit good biocompatibility over a large concentration range, characteristic confirmed in many studies [23].

Most of the inconvenient of micellar systems as drug delivery systems are related to the intrinsic toxicity due to the large content of surfactant required to produce micellar aggregates even after dilution suffered after administration. In this respect, a mixture of surfactants is investigated as a possible solution to prepare mixed micelles with superior stability. When classic surfactants are added to Pluronic micelles depending on the molecular interactions taking place in the system, size and morphologies of the formed aggregates are modified [24], significantly modifying the encapsulation and release capacity of the drug. Forming mixed micelles with Pluronics is especially used to decrease the critical micellar concentration of the systems. Extensive research is available on the synergistic effects in the micellization process in mixtures containing various ionic surfactant and polymeric surfactants, while very few studies report synergism in mixed micelles of Pluronics and nonionic surfactants used in drug delivery systems formulation [25,26].

Mixed micelles are used especially to enhance the drug encapsulation and delivery parameters and have great potential as efficient drug carrier [27]. Beyond the reduction of CMC value, mixed micelles show other synergistic properties, such as increased drug loading capacity and micelle stability, higher than of the individual components. According to some reports mixed micelles that include Pluronic F127 exhibit higher solubilization capacity compared to pure F127 micelles [21]. In a study is reported a polymeric mixed micellar formulation at 1:1 Poloxamer 407/Pluronic P123 ratio, that exhibits a slower and controlled release of the drug, in contrast to the pure polymer micellar system. This behavior minimized the adverse effects associated with exceeding the safe concentration of the drug [28].

Although polymeric micelles are known to be very efficient drug carriers, little attention has been paid in using them as nanosized formulations for antibiotics. In a study carried by Khanal [29], a drug delivery system was developed by encapsulate the anionic drug cloxacillin sodium in a polyvinyl pyridine block of polystyrene-b-2-vinyl pyridine-b-ethylene oxide in order to investigate the possibility of micelles being a suitable antibiotic delivery system. Polymeric micelles were also proposed as carrier to ensure the drug transport across the blood brain barrier (BBB). Micelles prepared from cholesterol-conjugated PEG and anchored with a transactivator of transcription (TAT) peptide (TAT-PEG-b-Col) were prepared to encapsulate Ciprofloxacin and prove sustained antibacterial activity against *B. subtilis* and *E. coli*. The in vivo study evidenced that the polymeric micelles pass the BBB [30].

The aim of the present study was to prepare mixed micellar systems containing a well-known nonionic surfactant, i.e., Cremophor EL and Pluronic F127 to encapsulate a poorly soluble antibiotic Norfloxacin. The self-assembling properties in mixed surfactant systems were systematic investigated to prove the possibility of synergistic effects in micelle forming behavior. The optimization of the composition ensures the minimum surfactant amount in formulation and the use of reduced quantity of Cremophor EL, to decrease the side effects associated with it. The antibacterial activity of Norfloxacin loaded mixed micelles was evaluated, in order to consider these novel colloidal vectors as possible nanocarriers for poorly soluble antibiotics.

2. Materials and Methods

2.1. Materials

Micelle forming polymeric surfactants Pluronic® F127 (BioReagent MW = 12,600 g/mol), Cremophor EL (Millipore, Burlington, MA) and model drug Norfloxacin (≥98% TLC) were purchased from Sigma-Aldrich (Merck Group, Darmstadt, Germany). Pyrene (99% purity) and the solvents absolute ethanol (99.9%), dimethyl sulfoxide (DMSO), benzene (99% purity), chloroform (99% purity), phosphate Buffer Solution (99% purity), and hydrochloric acid (36.5 g/mol, 99% purity) were also obtained from Sigma-Aldrich (Merck Group, Darmstadt, Germany). All used reagents and chemicals were used as received without further modifications.

Pluronic F127 (Pl F127)   Norfloxacin (NFLX)   Cremophor EL (Cr EL)

2.2. Preparation of Micelles

A simple thin-film rehydration method was used to prepare micelles of Pluronic F127 and Cremophor EL. The procedure is schematically presented in the Figure 1.

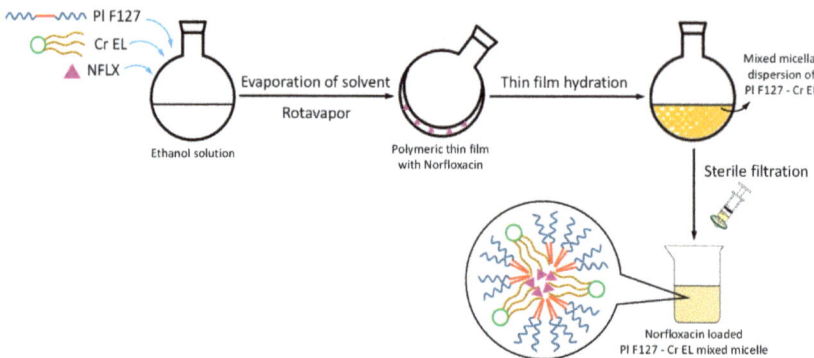

Figure 1. Schematic representation of the obtaining procedure for the Norfloacin loaded Pluronic F127—Cremophor EL mixed micelles.

Suitable amounts of surfactants or surfactant mixtures were dissolved in ethanol in a round-bottom flask. The vial was attached to a rotatory evaporator (Rotavapor-R-300®, Buchi Labortechnik AG, Flawil, Switzerland) and heated at 45 °C under vacuum to produce a thin film of micelle forming material deposited on the walls. After the total removal of the solvent, the required volume of distilled water was added to rehydrate the film under moderate magnetic stirring at 45 °C, for 30 min. The as prepared micellar dispersion was further filtered through sterile syringe filter Minisart® 0.2 μm (Sartorius, Gottingen,

Germany). For the mixed micelles, the two surfactants were added in ethanol solvent to obtain molar ratio 0.2, 0.4, 0.6 and 0.8 in the final aqueous dispersions.

The drug loaded pure and mixed micelles were prepared following the same procedure and Norfloxacin was dissolved together with the polymeric surfactants in alcohol. The dissolution of the Norfloxacin in the deposited thin film before the rehydration step ensure the maximum solubilization of the drug inside the micelle core.

2.3. Characterization of Mixed Micelles

CMC values of the pure and mixed surfactant systems were evaluated using the fluorescence method with pyrene as fluorescence probe [31]. Briefly, the fluorescence spectra of pyrene incorporated into the studied micelles (pure Cremophor EL, Pluronic F127 or mixed in various molar ratio) were recorded. A sharp variation of the slope in the graphic representation of the I3/I1 ratio (first and third vibronic peaks) indicate the CMC. For the sample preparation, pyrene was dissolved in acetone, a required volume was added in a graduate flask and the solvent was removed. Then, the surfactant solution was added to pyrene to reach a concentration of 1×10^{-6} M. The concentrations of the analyzed solutions ranked from 2.5×10^{-4} M to 2.5×10^{-6} M for all surfactants and their mixtures. The spectrofluorimetric measurements were performed using a Jasco FP8200 instrument (JASCO Corporation, Tokyo, Japan). The excitation wavelength for pyrene was 334 nm and its emission was recorded between 350 and 600nm. The intensity ratio between the first peak (373 nm) and the third peak (384 nm) was plotted against the concentration of the analyzed solutions and analyzed for the calculation.

Particle Size, Polydispersity Index (PI), and Zeta Potential: The pure and mixed polymeric micelles size and size distribution were measured using the dynamic light scattering (DLS) method. The data was analyzed by number and intensity weighted distributions. The zeta potential was calculated by Laser Doppler Velocimetry (LDV). The measurements were performed on a Nano ZS ZEN3600 Zetasizer (Malvern Instruments Ltd., Malvern, UK) equipment. The measurements were carried out on pristine and diluted samples, and the dilution was made with distilled water or PBS. In order to evidence the stability against aggregation and detect the presence of precipitated drug nanocrystals the samples were measured before and after filtration.

The micropolarity of the micelles was evaluated from the value of the I3/I1 ratio calculated for pyrene spectra in micellar solutions, compared to the values obtained in water and nonpolar solvent as reference.

The stability of micellar systems against dilution was evaluated by changes in size and size distribution when sample were diluted 10 time in either water or PBS. The resistance of micellar aggregates at different pH was also investigated by DLS measurements in surfactant solutions at pH = 4, pH = 6 and pH = 7.4 values.

The physicochemical stability of drug-containing micelles was evaluated by measuring the variation of the size and size distribution on samples stored at room temperature over four weeks.

2.4. Drug-Surfactant Interaction

The interaction of Norfloxacin with micelle forming surfactants was investigated using FTIR. The measurements were performed as follows. The spectra were recorded with a Tensor 37 Bruker equipment (Woodstock, NY, USA), using 32 scans with 4 cm^{-1} resolution in the 4000–400 cm^{-1} spectral range.

The sample pellets were prepared by adding pure components (NFLX, Pluronic or Cremophor) and drug loaded micellar solution in KBr powder, further subjected to extensive drying procedure to remove the solvent.

2.5. Drug Solubility and Entrapment Efficiency

For the measurement of the maximum solubility of Norfloxacin in surfactant solutions pure and mixed micelles were prepared with Cremophor EL, Pluronic F127 and binary mixture of Cremophor and Pluronic F127 with the molar ratio $\alpha = 0.2$, all samples at concentrations five time their CMC value. Excess amounts (2 mg) of Norfloxacin were added in flasks and dissolved with 1 mL of ethanol. The solvent was removed in a rotaevaporator and the drug was further dissolved in 1 mL of each micellar solution. The drug—micellar systems were left to equilibrate for 12 h and the obtained dispersions were centrifuged and filtered using 0.22 μm regenerated cellulose syringe filters.

The drug amount was quantified using fluorescence method adapted in our laboratory from literature [32]. Briefly, fluorescence spectra were recorded in acidic solution of 0.1 N HCl, with λ_{ex} = 330 nm and λ_{em} = 450 nm. Concentration of Norfloxacin in micellar systems tested for calibration was: 100 μg/mL, 50 μg/mL, 25 μg/mL, 12.5 μg/mL, 6.25 μg/mL and 3.125 μg/mL. Calibration curves were obtained by plotting the fluorescence intensity at 450 nm against the concentration of Norfloxacine.

Good linearity was obtained for the concentration range 50–3.125 μg/mL for all micellar systems with R^2 = 0.9961 for Cremophor micelles, R^2 = 0.9903. For Pluronic F127 micelles and R^2 = 0.9908 for the binary mixture of Cremophor and Pluronic F127 with the molar ratio, $\alpha = 0.2$.

The encapsulation efficiency (EE%) was calculated as the weight ratio of encapsulated drug NFLX to the drug in feed at drug-loaded micelles:

$$EE\ (\%) = \text{Experimental drug loading} / \text{Theoretical drug loading} \times 100$$

2.6. In Vitro Drug Release

The release of Norfloxacin from pure micelles of Cremophor and Pluronic and mixed micelles of binary mixture of Cremophor and Pluronic at selected molar ratio $\alpha = 0.2$ was studied using the dialysis bag method under physiological conditions. A volume of 2 mL of Norfloxacin encapsulated (100μg/mL) in Pluronic F127 (1.5×10^{-3} M), Cremophor EL (8×10^{-4} M) and a binary mixture of Cremophor EL and Pluronic F127 with the molar ratio, $\alpha = 0.2$ (1×10^{-3} M) were added to the pre-swelled dialysis bag with two ends sealed with plastic sealing clips. The systems were weighted before and after adding the NFLX micellar solution. Each bag was placed in PBS release medium at room temperature, under constant stirring (50 rpm). Aliquotes of 0.5 mL were withdrawn from the release medium at predetermined time intervals (15 min, 30 min, 45 min, 1–8 h, 24 h) and replaced with the same amount of fresh medium.

All aliquots were diluted 1:10 (v/v) with 0.1N HCl and quantified by means of fluorescence spectrophotometry. The spectrofluorimetric measurements were performed using a Jasco FP8200. The excitation wavelength was 330 nm, and its emission was recorded between 350–600 nm. The intensity of the peak at 450 nm was recorded and further used to calculate the cumulative % of drug release.

The influence of the temperature and pH of the media on drug release was tested and the experiment were performed at 25 °C and 37 °C, in PBS buffer with pH values of 7.4, 6 and 4.

2.7. Cells Viability Assay

Cell culture: Human lung fibroblasts MRC-5 (ATCC CCL-171) were grown in complete Eagle's minimal essential medium (Invitrogen, USA) containing 10% fetal bovine serum (Gibco, Carlsbad, CA, USA) at 37 °C in a humidified atmosphere with 5% CO_2. The cells were seeded at a cell density of 5×10^4 cells/cm^2 and left to adhere for 24 h. Then, the fibroblasts were incubated for the next 24 or 48 h with different concentrations of surfactants in the range 1×10^{-6}–1×10^{-3} M, which were previously sterilized by filtration with 0.2 μm pore size filter membrane. Untreated cells were used as control for all in vitro experiments.

MTT assay: The cellular viability was measured using the 3-(4,5-dimethylthiazol-2-yl)-2,5-diphenyltetrazolium bromide (MTT; Sigma-Aldrich, St. Louis, USA) assay. After 24 h of incubation, the culture medium was removed, and the cells were incubated with 1 mg/mL MTT for 2 h at 37 °C. The purple formazan crystals formed in the viable cells were dissolved with 2-propanol (Sigma-Aldrich, St. Louis, USA) and the absorbance was measured at 595 nm using a microplate reader (Flex Station, Molecular Devices).

Griess assay: The concentration of nitric oxide (NO) in the collected culture medium after the 24 h of incubation was performed with the Griess reagent, a stoichiometric solution (v/v) of 0.1% naphthylethylendiamine dihydrochloride and 1% sulphanilamide in 5% H_3PO_4). Increased levels of NO are related with cytotoxic effects as this molecule relates to inflammation and apoptosis. The absorbance of mix formed by equal volumes of medium supernatants and Griess reagent was read at 550 nm using the FlexStation 3 microplate reader and the NO concentration was calculated from the $NaNO_2$ standard curve.

Statistical analysis: The in vitro assays were performed in triplicates and the results were presented as mean ± standard deviation (SD) of three independent experiments. The statistical significance was analyzed by Student t-test. A value of p less than 0.05 was considered significant.

2.8. Antibacterial Activity

The antimicrobial assays were performed using standard and clinical bacterial strains that were included in the microbial collection of University of Bucharest, Faculty of Biology, Microbiology Department: *Staphylococcus aureus* ATCC 25923 and *Staphylococcus aureus* MRSA clinical strain, *Enterococcus faecalis* ATCC 29213 and *Enterococcus faecalis* VRE clinical strain, *Pseudomonas aeruginosa* ATCC 27853 and *Pseudomonas aeruginosa* 5399 clinical strain, and *Escherichia coli* ATCC 25922 and *Escherichia coli* ESBL 135 clinical strain. To perform the experiment, two successive passages were made by passing the microbial strains on nutritious agar medium and incubating for 24 h, at 37 °C.

The qualitative screening of the anti-microbial properties was performed by an adapted spot diffusion method, according with CLSI standard (Clinical Laboratory Standard Institute, 2021). Bacterial suspensions of 1.5×10^8 CFU/mL (corresponding with 0.5 McFarland standard density) obtained from 24 h microbial cultures developed on Muller Hinton agar (MHA) were used in the experiments. Petri dishes with MHA were seeded with microbial inoculums and an amount of 10 µL solution of each sample was spotted, the calculated concentration of norfloxacin being 20 µg/mL. The standard disks with 30 µg of norfloxacin were used as control for the strain's sensitivity. The plates were left at room temperature to ensure the equal diffusion of the compound in the medium and then incubated at 37 °C for 24 h. Sensitivity was evaluated by measuring the diameters of the inhibition zones that appeared around the spot and expressed in mm.

For establishing the MIC (minimum inhibitory concentration) values of the obtained compounds we utilized a serial microdilution method performed in nutritive broth. The sterile broth was added in sterile 96 well plates and binary dilutions of each tested compound were performed in a final volume of 150 µL, starting with 20 µg/mL concentration calculated for Norfloxacin, in the first well. Further, 15 µL of microbial suspension adjusted to 1.5×10^7 CFU/mL, were added in each well. The MIC values were established by spectrophotometric measurement (absorbance reading at 600 nm using BIOTEK SYNERGY-HTX ELISA multi-mode reader). Each experiment was performed in triplicate and repeated on at least three separate occasions.

Statistical analysis: For biological tests, significant differences between the means of triplicate experiments and the control were determined by using one-way ANOVA statistical analysis (significance difference was noted as * for $p < 0.05$, and ** for $p < 0.01$). All data are presented as mean values ± the standard deviations (SD).

3. Results and Discussion

3.1. Mixed Micelles Preparation and Non-Ideal Behavior in Mixed Pluronic F127-Cremophor EL Aqueous Solutions

In this study, a novel carrier from mixtures of two nonionic polymeric surfactants Cremophor EL and Pluronic F127 is proposed, in order to obtain a controlled drug delivery for Norfloxacin with extended release and higher permeability through cell membranes.

The adequate composition of the mixed polymeric micelles to ensure the minimum content of surfactants and a low value of CMC was evaluated from the non-ideal behavior of surfactant mixture, using Rubingh model. The self-assembling properties of the aqueous solution of Cremophor EL and Pluronic F127 have been studied and CMC values were calculated from the variation of pyrene fluorescence spectra, i.e, variation of the I3/I1 ratio with concentration of surfactant, as described in the previous section. The point where two linear fitting curves in premicellar (low concentration) and micellar region intersect is considered as CMC value. To evaluate the ideal or non-ideal behavior in mixed micelles, CMC theoretical values were calculated from the Clint Equation (1):

$$\frac{1}{C^*} = \frac{\alpha_1}{C_1} + \frac{1-\alpha_1}{C_2} \tag{1}$$

where C^* represents the CMC of the binary mixture of Surfactant 1 and 2, α is the mole fraction of surfactant 1 in the mixed solution and C_1 and C_2 are the individual CMCs of Surfactant 1 and Surfactant 2.

In order to calculate the intensity of interaction between the two surfactants from the binary mixture, one can use a parameter, β, calculated using Equation (2), from the model proposed by Rubingh [33]:

$$\beta_{12} = \frac{\ln \frac{\alpha_1 C^*}{x_1 C_1}}{(1-x_1)^2} \tag{2}$$

where α_1 is the mole fraction of surfactant (Cremophor EL) in the mixed micellar solution, C^* is CMC of mixed micelles, C_1 is the CMC of Surfactant 1 and x_1 is the micellar mole fraction of Surfactant 1.

The micelle mole fraction x_1 can be calculated by iteratively solving Equation (3):

$$\frac{x_1^2 \cdot \ln \frac{\alpha_1 C^*}{x_1 C_1}}{(1-x_1)^2 \cdot \ln \frac{(1-\alpha_1)C^*}{(1-x_1)C_1}} = 1 \tag{3}$$

The value of parameter of interaction β quantifies the interactions between the molecules of surfactant. When attractive forces between the two surfactants are present, the value of this parameter is negative, meaning that synergism is present in the mixed micelles. Positive values for parameter β indicate an antagonistic effect, whereas in the case of $\beta = 0$ the mixed micelles formation is considered ideal. The larger the value of β (both positive or negative) the stronger the interaction (repulsion or attraction) between the two surfactants. The determination of β values allow to select mixture where synergistic behavior is present, leading to the formation of micellar aggregates at lower concentration that corresponding pure surfactants. More stable micellar systems with low surfactant content could be obtained, with a certain advantage for pharmaceutical formulation.

In Table 1, the theoretical and experimental values of CMC, together with the molar fraction in mixed micelles and parameter of interaction β are summarized for the mixture containing Cremophor EL and Pluronic F127 in various molar ratio (α is expressed relative to Cremophor EL as Surfactant 1 and Pluronic F127 as Surfactant 2).

As it is expected for a mixture with nonionic surfactants, a moderate synergistic effect is observed [25], with low values of interaction parameter, ranging from -0.22 to -1.54.

Negatives values for β were obtained for all molar fractions of 0.2, 0.6 and 0.8, but the higher value is recorded for the molar fraction 0.2, where the higher synergistic effect appears. For further experiments mixture with molar ratio $\alpha = 0.2$ was selected since contain the smallest amount of Cremophor EL and the CMC value for the mixture is very low.

Table 1. The micellization parameters in binary mixtures Cremophor EL and Pluronic F127 in various molar ratio obtained from the Rubingh model.

A	Experimental CMC * (M)	Calculated CMC * (M)	X	β
0	8×10^{-5}	-	-	-
0.2	4×10^{-5}	6.0×10^{-5}	0.46	−1.54
0.4	4.5×10^{-5}	4.8×10^{-5}	0.57	−0.82
0.6	3.0×10^{-5}	4.0×10^{-5}	0.69	−0.45
0.8	2.8×10^{-5}	3.4×10^{-5}	0.83	−0.22
1	3×10^{-5}	-	-	-

* using Equation (1).

3.2. Micelles Characterization

The size and size distribution of the micelles formed in Cremophor EL, Pluronic F127, and their mixture in aqueous solution was evaluated from DLS measurements (Figure 2).

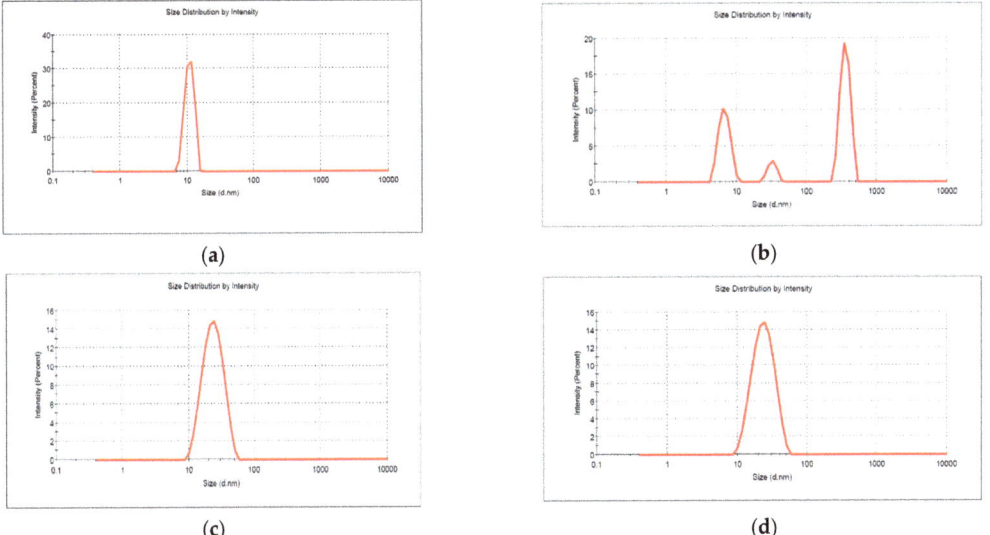

Figure 2. Size and size distribution of the micelles: (**a**) Cremophor EL, (**b**) Pluronic F127, (**c**) Mixed Cremophor EL-Pluronic F127 micellar system, (**d**) Norfloxacin loaded mixed Cremophor EL-Pluronic F127 micellar system.

At 25 °C the DLS diagram for 6×10^{-4} aqueous solution of Cremophor EL shows a single population of scattering units, the surfactant micelles, with an average diameter of 12.4 ± 2.4 nm and zeta potential -0.98 ± 0.4 mV. The polydispersity index PdI is 0.157 indicating high monodispersity of the sample. In contrast, the solution of Pluronic F127 exhibits trimodal distribution, with three signals in intensity mode representation. The main diameter of the empty micelles is 31.91 ± 4.4 nm, within the range of reported values [22]. The strong intensity signal at 6.88 nm is due to the presence of the polymeric macromolecules unassociated, in equilibrium with the micellar aggregates and the signal around 354 nm is probably due to some larger micelle—micelle aggregates, which have been reported in other papers [34]. The polydispersity index of 0.669 is consistent with a trimodal distribution. The sizes of the mixed micelles range from 14.90 nm to 27.54 nm with the increase of Pluronic F127 in composition, and the presence of Pluronic non associated polymeric chain is no longer evidenced. Also, the large aggregates disappear, that confirm the increase in micellization tendency in binary mixtures as it is observed from the synergistic behavior discussed in the previous section. The size of mixed micelles is lower that is expected from an ideal mixing, and it is also consistent with the data obtained from Rubing model (Table 1), where the molar fraction of Cremophor EL in mixed micelle is always higher than the one in mixed solution.

The solubilization of the drug in mixed micelle in a concentration of 100 µg/mL produced a slightly increase in the micellar size, from 27.54 ± 8.4 nm for empty Cremophor EL—Pluronic F127 mixed micelles F127 at $\alpha = 0.2$ molar ratio to 28.42 ± 7.9 nm for Norfloxacin loaded micelles. The solubilization of hydrophobic drugs inside the inner core of the micelles results in most of the case in more obvious increase of the loaded micelles [35]. Sometimes the encapsulation of the more complex molecule, such as Norfloxacin is simultaneously accompanied by a dehydration of the polymeric aggregate that produce a thinning of the hydrophilic polyoxiethylene corona [36], thus the modification of the micelle size is less evidenced.

The drug release from micelles do not produce observable changes in the size of mixed aggregates (average size before the experiment 26.42 ± 0.95 nm compared to samples after release experiment 26.90 ± 2.53 nm).

The micropolarity of the micelles was determined by using Pyrene as fluorescence probe, as recommended in literature [37]. The intensity of the vibronic bands in the fluorescence spectrum of monomeric Pyrene are reported to be very strong dependent with de polarity of the microenvironment. The ratio $I3/I1$ (where $I1$ is the first maximum emission peak at 372 nm and $I3$ the third one, at 384 nm) are considered as micropolarity index [38].

The $I3/I1$ value obtained from pyrene in water is very high, in the range 1.79–1.82, while smaller values in the range of 0.80–0.90 were determined for fluorescent probe inside micelles of various surfactants, indicating that pyrene molecules are located in a less polar environment, i.e., the hydrocarbonate core of the micellar aggregate.

For the evaluation of the microenvironmental polarity in the micelles, the ratio $I3/I1$ (first to third vibronic peaks) at the plateau region in the $I3/I1$ versus surfactant concentration curve was used, which is consistent with micellar domain.

From the spectra of pyridine recorded in pure Cremophor, pure Pluronic and mixed Cremophor-Pluronic micelles, the $I3/I1$ values were found 0.89, 0.96, and 0.90, respectively. The value of $I3/I1$ ratio of 0.89 for the Cremophor micellar system is consistent with the chemical structure of surfactant, which can produce a nonpolar core resembling to the hydrocarbon media to accommodate pyrene molecules. In contrast, the higher value, 0.96 found for Pluronic F127 micelles suggests that these micelles provide a microenvironment for the pyrene probe more polar than usual surfactants (in the domain of moderate polarity), due to the tendency of water penetration at the core-corona border [37]. The mixed Cremophor-Pluronic micelle exhibits an $I3/I1$ value similar to the pure Cremophor micelles, probably due to the higher molar ratio of Cremophor inside the mixed micelles than the actual molar ratio in the bulk surfactant solution.

The resistance of the micelles against dilution and pH changes was also checked.

The samples of pure and mixed micelles diluted 10 times show similar values of surfactant aggregates after dilution compared to concentrated ones. For drug loaded Cremophor EL-Pluronic F127 mixed micelles at $\alpha = 0.2$, for example, average size of concentrated dispersion (1×10^{-3} M) in PBS was 26.41 ± 0.95 nm while after a tenfold dilution, the size was 26.33 ± 0.95 nm.

The pH value of the dispersion media is expected to show negligible influence on the micellar size and shape, since both surfactants are nonionic. Thus, the values of the average size of mixed micelles Cremophor EL-Pluronic F127 at $\alpha = 0.2$ are found 26.97 ± 1.41 nm at pH = 4, 26.94 ± 2.54 at pH = 6, and 26.41 ± 0.95 nm at pH = 7.4, respectively. The mixed micelles prove to be resistant to dilution and no effect of pH variation in the range 4–7.4 affect the aggregation.

The DLS measurements were also applied to the samples after four weeks storage at room temperature. No significant changes were recorded in the size and size distribution of the void and NFLX.

3.3. Drug—Polymeric Micelle Interactions

To investigate the interaction of Norfloxacin molecules with the polymeric surfactants in micelles Fourier transformed infrared spectroscopy were used. In Figure 3, the FTIR spectra of pure Norfloxacin (1), Cremophor EL (2), Pluronic F127 (3), Norfloxacin in Cremophor EL micelles 100 µg/mL (4), Norfloxacin in mixed micelles Cremophor EL-Pluronic F127 (5) and Norfloxacin in Pluronic F127 micelles 100 µg/mL (6) are displayed.

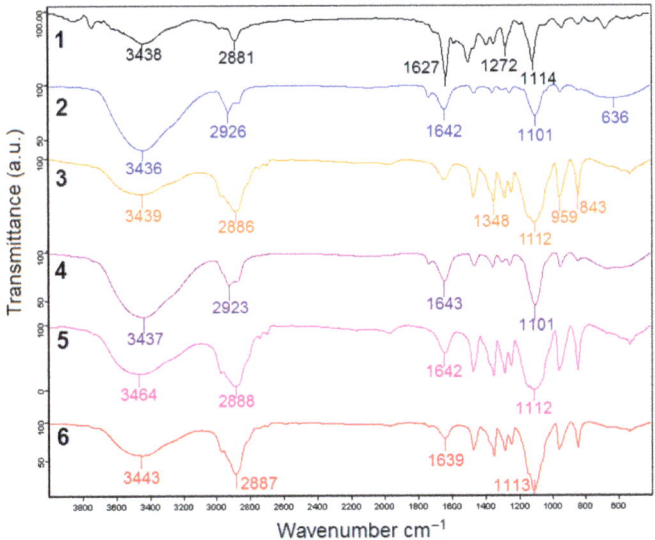

Figure 3. FTIR spectra of (1) Norfloxacin, (2) Cremophor EL, (3) Pluronic F127, (4) Norfloxacin in Cremophor EL micelles 100 µg/mL, (5) Norfloxacin in mixed micelles Cremophor EL-Pluronic F127 and (6) Norfloxacin in Pluronic F127 micelles 100 µg/mL.

The FTIR spectrum of Norfloxacin shows specific absorption peaks, similar to those reported in literature [13] as follows: the wide band centered at 3438 cm^{-1} is produced by both imino moiety of piperazinyl groups (–NH stretching vibration) and –OH group from acid and the band at 2881 cm^{-1} correspond to C–H stretching vibrations. The absorptions at 1627 cm^{-1} are characteristic for quinolones (–NH bending vibration) and the region between 1500–1450 cm^{-1} for =O–C–O– group of acid (v_s stretching vibration). The bending vibration of –OH was found at 1272 cm^{-1} and the strong absorption at 1114 cm^{-1} was related to C–F group.

For Cremophor EL were registered a broad band at 3436 cm^{-1} for the –OH group, the band at 2926 cm^{-1} attributed to C-H stretch and the very small absorption band between 1715–1730 cm^{-1} characteristic to C=O stretch for esters. The stretching band of C=C was found at 1642 cm^{-1}, the band from 1101 cm^{-1} was attributed to C-O stretch from alcohols and the wide absorption of 636 cm^{-1} to =C-H bend, similar to reported data in the literature [39]. In the spectra of Pluronic F127 micellar systems specific signal were observed as broad band at 3439 cm^{-1} for the –OH group, the bend of 2886 cm^{-1} was attributed to C-H stretch, 1348 cm^{-1} (in-plane O-H bend) and 1112 cm^{-1} (C-O stretch) [40].

For the sample with Norfloxacin in Cremophor EL micelles, FTIR spectrum absorptions at 2923 cm^{-1} attributed to C-H stretch, 1643 cm^{-1}, stretching band of C=C, 1101 cm^{-1} attributed C-O stretch from alcohols (identical to that of Cremophor), 950 cm^{-1} attributed to *trans*-CH=CH- group and 669 cm^{-1} attributed to =C-H bend. The most evident change is the broadening and increase intensity of the absorption band at 3438 cm^{-1}, probably due to the formation of numerous hydrogen bonding with OH group from acid (Norfloxacin) and from alcohol (Cremophor) and other interactions with the imino moiety of piperazinyl groups (NH stretching vibration).

As a result of the encapsulation of the Norfloxacin in Pluronic F127 micelles no significant changes were observed in the peak intensities and positions, with the exception of the wide absorption band in the 3500 cm^{-1} region, which is wider and more intense, due to the formation of hydrogen bonds between drug and polymer molecules. In the spectra of encapsulated Norfloxacin in the mixed micelles changes in shape and position of peaks could not be observed, except the same broadening and shifting to higher wavenumber of the peak at 3438 cm^{-1} to 3464 cm^{-1} and a minor shift to higher wavenumber of the peak corresponding to C-F bending. These changes are due to the interactions of the Norfloxacin with Cremophor and Pluronic F127, as a result of encapsulation of the Norfloxacin in the mixed micelles.

3.4. Drug Solubility and Encapsulation Efficiency

The maximum solubility of NFLX in micelles and encapsulation efficiency are tabulated in Table 2.

Table 2. Amount of Norfloxacin (NFLX) solubilized in polymeric micelles and encapsulation efficiency at 25 °C.

Micellar Dispersion	NFL Solubilized (µg/mL)	EE (%)
Cremohor EL	99.2	48.5 ± 3.3
Pluronic F127	93.5	45.7 ± 1.5
Mixed CrEL-Pl F127	93.8	52.2 ± 2.1

The concentration in the micellar dispersion were selected to represent 20 time the CMC value, in order to compare the solubility in micelle aggregates rather than conventional procedure versus weight of the polymeric material. The drug loading capacity expressed as % of NFLX from the weight of drug and micelle forming materials is 5% for Cremohor EL, 4.67% for Pluronic F127 and 4.89% for mixed micelles Cremohor EL-Pluronic F127 with molar ration $\alpha = 0.2$ (thus low content of Cremophor). One can conclude that a high loading capacity is maintained in mixed micelles, even at a significantly decreased surfactant concentration at the molar ratio where the synergistic effect is present, due to the favored micellization process.

3.5. In Vitro Drug Release

The release kinetics of Norfloxacin from various micellar dispersions was evaluated using PBS as receiving media and the results are presented in Figure 4.

The drug release profile is significantly dependent to the composition of micelles. Norfloxacin encapsulated in Cremohor EL micelles exhibit a cumulative release less than 20% up to 48 h, probably due to the compact packing of the hydrophobic chains of the surfactant inside the inner core and higher tendency of drug retention. The release profile show a burst in the first hour, then a decrease in the release rate. The burst region is present also in the Pluronic F127 micellar dispersion for the first 2.5 h, but cumulative release is far more important, up to 64%. The Norfloxacin molecules could be located both in the hydrophobic inner region of polypropylene oxide (PPO) and embedded in the hydrophilic corona of polyoxyethylene (POE) groups in the Pluronic micellar aggregate and lead to a higher extent of drug released than from Cremophor EL micelles. The release from the mixed micelles retains the burst segment, less pronounced compared to the situation in Cremophor micelles, due to the small amount of this polymeric surfactant in $\alpha = 0.2$ selected composition. The cumulative release is improved compared to Cremophor EL micelles, due to the influence of the large Pluronic, content up to 49% at 48 h.

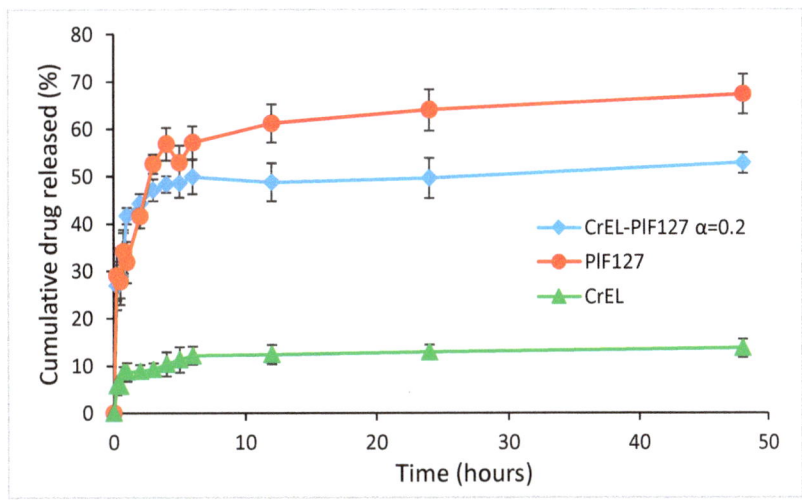

Figure 4. In vitro drug release profile for NFLX in Cremohor EL, Pluronic F127 and CrEL-Pl F127 (α = 0.2) mixed micelles.

The influence of the temperature and pH on the release profile of NFLX in selected mixed micelles (Cremophor-Pluronic F127 at molar ratio 0.2) is presented in Figure 5.

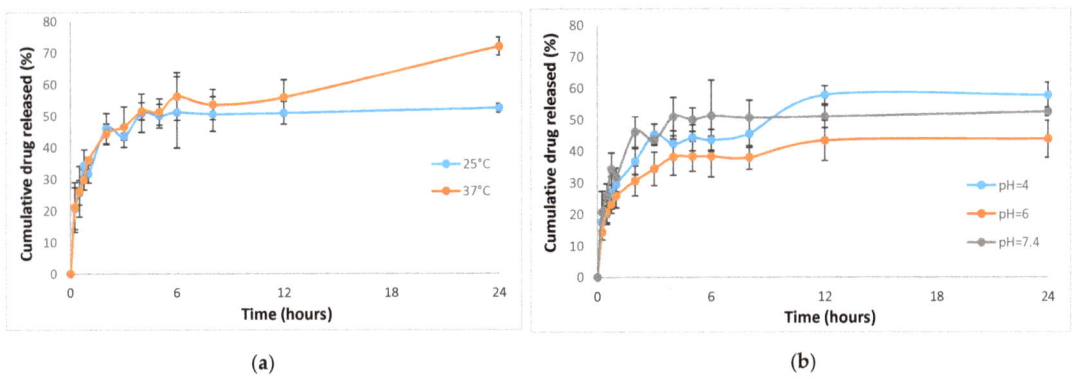

Figure 5. In vitro drug release profile for NFLX in mixed CrEL-Pl F127 (α = 0.2) micelles at various temperature (**a**) and pH values (**b**).

Since both Cremophor EL and Pluronic F127 are nonionic surfactants the effect of temperature up to 50 °C is negligible on the size and morphology of the micellar aggregates, thus the release of Norfloxacin encapsulates in either pure or mixed micelles is not significantly affected by the increase of the temperature from 25 °C to 37 °C. The kinetic profile is similar for the two temperatures investigated up to 12 h, with a moderate increase (from 51.8% at 25 °C to 72.0% at 37 °C) at 24 h, probably due to the increase in the aqueous solubility of drug when rise the temperature.

The release profile at various pH values shows an increase of the cumulative drug release at 24 h up to 60.80% at pH = 4, while at the pH = 6 a decrease of the total NFLX release to 47% is observed. This unexpected variation could be the result of the complex equilibrium of the drug species inside the micelles and release media, due to the peculiar variation of the solubility of Norfloxacin with pH.

This behavior is not the result of changes in micelle properties, but of the intrinsic properties of the drug. Size and size distribution of the Cremophor-Pluronic F127 (α = 0.2) micelles mixed micelles, as well as those for pure Cremophor or Pluronic micelles is not affected by the modification of the pH, according to the DLS measurements presented in Section 3.2.

The chemical structure of Norfloxacin produces amphiphilic, ionized and neutral species with variation of the pH, i.e at pH = 7.4 existence of both neutral NFLX^0 and zwitterionic NFLX$^\pm$ was evidenced, at pH = 6 a quasi-equimolecular mixture of zwitterionic NFLX$^\pm$ and ionic NFLX$^+$ is present and at pH = 4 only the ionic NFLX$^+$ is observed. This ionization behavior is consistent with the dramatic changes in solubility of NFLX with the pH, from 0.3 M at pH = 5 to 2.9×10^{-3} M at pH = 6 and 1.3×10^{-3} M at pH = 7 [41].

From the significant increase of the aqueous solubility of Norfloxacin at pH = 4, one can expect a more obvious increase in the drug released. However, the fully charged species NFLX$^+$ is stronger retained inside the micelles due to the interaction with the –OH and –COOH groups from the Pluronic and Cremophor molecules. At pH = 6 the coexistence of both zwitterionic and protonated Norfloxacin species results in a lower content of drug released.

The combination of the two polymeric surfactants results in a sustained release of NFLX form micelles that can ensure a long-term delivery of the antibiotic.

3.6. Biocompatibility of Mixed Micelles

The effect of surfactants on normal cells was studied in terms of cell viability by MTT assay and cellular inflammation and membrane damage with nitric oxide (NO) release test. The study was performed on human lung fibroblasts MRC-5 cells selected as model normal cells with moderate sensibility to dispersions. The results are shown in Figures 6 and 7.

As shown in Figure 6, the Cremophor EL micellar solution in the range 5×10^{-6}–2×10^{-4} M did not affect the number of viable cells after 24 h of incubation compared with the control. Although no change in cell viability was measured for sample Cremophor EL even at concentration approximative 5 times higher the CMC, a significant decrease was noticed for the 3.2×10^{-4} M concentration, after both time intervals of incubation with surfactants.

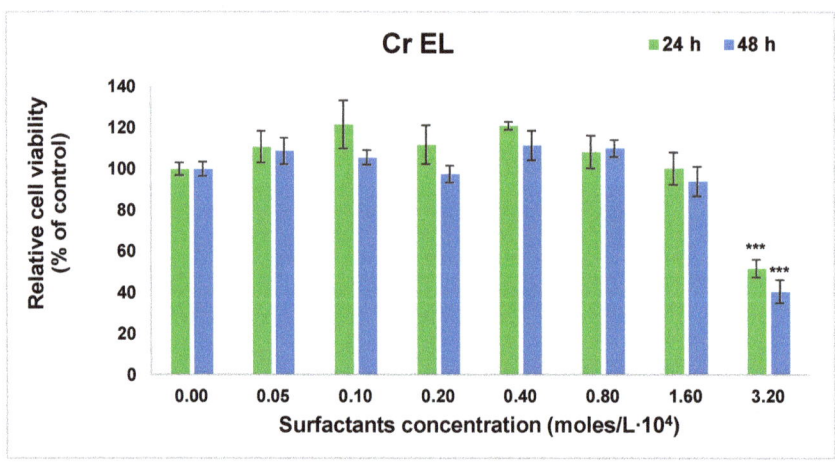

Figure 6. Cont.

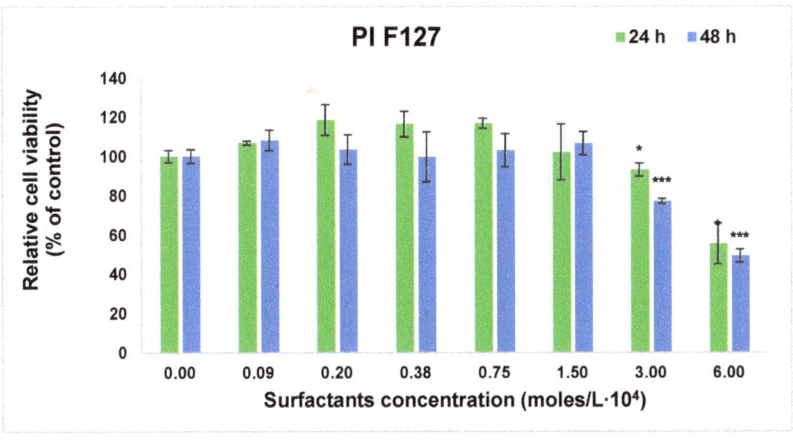

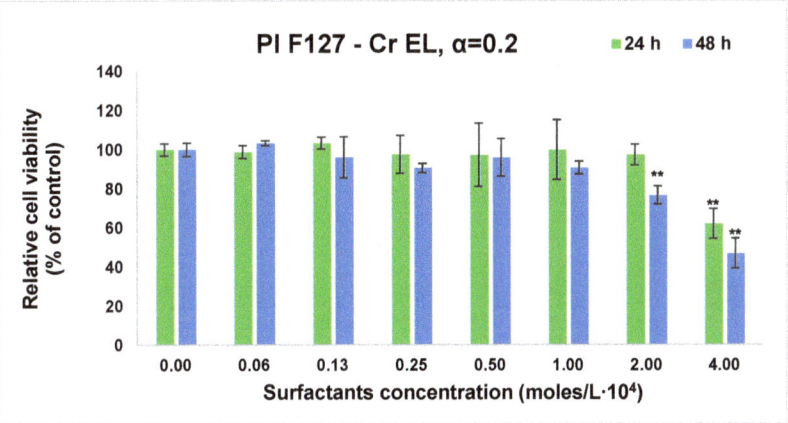

Figure 6. Cell viability results obtained by MTT assay after 24 and 48 h of cell growth in the presence of surfactants. Results are presented as mean ± standard deviation of three independent experiments (* $p < 0.05$, ** $p < 0.01$ and *** $p < 0.001$ compared with control).

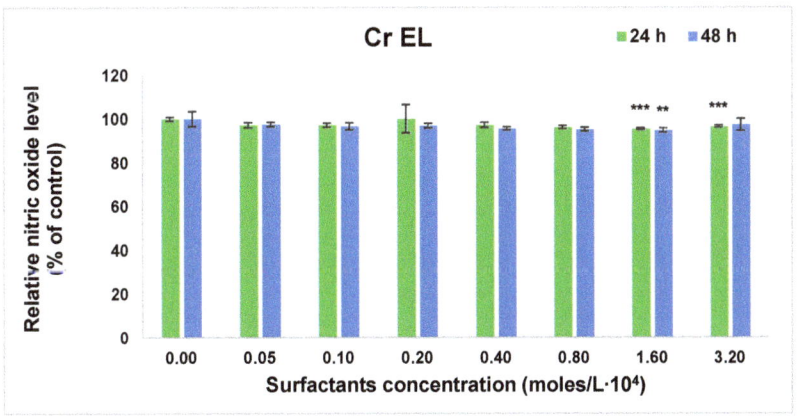

Figure 7. *Cont.*

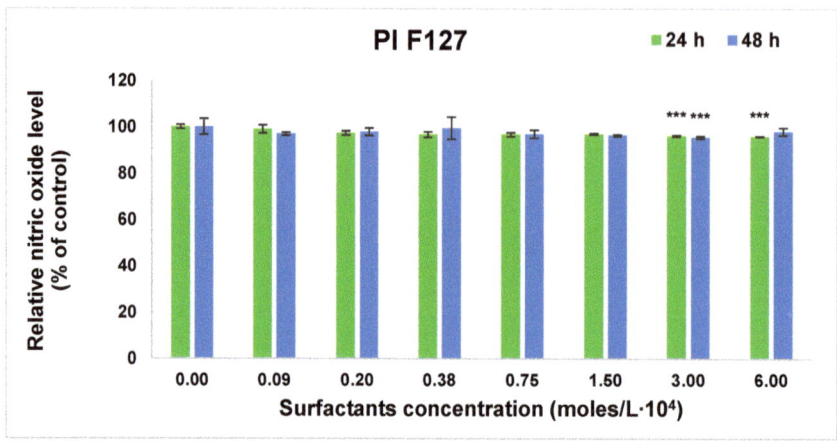

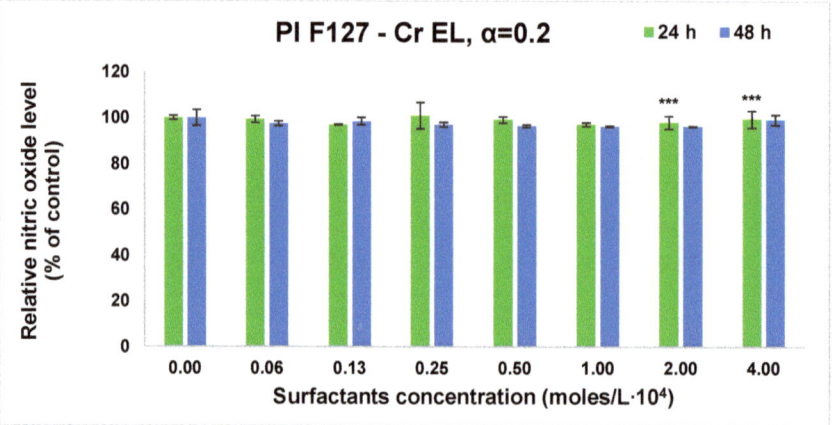

Figure 7. NO release measured by Griess assay after 24 and 48 h of cell growth in the presence of surfactants. Results are presented as mean ± standard deviation of three independent experiments (** $p < 0.01$ and *** $p < 0.001$ compared with control).

The micellar dispersions based on Pluronic F127 show lack of cytotoxicity up to 1.5×10^{-4} M, as it is reported in most paper for low concentrated polymeric solutions below 8×10^{-6} M, in premicellar region [42]. An unexpected dose-dependent decrease was obtained for Pluronic concentrated micellar dispersions from 3×10^{-4} M to 6×10^{-4} M, where the cellular viability decreased to 49% compared to control value after 48 h of exposure.

In the mixed micelle system with molar ratio Cremophor EL- Pluronic F127 $\alpha = 0.2$, the dose dependent variation of the cytotoxicity is observed similar to Pluronic F127 micellar dispersion, probably due to the small amount of the Cremophor in the mixture. Significant decrease in the cellular viability is recorded after 24 and 48 h at higher concentration than 2×10^{-4} M of mixed surfactants.

Since the synergistic molar ratio $\alpha = 0.2$ exhibits the low value of CMC 4×10^{-5} M, solutions with concentration 3-fold CMC will ensure the existence of the micellar aggregates and remains in the region without evident toxicity.

The amount of NO released in the culture medium was assessed as a valuable indicator of inflammation produced by the contact with surfactant solutions in premicellar and micellar regions. As it is shown in Figure 7, no significant changes in NO release after cell exposure to surfactants over whole range of studied concentrations could be observed. Thus, it was concluded that even in the case of the Cremohore EL presence, the surfactant micelles did not induce inflammation in human fibroblast cell cultures.

3.7. Antibacterial Activity

The qualitative screening of the antimicrobial activity evaluated the efficiency of the Norfloxacin encapsulated in Cremophor EL and Pluronic F127 micellar carriers, by measuring the diameters of the inhibition zone expressed by each tested bacterial strain. The value of the diameters of the inhibition zones demonstrated the achievement of a concentration gradient around the spot following the release of the antibiotic from the micellar carrier (20 µg in 10 µL micellar solution), by comparison with the concentration gradient achieved by the release of antibiotics from the standard disc (30 µg/disk) (Figure 8).

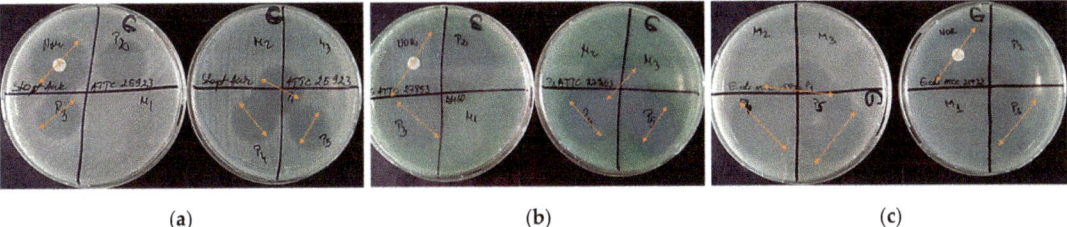

Figure 8. Aspect of the inhibition zones for microorganisms (**a**) *Staphylococcus aureus* ATCC 25923, (**b**) *Pseudomonas aeruginosa* ATCC 27853 and (**c**) *Escherichia coli* ATCC 25922. The samples are denoted P1 = NFLX in water; P2 = NFLX in DMSO; P3 = NFLX in Cremophor EL micellar solution; P4 = NFLX in Pluronic F127 micellar solution; P5 = NFLX in mixed micellar solution, while M1, M2 and M3 are empty micelles of Cremophor EL, Pluronic F127 and mixed micelles, respectively.

It cannot be observed significant difference between Cremophor and Pluronic micellar carriers (P3 and P4) or combination of them (P5) on the growth of standard bacterial strains.

In Figure 9 the values of the diameter of inhibition zone recorded for both clinical and standard bacterial strains are presented.

As shown in Figure 9, different behaviors for the clinical and the standard bacterial strains exposed to NFLX are recorded, with the clinical strains expressing larger diameters of the inhibition zones in both cases standard disc and micellar carriers. The exception is the *P. aeruginosa* 5399 clinical strain which shows low sensitivity to Norfloxacin in all the tested systems. It seems that this bacterial strain is resistant to fluoroquinolone, given the diameter of the inhibition zone for the norfloxacin (16 mm < 18 mm, according with CLSI 2021) and by using the micellar carrier for antibiotic the sensitivity pattern has not changed when NFLX was encapsulated in Cremophor and mixed micelles compared to NFLX in aqueous solution. A rather higher sensibility is recorded to the NFLX encapsulated in Pluronic F127 (15 mm), probably due to the cellular membrane permeability induced by the tri-block copolymer micelles.

For the *E. coli* strains, both standard and clinical strains, the diameter of inhibition zones produced by NFLX encapsulated in micelles were larger than the antibiotic in aqueous solution.

The quantitative results expressed by minimal inhibitory concentration values allowed the quantitative evaluation of the carriers' efficiency in terms of antibiotic release capacity in the liquid medium (Figure 10).

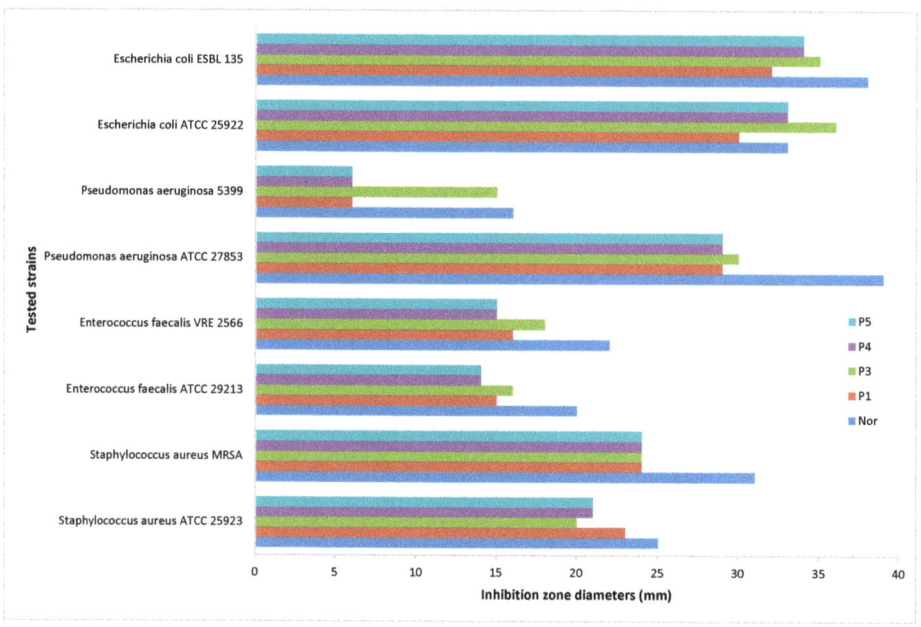

Figure 9. Graphic representation of inhibition zone diameters (mm).

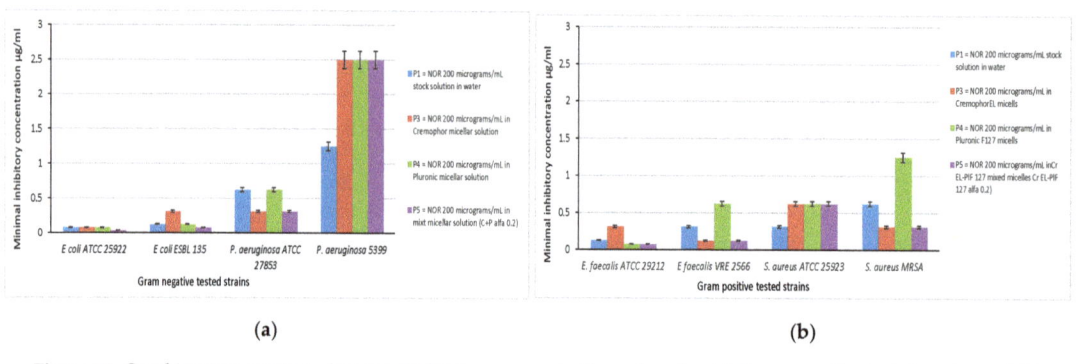

Figure 10. Graphic representation of minimal inhibitory concentration values for: (**a**) Gram negative tested strains and (**b**) Gram positive tested strains.

For *E. coli* ATCC 25922 strains the minimal inhibitory concentrations were similar for the reference aqueous solution of NFLX and the drug encapsulated in various micellar systems, with the exception of NFLX in mixed Cremophor EL- Pluronic F127 micelles, which exhibited a lower MIC of 0.039 µg/mL compared to 0.078 µg/mL. The clinical strain *E. coli* is less susceptible to NFLX encapsulated in Cremophor EL (MIC of 0.31 µg/mL) and again the highest activity was observed for the formulation with mixed surfactants (MIC 0.078 µg/mL).

In the case of *P. aeruginosa* ATCC 27853, a similar efficiency was observed for NFLX in aqueous solution and Pluronic micelles (MIC 0.625 µg/mL), while the presence of Cremophor EL in pure and mixed micelles reduced the MIC value to 0.312 µg/mL. As observed in the qualitative test, *P. aeruginosa* clinical strain proved to be more resistant to NFLX, and the encapsulation in micelles leads to an unexpected increase of the MIC values for all surfactants.

In the case of the Gram-positive microorganisms there were also differences in the results recorded for standard and clinical strains depending on the composition of the micellar carrier. For standard *E. fecalis* ATCC 29212 the lowest efficiency was demonstrated by the NFLX loaded Cremophor EL micelle dispersion (MIC value 0.312 µg/mL), while the encapsulation in Pluronic F127 and in the mixed micelles reduced the MIC value to quarter. The clinical *E. fecalis* VRE 2566 strain developed a high value of MIC in the case of NFLX in Pluronic micelles (MIC value 0.625 µg/mL). Again, the encapsulation in mixed micelles decreased the value of MIC up to 0.125 µg/mL.

For *S. aureus* standard strain ATCC 25923 the MIC values for NFLX in all micellar systems proved to be double compared to the value recorded for aqueous solution (0.625 µg/mL compared to 0.312 µg/mL).

In the case of resistant *S. aureus* strain, no significant improvement was observed with the Pluronic F127 micelles, on the contrary the MIC value obtained is the higher in our study (1.25 µg/mL) for Gram positive microbial cultures. The presence of Cremohor EL as pure micelles or in combination with Pluronic F127 increased the antibacterial efficiency of the encapsulated drug.

The micelles of two polymeric surfactants used in this study had different effects on the Norfloxacin antibacterial efficiency on different microorganisms, and a variation in behavior could also observed between standard and clinical strains. A possible explanation is the specific interaction between the cellular membrane and micelle forming surfactants, that should be investigated in detail in order design drug delivery systems for NFLX with enhanced activity against resistant microbial strains.

Pluronic polymeric surfactants have begun to be investigated to elucidate their role in management of biofilm formation, but relevant data and explanations about the complex interactions with the microbial cellular membrane are still lacking [43].

4. Conclusions

Polymeric micelles were prepared as drug delivery systems for model poorly soluble antibiotic Norfloxacin in order to achieve better stability and controlled delivery of drug. Two polymeric surfactants Cremophor EL and POE-PPO-POE triblock copolymer Pluronic F127 and their mixtures in various molar ratio were studied. The non-ideal behavior of the self-assembling process in surfactant mixtures reveal the existence of synergistic effects over the whole range of composition, with a maximum value of interaction parameter in mixed micelle for the molar ratio $\alpha = 0.2$. The micelles were characterized in term of size, size distribution and drug solubilization, and the selected composition with low content of Cremophor EL show suitable performance to be used as Norfloxacin carrier.

The mixed micelles selected exhibit resistance against dilution and pH changes in the range of 4–7.4. The encapsulation efficiency of NFLX in mixed CrEL—Pl F127 micelles was $52.2 \pm 2.1\%$ and do not significantly change the size of nanocarrier after the drug encapsulation.

The drug release profile exhibited an initial burst (more obvious in Cremophor EL micelles) in all micellar dispersion, with a cumulative release up to 51.8% in mixed Cremophor EL—Pluronic F127 system at 25 °C, intermediate from the value obtained for Cremphor EL and Pluronic F127 pure micelles. The total amount released in 24 h was increased to 72% at temperature of 37 °C. The results of cytotoxicity and inflammation tests on normal fibroblast cells indicate that both studied surfactants and their mixtures prove high biocompatibility for concentrations below $2-3 \times 10^{-4}$ M.

The analysis of qualitative and quantitative results showed an improvement of the antibacterial properties of Norfloxacin against the majority of the tested bacterial strains, both Gram positive and Gram negative, when the polymeric micelles were used as carriers.

The sample with NFLX encapsulated in the novel carrier prove to be effective on both *E. coli* ATCC 25922 and clinical strains, with MIC value of 0.039 µg/mL and 0.078 µg/mL, respectively. The minimum inhibitory concentrations were found to vary greatly with nature and provenience of the microbial strain and with the surfactant composition of the formulation. As a general conclusion, the drug loaded mixed micellar formulation exhibits good activity against clinical isolated strains, compared with the CLSI recommended standard strains, thus Cremophor EL-Pluronic F127 mixed micelles can be considered as novel controlled release delivery systems for hydrophobic antimicrobial drugs.

Author Contributions: Conceptualization, L.O.C. and C.P.; methodology, C.L.N.; validation, L.O.C. formal analysis, C.P.; investigation, M.A.T., A.R., P.O. spectroscopy, L.M.D. microbiology, M.S. biocompatibility, C.S., C.M.N. FTIR; writing—original draft preparation, L.O.C. and M.A.T.; writing—review and editing L.O.C. and C.P., project administration, L.O.C. All authors have read and agreed to the published version of the manuscript.

Funding: This research was funded by Romanian Ministry of Education and Research, CCCDI—UEFISCDI, project number PN-III-P2-2.1-PED-2019-4657, within PNCDI III.

Institutional Review Board Statement: Not Applicable.

Informed Consent Statement: Not Applicable.

Data Availability Statement: Not Applicable.

Conflicts of Interest: The authors declare no conflict of interest. The funders had no role in the design of the study; in the collection, analyses, or interpretation of data; in the writing of the manuscript, or in the decision to publish the results.

References

1. Kalhapure, R.S.; Suleman, N.; Mocktar, C.; Seedat, N.; Govender, T. Nanoengineered Drug Delivery Systems for Enhancing Antibiotic Therapy. *J. Pharm. Sci.* **2015**, *104*, 872–905. [CrossRef]
2. Bush, N.G.; Diez-Santos, I.; Abbott, L.R.; Maxwell, A. Quinolones: Mechanism, Lethality and Their Contributions to Antibiotic Resistance. *Molecules* **2020**, *25*, 5662. [CrossRef]
3. Maxwell, A.; Bush, N.G.; Evans-Roberts, K. DNA Topoisomerases. *EcoSal Plus* **2015**, *6*. [CrossRef]
4. Purushothaman, S.; Cama, J.; Keyser, U.F. Dependence of Norfloxacin Diffusion across Bilayers on Lipid Composition. *Soft Matter* **2016**, *12*, 2135–2144. [CrossRef]
5. Faccendini, A.; Ruggeri, M.; Miele, D.; Rossi, S.; Bonferoni, M.C.; Aguzzi, C.; Grisoli, P.; Viseras, C.; Vigani, B.; Sandri, G.; et al. Norfloxacin-Loaded Electrospun Scaffolds: Montmorillonite Nanocomposite vs. Free Drug. *Pharmaceutics* **2020**, *12*, 325. [CrossRef] [PubMed]
6. Kłosińska-Szmurło, E.; Pluciński, F.A.; Grudzień, M.; Betlejewska-Kielak, K.; Biernacka, J.; Mazurek, A.P. Experimental and Theoretical Studies on the Molecular Properties of Ciprofloxacin, Norfloxacin, Pefloxacin, Sparfloxacin, and Gatifloxacin in Determining Bioavailability. *J. Biol. Phys.* **2014**, *40*, 335–345. [CrossRef] [PubMed]
7. Gadade, D.; Sarda, K.; Shahi, S. Investigation and Optimization of the Effect of Polymers on Drug Release of Norfloxacin from Floating Tablets. *Polym. Med.* **2017**, *46*, 117–127. [CrossRef]
8. Oliveira, P.R.; Mendes, C.; Klein, L.; da Sangoi, M.S.; Bernardi, L.S.; Silva, M.A.S. Formulation Development and Stability Studies of Norfloxacin Extended-Release Matrix Tablets. *BioMed Res. Int.* **2013**, *2013*, 1–9. [CrossRef] [PubMed]
9. Dave, V.; Yadav, R.B.; Kushwaha, K.; Yadav, S.; Sharma, S.; Agrawal, U. Lipid-Polymer Hybrid Nanoparticles: Development & Statistical Optimization of Norfloxacin for Topical Drug Delivery System. *Bioact. Mater.* **2017**, *2*, 269–280. [CrossRef]
10. Ahmad, I.; Arsalan, A.; Ali, S.A.; Bano, R.; Munir, I.; Sabah, A. Formulation and Stabilization of Norfloxacin in Liposomal Preparations. *Eur. J. Pharm. Sci.* **2016**, *91*, 208–215. [CrossRef] [PubMed]
11. Mendes, C.; Meirelles, G.C.; Barp, C.G.; Assreuy, J.; Silva, M.A.S.; Ponchel, G. Cyclodextrin Based Nanosponge of Norfloxacin: Intestinal Permeation Enhancement and Improved Antibacterial Activity. *Carbohydr. Polym.* **2018**, *195*, 586–592. [CrossRef] [PubMed]
12. Dong, Z.; Xie, S.; Zhu, L.; Wang, Y.; Wang, X.; Zhou, W. Preparation and in Vitro in Vivo Evaluations of Norfloxacin-Loaded Solid Lipid Nanopartices for Oral Delivery. *Drug Deliv.* **2011**, *18*, 441–450. [CrossRef]
13. Salahuddin, N.; Abdelwahab, M.; Gaber, M.; Elneanaey, S. Synthesis and Design of Norfloxacin Drug Delivery System Based on PLA/TiO2 Nanocomposites: Antibacterial and Antitumor Activities. *Mater. Sci. Eng. C* **2020**, *108*, 110337. [CrossRef] [PubMed]
14. Gao, W.; Chen, Y.; Zhang, Y.; Zhang, Q.; Zhang, L. Nanoparticle-Based Local Antimicrobial Drug Delivery. *Adv. Drug Deliv. Rev.* **2018**, *127*, 46–57. [CrossRef]
15. Gopala Kumari, S.V.; Manikandan, N.A.; Pakshirajan, K.; Pugazhenthi, G. Sustained Drug Release and Bactericidal Activity of a Novel, Highly Biocompatible and Biodegradable Polymer Nanocomposite Loaded with Norfloxacin for Potential Use in Antibacterial Therapy. *J. Drug Deliv. Sci. Technol.* **2020**, *59*, 101900. [CrossRef]

16. Mirzaie, A.; Peirovi, N.; Akbarzadeh, I.; Moghtaderi, M.; Heidari, F.; Yeganeh, F.E.; Noorbazargan, H.; Mirzazadeh, S.; Bakhtiari, R. Preparation and Optimization of Ciprofloxacin Encapsulated Niosomes: A New Approach for Enhanced Antibacterial Activity, Biofilm Inhibition and Reduced Antibiotic Resistance in Ciprofloxacin-Resistant Methicillin-Resistance Staphylococcus Aureus. *Bioorg. Chem.* **2020**, *103*, 104231. [CrossRef] [PubMed]
17. Taha, E.I.; Badran, M.M.; El-Anazi, M.H.; Bayomi, M.A.; El-Bagory, I.M. Role of Pluronic F127 Micelles in Enhancing Ocular Delivery of Ciprofloxacin. *J. Mol. Liq.* **2014**, *199*, 251–256. [CrossRef]
18. Knemeyer, I.; Wientjes, M.G.; Au, J.L.-S. Cremophor Reduces Paclitaxel Penetration into Bladder Wall during Intravesical Treatment. *Cancer Chemother. Pharmacol.* **1999**, *44*, 241–248. [CrossRef]
19. Szebeni, J.; Alving, C.R.; Muggia, F.M. Complement Activation by Cremophor EL as a Possible Contributor to Hypersensitivity to Paclitaxel: An In Vitro Study. *JNCI J. Natl. Cancer Inst.* **1998**, *90*, 300–306. [CrossRef] [PubMed]
20. Dahmani, F.Z.; Yang, H.; Zhou, J.; Yao, J.; Zhang, T.; Zhang, Q. Enhanced Oral Bioavailability of Paclitaxel in Pluronic/LHR Mixed Polymeric Micelles: Preparation, in Vitro and in Vivo Evaluation. *Eur. J. Pharm. Sci.* **2012**, *47*, 179–189. [CrossRef]
21. Pitto-Barry, A.; Barry, N.P.E. Pluronic®Block-Copolymers in Medicine: From Chemical and Biological Versatility to Rationalisation and Clinical Advances. *Polym. Chem.* **2014**, *5*, 3291–3297. [CrossRef]
22. Almeida, H.; Amaral, M.H.; Lobão, P.; Lobo, J.M.S. Pluronic®F-127 and Pluronic Lecithin Organogel (PLO): Main Features and Their Applications in Topical and Transdermal Administration of Drugs. *J. Pharm. Pharm. Sci.* **2012**, *15*, 592. [CrossRef]
23. Soliman, K.A.; Ullah, K.; Shah, A.; Jones, D.S.; Singh, T.R.R. Poloxamer-Based in Situ Gelling Thermoresponsive Systems for Ocular Drug Delivery Applications. *Drug Discov. Today* **2019**, *24*, 1575–1586. [CrossRef]
24. Bayati, S.; Anderberg Haglund, C.; Pavel, N.V.; Galantini, L.; Schillén, K. Interaction between Bile Salt Sodium Glycodeoxycholate and PEO–PPO–PEO Triblock Copolymers in Aqueous Solution. *RSC Adv.* **2016**, *6*, 69313–69325. [CrossRef]
25. Löf, D.; Tomšič, M.; Glatter, O.; Fritz-Popovski, G.; Schillén, K. Structural Characterization of Nonionic Mixed Micelles Formed by C12 EO6 Surfactant and P123 Triblock Copolymer. *J. Phys. Chem. B* **2009**, *113*, 5478–5486. [CrossRef]
26. Ćirin, D.; Krstonošić, V.; Poša, M. Properties of Poloxamer 407 and Polysorbate Mixed Micelles: Influence of Polysorbate Hydrophobic Chain. *J. Ind. Eng. Chem.* **2017**, *47*, 194–201. [CrossRef]
27. Yang, C.; Liu, W.; Xiao, J.; Yuan, C.; Chen, Y.; Guo, J.; Yue, H.; Zhu, D.; Lin, W.; Tang, S.; et al. PH-Sensitive Mixed Micelles Assembled from PDEAEMA-PPEGMA and PCL-PPEGMA for Doxorubicin Delivery: Experimental and DPD Simulations Study. *Pharmaceutics* **2020**, *12*, 170. [CrossRef]
28. Jindal, N.; Mehta, S.K. Nevirapine Loaded Poloxamer 407/Pluronic P123 Mixed Micelles: Optimization of Formulation and in Vitro Evaluation. *Colloids Surf. B Biointerfaces* **2015**, *129*, 100–106. [CrossRef] [PubMed]
29. Khanal, A.; Nakashima, K. Incorporation and Release of Cloxacillin Sodium in Micelles of Poly(Styrene-b-2-Vinyl Pyridine-b-Ethylene Oxide). *J. Control. Release* **2005**, *108*, 150–160. [CrossRef] [PubMed]
30. Liu, L.; Venkatraman, S.S.; Yang, Y.-Y.; Guo, K.; Lu, J.; He, B.; Moochhala, S.; Kan, L. Polymeric Micelles Anchored with TAT for Delivery of Antibiotics across the Blood-Brain Barrier. *Biopolymers* **2008**, *90*, 617–623. [CrossRef]
31. Stopková, L.; Gališinová, J.; Šuchtová, Z.; Čižmárik, J.; Andriamainty, F. Determination of Critical Micellar Concentration of Homologous 2-Alkoxyphenylcarbamoyloxyethyl-Morpholinium Chlorides. *Molecules* **2018**, *23*, 1064. [CrossRef]
32. Chierentin, L.; Salgado, H.R.N. Review of Properties and Analytical Methods for the Determination of Norfloxacin. *Crit. Rev. Anal. Chem.* **2016**, *46*, 22–39. [CrossRef]
33. Holland, P.M.; Rubingh, D.N. (Eds.) *Mixed Surfactant Systems*; ACS Symposium Series; American Chemical Society: Washington, DC, USA, 1992; Volume 501, ISBN 978-0-8412-2468-1.
34. Thapa, R.K.; Cazzador, F.; Grønlien, K.G.; Tønnesen, H.H. Effect of Curcumin and Cosolvents on the Micellization of Pluronic F127 in Aqueous Solution. *Colloids Surf. B Biointerfaces* **2020**, *195*, 111250. [CrossRef]
35. Basak, R.; Bandyopadhyay, R. Encapsulation of Hydrophobic Drugs in Pluronic F127 Micelles: Effects of Drug Hydrophobicity, Solution Temperature, and PH. *Langmuir* **2013**, *29*, 4350–4356. [CrossRef]
36. Sharma, R.K.; Shaikh, S.; Ray, D.; Aswal, V.K. Binary Mixed Micellar Systems of PEO-PPO-PEO Block Copolymers for Lamotrigine Solubilization: A Comparative Study with Hydrophobic and Hydrophilic Copolymer. *J. Polym. Res.* **2018**, *25*, 73. [CrossRef]
37. Croy, S.R.; Kwon, G.S. The Effects of Pluronic Block Copolymers on the Aggregation State of Nystatin. *J. Control. Release* **2004**, *95*, 161–171. [CrossRef]
38. Kalyanasundaram, K.; Thomas, J.K. Environmental Effects on Vibronic Band Intensities in Pyrene Monomer Fluorescence and Their Application in Studies of Micellar Systems. *J. Am. Chem. Soc.* **1977**, *99*, 2039–2044. [CrossRef]
39. Elkordy, A.A.; Essa, E.A.; Dhuppad, S.; Jammigumpula, P. Liquisolid Technique to Enhance and to Sustain Griseofulvin Dissolution: Effect of Choice of Non-Volatile Liquid Vehicles. *Int. J. Pharm.* **2012**, *434*, 122–132. [CrossRef]
40. Liu, Y.; Fu, S.; Lin, L.; Cao, Y.; Xie, X.; Yu, H.; Chen, M.; Li, H. Redox-Sensitive Pluronic F127-Tocopherol Micelles. Synthesis, Characterization, and Cytotoxicity Evaluation. *Int. J. Nanomed.* **2017**, *12*, 2635–2644. [CrossRef]
41. Otalvaro, J.O.; Avena, M.; Brigante, M. Adsorption of Norfloxacin on a Hexagonal Mesoporous Silica: Isotherms, Kinetics and Adsorbent Reuse. *Adsorption* **2019**, *25*, 1375–1385. [CrossRef]
42. Meng, X.; Liu, J.; Yu, X.; Li, J.; Lu, X.; Shen, T. Pluronic F127 and D-α-Tocopheryl Polyethylene Glycol Succinate (TPGS) Mixed Micelles for Targeting Drug Delivery across The Blood Brain Barrier. *Sci. Rep.* **2017**, *7*, 2964. [CrossRef]
43. Aguirre-Ramírez, M.; Silva-Jiménez, H.; Banat, I.M.; Díaz De Rienzo, M.A. Surfactants: Physicochemical Interactions with Biological Macromolecules. *Biotechnol. Lett.* **2021**, *43*, 523–535. [CrossRef]

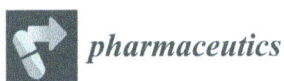

Article

Hybrid Nanoparticles of Poly (Methyl Methacrylate) and Antimicrobial Quaternary Ammonium Surfactants

Beatriz Ideriha Mathiazzi and Ana Maria Carmona-Ribeiro *

Biocolloids Laboratory, Departamento de Bioquímica, Instituto de Química, Universidade de São Paulo, Av. Prof. Lineu Prestes 748, 05508-000 São Paulo, Brazil; bemathi@usp.br
* Correspondence: amcr@usp.br; Tel.: +55-011-3091-1887

Received: 23 March 2020; Accepted: 8 April 2020; Published: 10 April 2020

Abstract: Quaternary ammonium surfactants (QACs) are microbicides, whereas poly (acrylates) are biocompatible polymers. Here, the physical and antimicrobial properties of two QACs, cetyl trimethyl ammonium bromide (CTAB) or dioctadecyl dimethyl ammonium bromide (DODAB) in poly (methyl methacrylate) (PMMA) nanoparticles (NPs) are compared to those of QACs alone. Methyl methacrylate (MMA) polymerization using DODAB or CTAB as emulsifiers and initiator azobisisobutyronitrile (AIBN) yielded cationic, nanometric, homodisperse, and stable NPs. NPs' physical and antimicrobial properties were assessed from dynamic light scattering (DLS), scanning electron microscopy, and viability curves of *Escherichia coli*, *Staphylococcus aureus*, or *Candida albicans* determined as log(colony-forming unities counting) over a range of [QACs]. NPs were spherical and homodisperse but activity for free QACs was higher than those for QACs in NPs. Inhibition halos against bacteria and yeast were observed only for free or incorporated CTAB in NPs because PMMA/CTAB NPs controlled the CTAB release. DODAB displayed fungicidal activity against *C. albicans* since DODAB bilayer disks could penetrate the outer glycoproteins fungus layer. The physical properties and stability of the cationic NPs highlighted their potential to combine with other bioactive molecules for further applications in drug and vaccine delivery.

Keywords: hybrid nanoparticles; biocompatible polymer; antimicrobial amphiphiles; dynamic light scattering; scanning electron microscopy; cell viability from counting of colony-forming unities; antimicrobial activity of nanoparticles; *Escherichia coli*; *Staphylococcus aureus*; *Candida albicans*

1. Introduction

Biocompatible synthetic or natural polymers can improve body functions without interfering with its normal functioning or triggering side effects [1–7]. They have been useful in tissue culture, tissue scaffolds, implants, artificial grafts, wound dressings, controlled drug release, prosthetic replacements for bones, dentistry, etc [8]. Some examples of biocompatible polymers are poly (lactic-co-glycolic acid) [9], poly (ε-caprolactone) (PCL) [10], poly (lactic acid) [11], poly (3- hydroxybutyrate-co-3-hydroxyvalerate) (PHBV) [12], chitosan [13,14], cellulose [15], and poly (acrylates) including poly (methyl methacrylate) (PMMA) [6,16–18]. Among the poly (acrylates), several cationic latexes and coatings obtained from additives such as cationic surfactants, lipids, antimicrobial polymers or co-polymers have been described [19–25]. In the case of PMMA, the discovery of PMMA biocompatibility occurred when an optical technician placed a PMMA scleral lens on his eye and found that it could be well tolerated. The first PMMA patent appearing in 1948 [16] was acquired by Bausch & Lomb in 1972 [26].

In our laboratory, the good compatibility between PMMA and some antimicrobial quaternary ammonium compounds (QACs) was first described both for PMMA/QAC coatings [19] and

PMMA/QACs nanoparticles (NPs) [27]. The QACs were apparently able to impart their antimicrobial activity [28–31] to the PMMA/QACs assemblies [19,27]. In the absence of PMMA, QACs in water dispersion self-assemble to yield micelles or bilayers depending on the QAC chemical structure and molecular shape [32,33]. Dioctadecyl dimethyl ammonium bromide (DODAB) assembles in water solution as bilayer vesicles or bilayer fragments (BF) depending on the dispersion method; sonication disrupts DODAB vesicles producing BF [34–36]. Cetyltrimethylammonium bromide (CTAB) assembles in water solution as micelles above the critical micellar concentration [32]. Ion–dipole interactions between the quaternary ammonium in DODAB and the carbonyl moiety in PMMA plus other weak but cooperative van der Waals interactions led to hybrid materials where DODAB was found well dispersed in the polymeric matrix [19]. This allowed for combining the bactericidal DODAB property [29–31,37–42] with excellent DODAB immobilization and distribution in the PMMA polymeric network [19]. Later on, determining the effect of QAC chemical structure on the antimicrobial activity of PMMA/QAC coatings revealed that DODAB and CTAB behaved differently; CTAB diffused through the film and reached bacteria in the outer medium, whereas DODAB impregnation in the polymeric matrix killed bacteria upon contact without leakage [20].

In this work, PMMA/QAC NPs synthesized by emulsion polymerization of methyl methacrylate (MMA) using azo-bis-isobutyronitrile (AIBN) as initiator and DODAB BF or CTAB as emulsifiers were evaluated regarding their physical properties and antimicrobial activity as compared to the free QACs. Scheme 1 illustrates the emulsion polymerization of MMA in the presence of DODAB BF or CTAB using AIBN as the initiator.

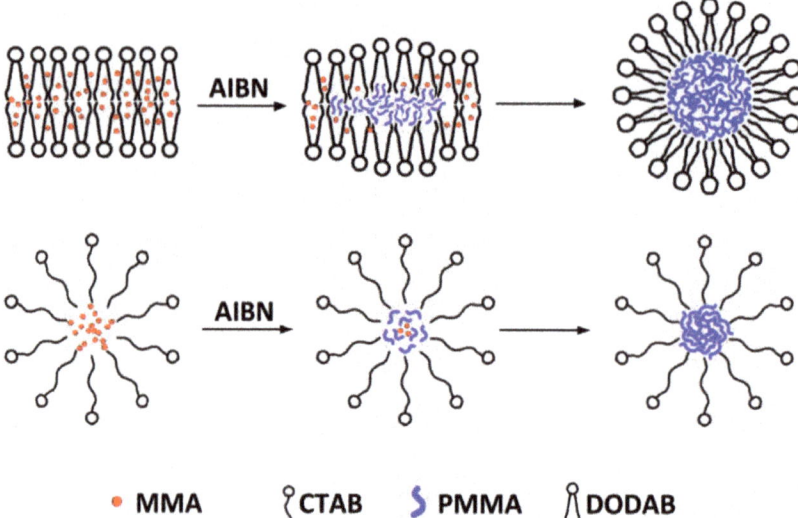

Scheme 1. Emulsion polymerization of methyl methacrylate (MMA) initiated by azobisisobutyronitrile (AIBN) using dioctadecyl dimethyl ammonium bromide (DODAB) or cetyltrimethylammonium bromide (CTAB) as emulsifiers. The cross sections of DODAB bilayer fragments (BF) and CTAB micelles were schematically represented as loaded with the MMA monomer (in red) before adding AIBN to initiate the polymerization.

Over a range of MMA or QAC concentrations, 0.4 M MMA and 2 mM QAC yielded optimal physical properties for the PMMA/DODAB and PMMA/CTAB NPs (nanometric size, low polydispersity, high and positive zeta-potential, high yield, and high colloidal stability). Inhibition halos by CTAB and PMMA/CTAB NPs against bacteria and yeast showed that PMMA/CTAB NPs behaved as reservoirs for the release of CTAB with time after dialysis. CTAB was able to move both through the dialysis membrane and the agar to inhibit microbial growth. In contrast, DODAB incorporated in the PMMA polymeric matrix did not move in the agar and did not cross the dialysis membrane. For PMMA/DODAB NPs or DODAB BF, inhibition halos were not observed due to the lack of DODAB diffusion in the agar medium. The incorporation of QACs in the PMMA/QAC NPs reduced antimicrobial activity in comparison to the QACs in dispersion. CTAB was the most active microbicidal agent against the three microbes tested (*E. coli*, *S. aureus*, and *C. albicans*) reducing cell viability countings by 7 logs at submicellar concentrations. CTAB mobility in hydrated medium favored its electrostatic interaction and penetration through the microbes' cell wall and membrane, imparting a lytic effect on the cells. DODAB BF revealed an important fungicidal activity against *C. albicans* not described before; similar to rod-like copolymers assemblies, the disk-like cationic DODAB BF possibly entered the outer glycoproteins layer of the fungus penetrating the cell and causing a 5-log reduction in yeast viability. Besides applications in antimicrobial chemotherapy, PMMA/QAC NPs here described may find interesting uses also as immunoadjuvants due to their nanometric size, positive zeta-potential, narrow size distribution, and high colloidal stability. They are expected to combine well with oppositely charged antigens, such as proteins [43], peptides [44,45], or DNA [46–48] for subunit vaccines design as many cationic adjuvants do.

2. Materials and Methods

2.1. Materials

Methyl methacrylate (MMA), hexadecyltrimethyl ammonium bromide (CTAB) dioctadecyldimethyl ammonium bromide (DODAB), azobisisobutyronitrile (AIBN), agarose, Mueller-Hinton agar (MHA), D-glucose, NaCl, ethanol 99.9%, and cellulose acetate membranes with a molecular weight cutoff around 12,400 g/mol were obtained from Sigma-Aldrich (Darmstadt, Germany) and used without further purification.

2.2. Preparation of CTAB or DODAB Dispersions in Water Solution

CTAB and DODAB are quaternary ammonium amphiphiles (QACs) that were separately weighted and added to a 1-mM NaCl solution (pH 6.3) to yield a stock dispersion at 10 mM amphiphile. Whereas CTAB yielded a homogeneous and transparent dispersion, typical of its assembly in water as micelles, DODAB had to be dispersed ultrasonically with a macroprobe. The DODAB BF were obtained from the DODAB powder added to the aqueous 1 mM NaCl solution dispersed by sonication with tip at 85 W for 15 min above 47 °C, before centrifuging the dispersion for precipitation of titanium ejected from the tip (9300× g for 1 h at 4 °C). This yielded the DODAB BF as a somewhat turbid dispersion. These DODAB dispersions were previously characterized as containing open bilayer fragments that did not enclose a water compartment, were nano-sized, and able to incorporate hydrophobic drugs in the bilayer or antimicrobial peptides or polymers [34,35,44,45,49–54]. Both CTAB and DODAB dispersions were diluted from the stock dispersions to obtain the final desired concentrations. The analytical CTAB or DODAB concentrations were determined from halide microtitration [55,56].

2.3. Synthesis of Waterborne PMMA/QACs Nanoparticles (NPs) by Emulsion Polymerization

The PMMA/CTAB or PMMA/DODAB hybrid and polymeric NPs were obtained by emulsion polymerization of MMA using AIBN as the initiator of the MMA polymerization, similar to the synthesis previously described using potassium persulfate (KPS) as the initiator [27]. The synthesis protocol was similar to the one previously described for the synthesis of PMMA/PDDA NPs using AIBN as the initiator [21–23]. In order to eliminate oxygen, a flow of nitrogen gas was applied for a few minutes to 10 mL DODAB or CTAB dispersions in 1 mM NaCl added of the desired MMA concentration and 0.0036 g AIBN. The reaction mixture inside the glass tube was then closed with a cap, heated, and kept at 80 °C in a water bath for 1 h under periodic vortexing. Thereafter, the capped tube containing the reaction mixture was withdrawn from the water bath and allowed to reach room temperature. The dispersions thus obtained were purified by dialysis against 2 L of ultrapure water (3×) for 24 h. Particle characterization took place after dialysis using dilutions of the original dispersion in 1 mM aqueous NaCl solution.

2.4. Determination of Sizes, Zeta-Potentials, and Polydispersity of PMMA/QAC Dispersions by Dynamic Light Scattering (DLS)

Size distributions, zeta-average diameters (Dz), and zeta potentials (ζ potentials) were obtained by dynamic light scattering (DLS) using a Zeta plus−Zeta potential Analyzer (Brookhaven Instruments Corporation, Holtsville, NY, USA) equipped with a 677-nm laser with measurements at 90°. The polydispersity of the dispersions was determined by dynamic light scattering (DLS) following well-defined mathematic equations [57]. The mean hydrodynamic diameters (mean Dz) were obtained from the log-normal distribution of the light-scattering intensity curve against Dz. The ζ potentials were determined from the electrophoretic mobility (μ) and the Smoluckowski equation, $\zeta = \mu\eta/\varepsilon$, where η and ε are the viscosity and the dielectric constant of the medium, respectively. Samples that underwent the DLS measurements were usually diluted from the original dispersions for optimal readings (50–100 μL PMMA/QAC dispersions in 2 mL of 1 mM NaCl). All measurements were performed in the DLS apparatus took place at 25 ± 1 °C.

2.5. Visualization and Morphology of PMMA/QAC NPs from Scanning Electron Microscopy (SEM)

Scanning electron microscopy (SEM) was performed using Jeol JSM-7401F equipment. Silicon <100> wafers were from Silicon Quest (Santa Clara, CA, USA) with a native oxide layer approximately 2 nm thick and used as substrates for casting the PMMA/QAC dispersions. The Si wafers with a native SiO_2 layer were cut into small pieces of ca 1 cm^2, cleaned with ethanol, and dried under an N_2 stream. Samples of 0.050 mL PMMA/QAC dispersions were deposited on clean Si/SiO$_2$ wafers and dried overnight in a desiccator. Then, the coatings were covered with a thin layer of gold before SEM analyses, as required for contrast and visualization. Mean diameters (D) for dry NPs were evaluated from ImageJ software Version 1.52u for 100 particles and presented as a mean value.

2.6. Microorganisms Cultures and Effect of CTAB, DODAB, or PMMA/QAC NPs on Cell Viability in the Presence of the Cationic Amphiphiles Solutions or Dispersions

Escherichia coli ATCC (American Type Culture Collection) 25922, *Staphylococcus aureus* ATCC 29213 or *Candida albicans* ATCC 90028 were cultured from previously frozen stocks (kept at −20 °C in the appropriate storage medium). Each microorganism was reactivated separately, seeded by streaking technique on the plates of Mueller-Hinton agar, and incubated for 18–24 h at 37 °C. The turbidity of either bacteria or fungus suspensions was adjusted according to tube 0.5 of the McFarland scale at 625 nm in isotonic 0.264 M D-glucose solution. The 0.264 M D-glucose solution was used instead of any culture medium because cationic molecules are inactivated by the relatively high ionic strength or negatively charged molecules, such as amino acids and polysaccharides. For the determination of cell viability, 0.1 mL of the cell suspensions (around 10^7–10^8 colony-forming unities per mL, CFU.mL^{-1}) were mixed with 0.9 mL of NPs dispersions diluted in the same D-glucose solution and interacted for 1 h. Thereafter, aliquots of 0.1 mL were withdrawn and either directly plated or diluted 10 to 10^6 times before plating on MHA plates. The plates were incubated at 37 °C for 24 h. The CFU were counted and plotted in a logarithmic or percentage scale as a function of QAC concentration (mM). When no counting was obtained, since the log function does not exist for zero, the CFU counting was taken as 1 so that log CFU.mL^{-1} could be taken as zero.

2.7. Determination of Growth Inhibition Zones by PMMA/QAC NPs

Escherichia coli ATCC (American Type Culture Collection) 25922, *Staphylococcus aureus* ATCC 29213, and *Candida albicans* ATCC 90028 from previously frozen stocks kept at −20 °C in an appropriate storage medium were grown as described above, and the bacterial suspension prepared in 0.264 M

D-glucose had its turbidity adjusted according to 0.5 of the McFarland scale, as previously described. A softer growth medium containing 2.3% Muller-Hinton broth and 0.64% agar was prepared and sterilized in steam autoclave at 121 °C for 20 min. In 50 mL of this growth medium, 0.5 mL of the microorganism suspension was added and then carefully homogenized. Plates containing MHA were previously prepared and used to place micropipette tips with their bases positioned on the MHA to form wells with a 9 mm diameter. Before withdrawing the tips, ca. 20 mL of the microorganism culture in the soft MHA was allowed to harden. After agar hardening, the tips were removed and, in each well, 100 µL of the QAC dispersions at 0.01, 0.1, 0.2, 0.5, 1, 1.5, 2, and 2.5 mM or of the NPs dispersions were added for incubation 18–24 h at 37 °C for determining the inhibition zones surrounding the wells. From the comparison between inhibition zones for the standard QAC dispersions and the PMMA/QAC NPs, the QAC concentration in the NPs dispersions was estimated.

2.8. Determination of QAC Concentration from Halide Microtitration

Bromide is the counterion of DODAB and CTAB. Similar to chloride, bromide can be determined by halide microtitration [55], as given in a detailed protocol for halide microtitration [56].

3. Results and Discussion

3.1. Synthesis of PMMA/QACs NPs by Emulsion Polymerization and their Physical Characterization from SEM and DLS

PMMA/QAC NPs' morphology, size, and homogeneity were assessed by SEM. Two different PMMA/QAC NPs were synthesized and observed after drying under SEM (Figure 1). The QAC was DODAB (Figure 1a) or CTAB (Figure 1b). Both syntheses employed 0.4 M MMA, 2 mM QAC, 0.0036 g AIBN and 1 mM NaCl in 10 mL of reaction mixture. The NPs were spherical, displayed a narrow size distribution and were homo dispersed. PMMA/DODAB and PMMA/CTAB mean diameters after drying (D) were obtained for at least 100 particles from the ImageJ software as 56 ± 7 and 85 ± 11 nm, respectively (Figure 1).

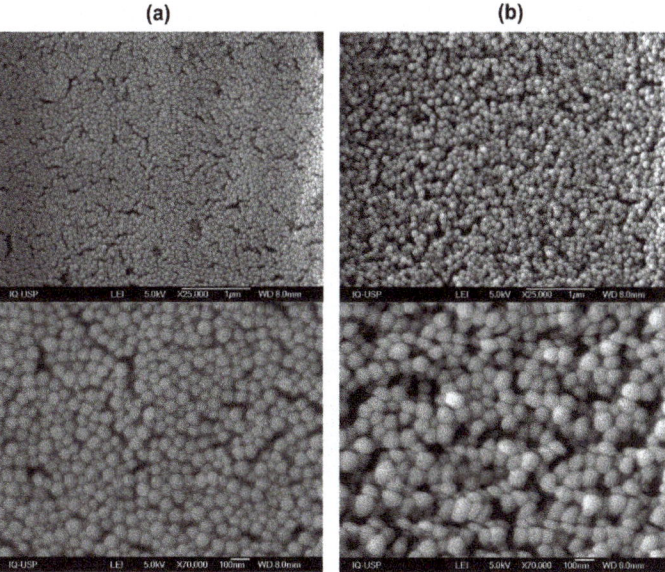

Figure 1. Scanning electron micrographs (SEM) of original dispersions of poly methyl methacrylate /dioctadecyldimethylammonium (PMMA/DODAB) (**a**) or PMMA/CTAB nanoparticles (NPs) on silicon wafers (**b**). The magnification was either 25,000× (on the top) or 70,000× (on the bottom).

The mean diameter of dry NPs (D) was compared to the one of NPs in water dispersion given by dynamic light scattering (DLS) as the mean hydrodynamic diameter (Dz) (Table 1).

Table 1. Dry mean diameter (D) and mean hydrodynamic diameter (Dz) for PMMA/QAC NPs. D was from scanning electron microscopy (SEM) and Dz was determined by dynamic light-scattering (DLS). The nanoparticles (NPs) were obtained from 0.4 M methyl methacrylate (MMA), 2 mM dioctadecyl dimethyl ammonium bromide (DODAB) or cetyl trimethylammonium bromide (CTAB), and 0.36 mg·mL^{-1} AIBN in 10 mL of 1 mM NaCl. The mean D was obtained using ImageJ software from 100 particles.

NPs	D (nm)	Dz (nm)
PMMA/DODAB	56 ± 7	75 ± 1
PMMA/CTAB	85 ± 11	81 ± 1

For NPs obtained from 0.4 M MMA, 2 mM DODAB, or CTAB using 0.0036 g AIBN, the mean hydrodynamic diameters (Dz) were 75 ± 1 and 81 ± 1 nm for PMMA/DODAB and PMMA/CTAB NPs, respectively. One would expect that the Dz values from DLS would be higher than D from SEM due to an eventual hydration layer surrounding each NP. Indeed, this occurred for the PMMA/DODAB NPs but did not occur for the PMMA/CTAB NPs. It is possible that the PMMA/CTAB NPs exhibited a less hydrophilic surface at the particle/water interface than the PMMA/DODAB NPs. This was possibly due to the mobile character of the CTAB molecules leaving the nanoparticles to the bulk water and the large affinity of the DODAB molecules for the PMMA polymeric matrix [19,20]. Whereas DODAB would improve the NP affinity for the surrounding water and the hydration layer, this would not be very significant for CTAB so that, for CTAB, the dry, dehydrated diameter D would not be significantly lower than the hydrodynamic diameter Dz. D was 56 ± 7 nm for PMMA/DODAB NPs and 85 ± 11 nm for PMMA/CTAB NPs.

Curiously, DODAB behaved as a better emulsifier than CTAB during the emulsion polymerization process remaining in the PMMA/DODAB NPs after polymerization due to its higher affinity for PMMA than the one exhibited by CTAB [19,20]. At this point, one should recall the nanostructures present in DODAB and CTAB dispersions in water: the DODAB bilayer fragments (DODAB BF) with Dz inside the 56–67 nm range, as determined by DLS or SEM [44,58,59] or CTAB micelles with 10–20 nm of diameter determined by small-angle neutron scattering (SANS) [60]. IT is possible that the higher amount of DODAB in DODAB BF as compared to the amount of CTAB in the micelle improved the emulsifying effect of DODAB and resulted in a smaller NP size for the PMMA/DODAB NPs than the one for the PMMA/CTAB NPs. Since CTAB has only one hydrocarbon chain, its hydrophilic–hydrophobic balance is larger than the one for DODAB with two long hydrocarbon chains. The resulting emulsifying effect during NP synthesis promoted by CTAB was inferior to the one promoted by the DODAB BF so that sizes for the resultant NPs were larger than those synthesized with DODAB BF.

3.2. Effects of MMA Concentration, QAC Concentration, and Initiator Type on Physico-Chemical Properties of PMMA/QAC NPs Obtained by Emulsion Polymerization

Over a range of [MMA] varying from 0.1 to 1 M MMA, PMMA/QAC dispersions exhibited variable colloidal stability after synthesis and before dialysis. Above 0.4 M MMA, at 2 mM QAC, aggregation and precipitation took place so that only the supernatants were dialyzed and used for DLS and solid contents analysis. From 0.1–0.4 M MMA, no precipitation took place after synthesis and before dialysis.

Table 2 and Figure 2 show the effect of [MMA] on the physical properties of PMMA/QAC NPs obtained by emulsion polymerization at 2 mM QAC.

The data on Table 2 reveal that increasing [MMA] from 0.1 to 0.4 M at 2 mM DODAB, slightly increased the Dz for the NPs, increased ζ, reduced P, increased the solid contents and conversion of monomer into polymer, and slightly increased number density (N_p) for the NPs, in absence of aggregation. Above 0.4M MMA, poor colloidal stability associated with low zeta-potential was depicted as precipitation at the bottom of the assay tubes (Table 2). For PMMA/CTAB NPs, similar behavior took place for the physical properties except for the zeta-potential that remained low and approximately constant 17–23 mV. These results for the compared zeta-potentials for PMMA/DODAB and PMMA/CTAB NPs, again, suggest that increasing [MMA] leads to increased incorporation of DODAB in the NPs, whereas the incorporation of CTAB remains low and practically unaffected by the increased amount of solid contents.

Table 2. Physical properties of PMMA/QAC NPs obtained by emulsion polymerization of MMA monomer over a range of [MMA] at 2 mM DODAB or CTAB using AIBN as the initiator. Zeta-average diameter (Dz), zeta potential (ζ), and polydispersity (P) were obtained by dynamic light scattering. The conversion of monomer into polymer was expressed in percentile. The particles' number density (N_p), in mL^{-1}, was calculated from nanoparticle size (Dz) and the mass of lyophilized dispersions. Solid contents, conversion, and N_p were determined as previously described in [27].

QAC	[MMA] /M	Dz /nm	ζ /mV	P	Solid Contents /mg·mL^{-1}	Conversion /%	N_p /mL^{-1}	Aggregates
DODAB	0.1	101 ± 1	+20 ± 2	0.355 ± 0.002	0.0051 ± 0.0001	51	8.35 × 10^{12}	No
	0.2	52 ± 1	+20 ± 1	0.265 ± 0.003	0.0081 ± 0.0001	40	9.52 × 10^{13}	No
	0.3	73 ± 1	+27 ± 1	0.038 ± 0.010	0.0183 ± 0.0009	61	7.76 × 10^{13}	No
	0.4	75 ± 1	+49 ± 5	0.037 ± 0.005	0.0317 ± 0.0001	79	1.26 × 10^{14}	No
	0.7	94 ± 1	+26 ± 2	0.033 ± 0.009	0.0479 ± 0.0008	68	1.04 × 10^{14}	Yes
	0.9	103 ± 1	+38 ± 2	0.013 ± 0.004	0.0697 ± 0.0001	77	1.07 × 10^{14}	Yes
	1.0	109 ± 1	+33 ± 1	0.020 ± 0.010	0.0781 ± 0.0005	78	1.02 × 10^{14}	Yes
CTAB	0.1	916 ± 56	+18 ± 1	0.477 ± 0.042	0.0021 ± 0.0004	20	4.43 × 10^{9}	No
	0.2	40 ± 1	+20 ± 1	0.291 ± 0.003	0.0105 ± 0.0004	53	2.82 × 10^{14}	No
	0.3	70 ± 1	+17 ± 1	0.078 ± 0.009	0.0197 ± 0.0019	65	9.52 × 10^{13}	No
	0.4	81 ± 1	+23 ± 1	0.041 ± 0.008	0.0320 ± 0.0019	80	1.01 × 10^{14}	No
	0.7	100 ± 1	+20 ± 1	0.032 ± 0.008	0.0363 ± 0.0014	52	6.10 × 10^{13}	Yes
	0.9	121 ± 1	+26 ± 1	0.012 ± 0.004	0.0692 ± 0.0013	77	6.52 × 10^{13}	Yes
	1.0	121 ± 1	+17 ± 1	0.046 ± 0.010	0.0702 ± 0.0005	70	6.52 × 10^{13}	Yes

Figure 2 gives an overview of the effect of [MMA] on the physical properties of the PMMA/DODAB and PMMA/CTAB NPs' dispersions. The green rectangle emphasizes the NPs obtained with desirable characteristics, such as low size, low polydispersity, high zeta-potential, high yield, high particle number density (N_p), and high colloidal stability (absence of aggregates and precipitates). The synthesis performed at 0.4 M MMA was selected as the one yielding the optimal NPs to be analyzed regarding their antimicrobial properties. One should notice that at 0.1 M [MMA] in the presence of DODAB BF, the high P and large sizes obtained might be explained from the intrinsically high polydispersity of the DODAB BF; polymerization took place inside the bilayer fragments, and NPs acquired their polydispersity.

The effect of [QAC] on the physical properties of the PMMA/QAC NPs is shown in Table 3. Increasing [QAC] reduced Dz, decreased the zeta-potential of PMMA/DODAB NPs and increased the one of PMMA/CTAB NPs, increased the polydispersity, and barely affected conversion or particle number density. The highest zeta-potentials for PMMA/DODAB NPs occurred at the lowest [DODAB], meaning that DODAB imparted high positive charges to the NPs but preferred to interact with other DODAB BF in dispersion when [DODAB] increased. For PMMA/CTAB, similar behavior to the one of PMMA/DODAB NPs was found except for the zeta-potential that decreased with [DODAB] and increased with [CTAB]. This means that the low affinity of CTAB for PMMA again explained the low incorporation of CTAB to this polymer over a range of low CTAB concentrations. Only when [CTAB] increased did it become possible to cause an increase in the zeta-potential of the PMMA/CTAB NPs from 15 to 40 mV due to increased CTAB incorporation in the NPs (Table 3). Increasing [QAC], affected the polydispersity that also increased for both types of NPs. QACs indeed tend to increase the size of their aggregates with increase in their concentration or on the ionic strength of the medium [60–62]. The selected concentration of MMA was 0.4 M because, above 0.4 M MMA, poor colloidal stability was depicted from a visual observation of precipitated material; in this case, the measurements were performed with the dialyzed supernatants. Below 0.3 M MMA, low MMA concentrations resulted in low conversion (yield %), high polydispersities (P), and comparatively low zeta-potentials (ζ). The green rectangle indicates the region of [MMA] yielding stable PMMA/QACs NPs at high conversion rates, maximal particles number densities (N_p), low P (0.03–0.06), high ζ (20–50 mV), and low Dz (70–75 nm).

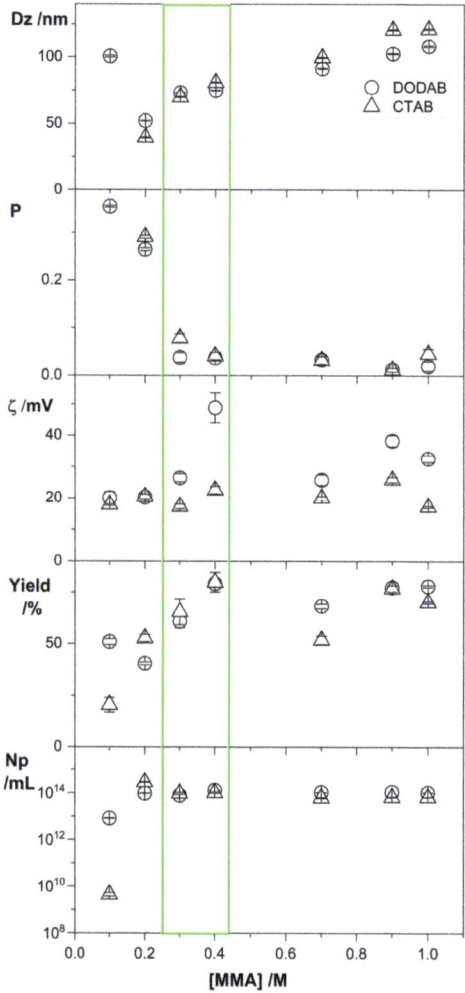

Figure 2. Physical properties of PMMA/QAC NPs obtained by emulsion polymerization over a range of [MMA] at 2 mM DODAB (○) or CTAB (Δ). All dispersions were exhaustively submitted to dialysis in pure water before measurements. Above 0.4 M MMA, poor colloidal stability was depicted from the visual observation of precipitated material; the measurements were performed with the dialyzed supernatants. Below 0.3 M MMA, low MMA concentrations resulted in low conversion (yield %), high polydispersities (P), and comparatively low zeta-potentials (ζ). The green rectangle indicates the region of [MMA] yielding stable PMMA/QACs NPs at high conversion rates, maximal particle number densities (N_p), low P (0.03–0.06), high ζ (20–50 mV), and low Dz (70–75 nm).

Table 3. Physical properties of PMMA/QAC NPs obtained by the emulsion polymerization of MMA monomer at 0.4 M MMA over a range of [QAC] using AIBN as the initiator. Zeta-average diameter (Dz), zeta potential (ζ), and polydispersity (P) were obtained by dynamic light scattering. The conversion of monomer into polymer was expressed in percentile. The particles number density (N_p), in mL^{-1}, was calculated from nanoparticle size (Dz) and the mass of lyophilized dispersions.

QAC	[QAC] /mM	Dz /nm	ζ /mV	P	Solid Contents /mg·mL^{-1}	Conversion /%	N_p /mL^{-1}
DODAB	0.3	99 ± 1	+50 ± 2	0.035 ± 0.009	0.0303 ± 0.0003	76	5.24 × 10^{13}
	0.5	93 ± 1	+44 ± 2	0.045 ± 0.014	0.0300 ± 0.0004	75	6.21 × 10^{13}
	1.0	85 ± 1	+33 ± 2	0.028 ± 0.008	0.0303 ± 0.0006	76	8.08 × 10^{13}
	2.0	75 ± 1	+49 ± 5	0.037 ± 0.005	0.0317 ± 0.0001	79	1.26 × 10^{14}
	4.0	69 ± 1	+31 ± 1	0.072 ± 0.008	0.0349 ± 0.0006	87	1.79 × 10^{14}
	5.0	62 ± 1	+29 ± 2	0.068 ± 0.010	0.0333 ± 0.0006	83	2.31 × 10^{14}
	8.0	58 ± 1	+32 ± 2	0.098 ± 0.010	0.0365 ± 0.0008	91	3.04 × 10^{14}
	10.0	59 ± 1	+35 ± 3	0.123 ± 0.007	0.0364 ± 0.0021	91	2.92 × 10^{14}
CTAB	0.3	126 ± 1	+15 ± 1	0.055 ± 0.013	0.0261 ± 0.0001	65	2.16 × 10^{13}
	0.5	115 ± 1	+15 ± 1	0.069 ± 0.016	0.0274 ± 0.0001	68	3.02 × 10^{13}
	1.0	103 ± 1	+27 ± 2	0.069 ± 0.013	0.0319 ± 0.0005	80	4.86 × 10^{13}
	2.0	81 ± 1	+23 ± 1	0.041 ± 0.008	0.0320 ± 0.0019	80	1.01 × 10^{14}
	4.0	67 ± 1	+24 ± 1	0.070 ± 0.011	0.0282 ± 0.0003	70	1.55 × 10^{14}
	5.0	67 ± 1	+31 ± 2	0.052 ± 0.012	0.0234 ± 0.0006	58	1.32 × 10^{14}
	8.0	60 ± 1	+34 ± 1	0.095 ± 0.011	0.0320 ± 0.0002	80	2.50 × 10^{14}
	10.0	57 ± 1	+41 ± 2	0.092 ± 0.008	0.0308 ± 0.0001	77	2.72 × 10^{14}

Figure 3 showed the desired properties for the PMMA/QAC dispersions at 2 mM QAC (green line), which was the concentration selected for the evaluation of antimicrobial activity. At 2 mM DODAB or CTAB, there was low size, low polydispersity, high zeta-potential, high yield, high Np and good colloidal stability for the PMMA/QAC NPs.

Two initiators were compared for the NPs synthesis: potassium persulfate (KPS) and AIBN. The initiator effect on NP properties is shown in Table 4. The MMA concentration selected for the comparison was identical to the one previously used in [27], where NPs had been synthesized with 0.56 M MMA using KPS as initiator.

Table 4. Comparison between nanoparticles of PMMA/QAC synthesized using either potassium persulfate (KPS) or azobisisobutyronitrile (AIBN) as initiators, at 0.56 M MMA and 2 mM QAC.

NPs	Initiator	Dz/nm	ζ/mV	P
PMMA/DODAB	KPS [1]	1260 ± 43	−10 ± 1	0.370
	AIBN	89 ± 1	+45 ± 2	0.027 ± 0.010
PMMA/CTAB	KPS [1]	395 ± 5	−38 ± 1	0.262
	AIBN	96 ± 1	+23 ± 1	0.033 ± 0.012

[1] Results taken from the reference [27].

Imparting the positive charge on the NPs was a difficult task in the presence of the negative sulfate charges on the PMMA/DODAB particles coming from the synthesis with KPS as the initiator; at 2 mM DODAB during the NPs synthesis, the zeta-potential was still negative (ζ = −10 ± 1 mV) and the particles were large (Dz = 1260 ± 43) and very polydisperse (P = 0.370), suggesting poor colloidal stability (Table 4). Naves and coworkers used large concentrations of the QACs, such as ca. 10 mM DODAB, to revert the KPS effect and obtain positively charged NPs [27]. AIBN was a much more convenient initiator since, when using only 2 mM DODAB, the dispersion contained small NPs (Dz = 89 ± 1) that were positively charged (ζ = +45 ± 2 mV) and homodispersed (P = 0.027 ± 0.010). Similar results were obtained from the comparison between PMMA/CTAB NPs synthesized with KPS and PMMA/CTAB NPs synthesized with AIBN (Table 4). In summary, at 2 mM QAC, the comparison between NPs synthesized using KPS or AIBN indicated that the low sizes, the high positive zeta-potentials, and the low polydispersities occurred only using AIBN.

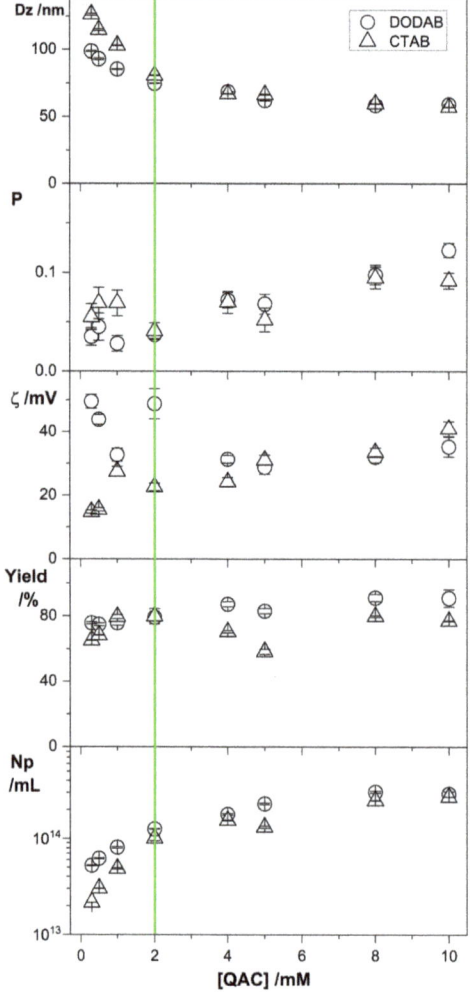

Figure 3. Physical properties of PMMA/QAC NPs obtained by emulsion polymerization over a range of [QAC] at 0.4 M MMA during particle synthesis where QAC is DODAB (○) or CTAB (Δ). All dispersions were exhaustively submitted to dialysis in pure water before measurements.

3.3. Incorporation of QACs in the PMMA/QAC NPs

DODAB and CTAB have a different hydrophobic–hydrophilic balance, as depicted from their chemical structure. The double-chained DODAB tends to prefer more hydrophobic environments than the single-chained CTAB. The determination of QAC incorporation in the PMMA polymeric matrix of the NPs showed the higher incorporation of DODAB in comparison to the one of CTAB (Table 5).

Table 5. Determination of QAC concentration [QAC] in PMMA/QAC NPs from halide microtitration in the supernatants of PMMA/DODAB and PMMA/CTAB NP water dispersions before and after dialysis. The PMMA/QAC dispersions were prepared in 2.0 mM QAC. The controls for the dialysis were QAC dispersions in water and 1 mM NaCl solution.

Dispersion or Solution	[QAC]/mM	
	Before Dialysis	After Dialysis
CTAB dispersion in water	2.5 ± 0.1	0.1 ± 0.1
DODAB bilayer fragments in water	2.3 ± 0.1	2.0 ± 0.1
NaCl water solution	1.2 ± 0.1	0.2 ± 0.1
Supernatant of PMMA/DODAB dispersion	2.0 ± 0.1	1.3 ± 0.1 [1]
Supernatant of PMMA/CTAB dispersion	2.0 ± 0.1	0.5 ± 0.1 [1]

[1] Microtitration done for supernatants of dialyzed dispersions 3 days after dialysis.

A CTAB control solution with 2.5 mM CTAB before dialysis permeated the dialysis membrane almost completely, yielding 0.1 mM CTAB just after dialysis (Table 5). DODAB BF at 2 mM DODAB, on the contrary, did not permeate the dialysis bag. Similarl to CTAB, NaCl permeated the dialysis membrane almost completely. On the third day after dialysis, the supernatants of centrifuged PMMA/DODAB dispersions contained 1.3 mM DODAB, suggesting that 0.7 mM DODAB was still incorporated by the PMMA/DODAB NPs. PMMA/CTAB NPs dispersions had contents of QAC determined after dialysis and centrifugation, revealing the absence of CTAB in the supernatants just after dialysis but its presence in the supernatant 3 days after dialysis showing its low affinity for the PMMA/CTAB NPs. In contrast, 3 days after dialysis, 0.5 mM CTAB was determined in the supernatant of PMMA/CTAB NPs showing CTAB leakage from the PMMA/CTAB NPs just after dialysis (Table 5). In summary, DODAB incorporation in the NPs was substantial, whereas the one of CTAB was transient and possibly almost lost after dialysis.

The evaluation of inhibition halos by CTAB against bacteria and yeast is in Figure 4. Just after dialysis, CTAB was not found in the supernatants of PMMA/CTAB NPs. This contrasted with 0.5 mM CTAB found in the supernatant 3 days after dialysis (Table 5). PMMA/CTAB NPs behaved as a reservoir for the release of CTAB with time after dialysis. The experiment using CTAB to determine the inhibition halos also showed that CTAB is able to move through the agar to inhibit microbial growth. Due to this property, inhibition halos against seeded bacteria and fungus could be determined on Petri dishes as a function of [CTAB] over a range of [CTAB] (0.01–2.5 mM CTAB) (Figure 4). Inhibition halos occurred for PMMA/CTAB NPs before (B) dialysis but did not occur just after dialysis (A), confirming the momentaneous absence of CTAB in the NPs supernatant. Estimated [CTAB] in the NPs' supernatant before dialysis resulted from the similarity with halo 3 against *S. aureus* (Figure 4b) or halo 3 against *C. albicans* (Figure 4c), yielding 0.3 mM CTAB outside the NPs. If the added CTAB during particle synthesis was 2 mM, after synthesis, 1.7 mM was incorporated in the NPs and 0.3 mM was in the outer solution. However, the NPs dialysis after synthesis eliminated non-incorporated CTAB from the dispersions, as depicted from the absence of halo in A (Figure 4). Regarding the antimicrobial activity that will be determined just after dialysis, one will have to consider 1.7 mM as the CTAB concentration in the NPs.

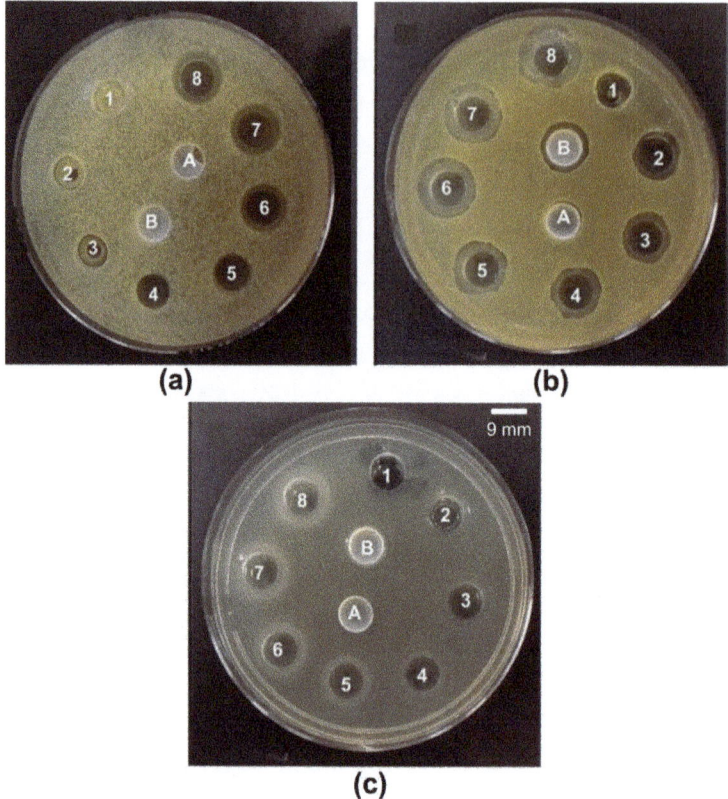

Figure 4. (a) *E. coli*, (b) *S. aureus*, and (c) *C. albicans* inhibition halos induced by CTAB alone (numbered from 1 to 8) or by PMMA/CTAB dispersions after (A) or before dialysis (B). From 1 to 8, [CTAB] inside the wells was 0.01, 0.2, 0.3, 0.5, 1.0, 1.5, 2.0, and 2.5 mM.

For PMMA/DODAB NPs, the experiment based on inhibition halos was not possible since DODAB BF are not able to diffuse in the agar medium as reported before [23].

3.4. Antibacterial and Antifungal Activity of QACs and PMMA/QAC NPs

A proper evaluation of the antimicrobial activity involves determining CFU counting over a range of [QAC] and expressing the CFU countings on a logarithmic scale so that the effective potency of the QACs becomes evaluated over ample range of magnitude.

Figure 5 shows the cell viability of *Escherichia coli* in the presence of CTAB (a), PMMA/CTAB NPs (b), DODAB BF (c), and PMMA/DODAB NPs (d). Just after dialysis, the inhibition halo experiment yielded an absence of free CTAB in the supernatant of PMMA/CTAB NPs and 1.7 mM CTAB in the NPs. This [CTAB] initially incorporated in the NPs decreased *E. coli* viability by 1.5 logs (Figure 5b), in contrast to free CTAB that reduced viability by 7 logs (Figure 5a). CTAB exhibited a remarkable activity against *E. coli* that could not be identified before from experiments expressing only % cell viability (limited to only 2 logs at most). CTAB incorporation in the PMMA/CTAB NPs reduced substantially its activity but may be useful for controlled release in biomedical prosthetic devices [63] or agar-based hydrogels [64].

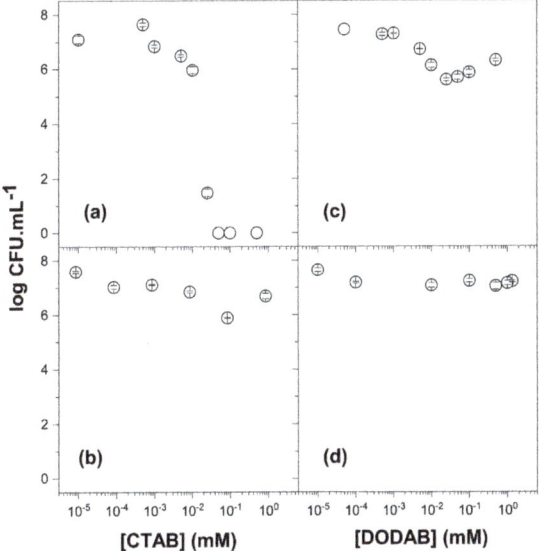

Figure 5. Viability of *Escherichia coli* in the presence of CTAB (**a**), PMMA/CTAB (**b**), DODAB (**c**), and PMMA/DODAB dispersions (**d**). The NP dispersions of PMMA/CTAB and PMMA/DODAB were used after dialysis. The counting of colony-forming unities (CFU) was expressed on a logarithmic scale.

The CTAB mechanism of action involves reaching the bacterial cell membrane causing its disruption and cell lysis [65]. Therefore, the large reduction in CTAB activity was due to its location in the PMMA/CTAB NPs instead of moving freely in the bulk solution to interact with the bacteria. In another report, CTAB adsorbed by BiOBr nanosheets showed lower toxicity than the same level of free CTAB, which was attributed to the adsorption or hindering effect of BiOBr nanosheets [66]. PMMA/CTAB NPs in this work released 0.5 mM CTAB on the third day after dialysis from an initial concentration in the NPs of 1.7 mM CTAB (Table 5; Figure 4). This behavior was similar to the one of the inorganic BiOBr nanosheets incorporating CTAB that exhibited a slow and sustained release of CTAB or benzalkonium chloride for 8 h [66].

Among the biocompatible polymers, PMMA was used in combinations with CTAB or DODAB to prepare spin-coated films able to kill bacteria upon release to the medium (CTAB) or upon contact on the surface of the coating (DODAB) [19]. In pharmaceutics, polymers are often be used as reservoirs of the active principle or drug so that the polymer can control the release of the active molecule over time in vivo [3,67,68].

DODAB BF reduced the viability of *E. coli* by 2 logs (Figure 5c), whereas PMMA/DODAB NPs reduced viability by 0.5 logs CTAB (Figure 5d). Possibly, the lack of mobility of the DODAB BF across the bacterial cell wall to reach the cell membrane resulted in the much lower activity of DODAB in comparison to the one of CTAB. In fact, no leakage of intracellular contents was detected for DODAB BF interacting with *E. coli* in comparison to the pronounced leakage determined for CTAB and the anionic sodium dodecylsulfate (SDS) [29].

The high affinity of DODAB for PMMA determined its incorporation in the NPs, which was 0.7 mM remaining 1.3 mM in the supernatant after dialysis and centrifugation (Table 5). For the PMMA/DODAB NPs, the activity was lower than the one of DODAB BF (Figure 5c,d). A possible explanation for this is that the DODAB incorporated in the NPs was not leaving them to kill the microbia; this meant that only DODAB BF outside the NPs was effective.

Figure 6 shows the compared activity of CTAB (Figure 6a) and PMMA/CTAB NPs (Figure 6b) against *S. aureus*. Similar to the effect of PMMA/CTAB NPs against *E. coli*, before dialysis there was

0.3 mM CTAB outside the PMMA/CTAB NPs with 1.7 mM incorporated in the NPs. The CTAB reservoir effect of the NPs reduced its effect against the bacteria, as compared to free CTAB. The compared effect for DODAB BF (Figure 6c) and PMMA/DODAB NPs (Figure 6d) revealed a similar and low activity. *Staphylococcus* sp. developed a sensor system for cationic antimicrobial peptides based on a sensor consisting of a short and negatively charged extracellular loop of amino acid residues able to interact with cationic antimicrobial peptides [69]. The transduction of this interaction signal would trigger the d-alanylation of teichoic acids and the lysylation of phosphatidylglycerol, resulting in a decreased negative charge of the bacteria. It is possible that DODAB BF (but not CTAB molecules) were possibly able to trigger this resistance mechanism in *S. aureus* due to the multipoint attachment of DODAB BF to the negatively charged loop. CTAB, on the other hand, would kill microorganisms as individual molecules below its critical micellar concentration (1 mM) [28,30], rapidly and extensively penetrating the cell wall to reach the cell membrane.

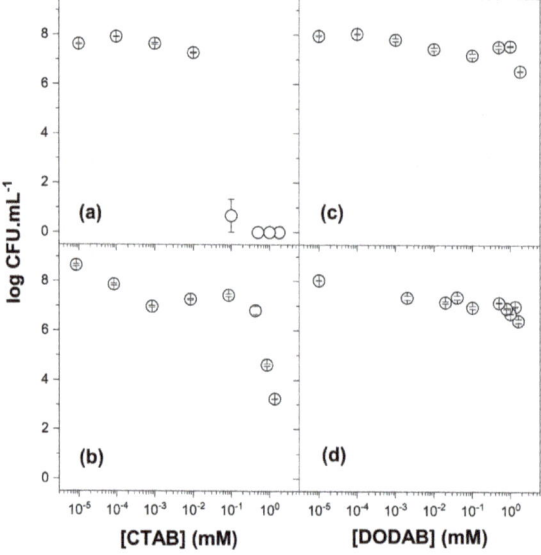

Figure 6. Viability of *Staphylococcus aureus* in the presence of CTAB (**a**), PMMA/CTAB (**b**), DODAB (**c**), and PMMA/DODAB dispersions (**d**). The NP dispersions of PMMA/CTAB and PMMA/DODAB were used after dialysis. The counting of colony-forming unities (CFU) was expressed on a logarithmic scale.

Against *Candida albicans*, free CTAB showed remarkable activity (Figure 7a) in contrast with the reduced activity of PMMA/CTAB NPs (Figure 7b). The NP dispersion just after dialysis was used to interact with the fungus so that no CTAB molecules were available outside the NPs to interact with the cells. However, some CTAB leakage from the NPs was probably taking place to yield the 1.5-logs reduction observed in Figure 7b. On the other hand, DODAB BF was surprisingly active against *C. albicans*, resulting in a reduction of ca. 5 logs at 1.2 mM DODAB after a 1-h interaction (Figure 7c). Neither Campanhã and coworkers [40] nor Vieira and coworkers [31] could observe the good antifungal activity of DODAB BF since they employed percentiles of viable cells to express the viability curves as a function of DODAB concentration. Consistently, Fukushima and coworkers [70] also reported a superior activity of supramolecular assemblies made of poly(lactide) (interior block) and cationic polycarbonates (exterior block); upon testing the spherical and rod-like morphologies for antimicrobial properties, they found that only the rod-like assemblies were effective against *Candida albicans*. This showed that the shape of the antimicrobial supramolecular assembly was important to determine antifungal activity. In the present case, the disk-like shape of the DODAB BF assemblies resulted in good antifungal activity that was not described before (Figure 7c). This can possibly be ascribed to the improved penetration of rod-like or disk-like nanostructures through the outer layer of glicoproteins on the fungus cell wall as compared to vesicles, liposomes, or nanoparticles [42,52,71].

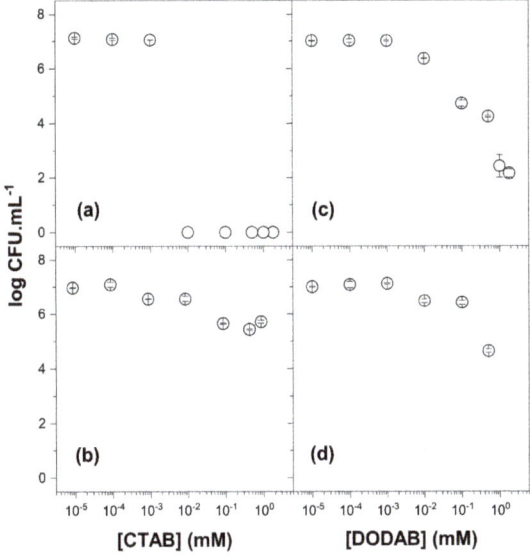

Figure 7. Viability of *Candida albicans* in the presence of CTAB (**a**), PMMA/CTAB (**b**), DODAB (**c**), and PMMA/DODAB dispersions (**d**). The NP dispersions of PMMA/CTAB and PMMA/DODAB were used after dialysis. The counting of colony-forming unities (CFU) was expressed in a logarithmic scale. The superior activity of QACs by themselves as compared to QACs in NPs is depicted from comparisons between (**a**,**b**) or (**c**,**d**). CTAB was active as a monomer at submicellar concentrations (**a**). DODAB was active as bilayer fragments (**c**).

In Figure 7d, the reduced activity of PMMA/DODAB NPs in comparison to the one of DODAB BF (Figure 7c), again, can be understood from the incorporation of DODAB in the NPs reducing its availability to interact with the fungus; there was 1.3 mM DODAB BF outside the NPs, whereas, in the DODAB BF, dispersion was 2.0 mM DODAB (Figure 7c; Table 5).

In Figure 8, the cell viability of *Candida albicans* as a percentile of viable cells (%) was obtained as a function of CTAB (Figure 8a) or DODAB concentration (Figure 8b) and compared with previous data from the literature [31]. There was a dependence of the viability curve on the initial concentration of viable cells: around 10^6 CFU.mL^{-1}, the sigmoidal curve occupied a range of lower QAC concentrations than the one around 10^7 CFU.mL^{-1}. This was consistent with the lower amounts of QAC required to kill lower concentrations of cells. In addition, one should notice that achieving a reduction of two logs in viable cells counting did not allow to discriminate whether the effect of the QACs reduced the counting by more than 2 logs. It is necessary to express CFU counting on a logarithmic scale in order to determine the complete effect of any antimicrobial, as done against *C. albicans* in Figure 7a,c. Consequently, the CTAB and DODAB BF effects were fully revealed, showing important reductions in CFU countings over 7 and 5 logs, respectively (Figure 7a,c).

Regarding the PMMA/CTAB NPs, the percentiles of viable countings plotted as circles in Figure 8c did not reveal the 5-logs reduction observed against *S. aureus* in Figure 6b. Only in the case of a small antimicrobial effect were the percentiles of viable cells sufficient to determine antimicrobial activity as was the case of the 1.0-logs reduction caused by PMMA/DODAB NPs in Figure 8d corresponding to Figure 6d expressed on a logarithmic scale.

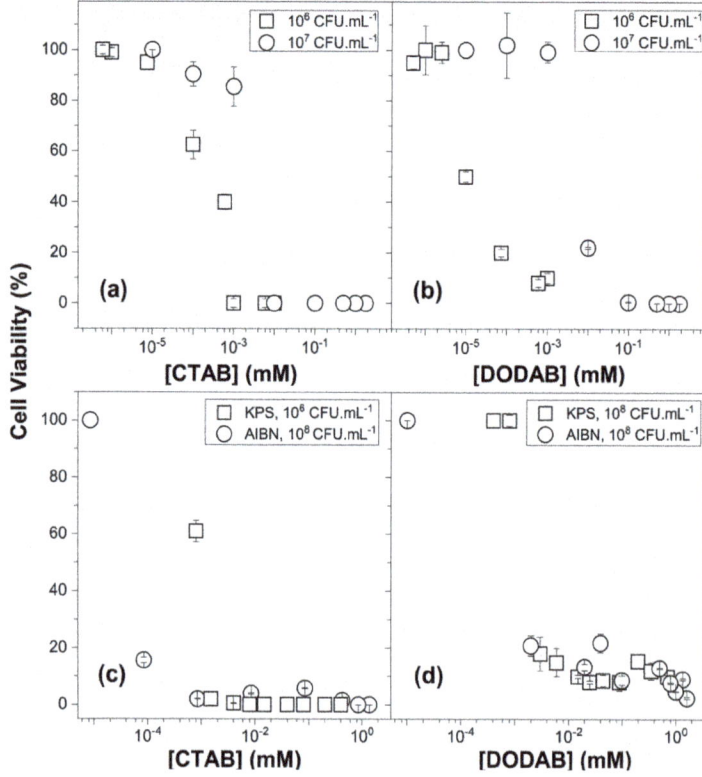

Figure 8. *Candida albicans* viability (%) (○) over a range of CTAB (**a**) or DODAB concentrations (**b**) in QAC dispersions in water as compared to data from [31] (□). *Staphylococcus aureus* viability (%) (○) over a range of CTAB (**c**) or DODAB concentrations (**d**) in the presence of PMMA/QAC NPs, as compared to data from [27] (□). QAC dispersions in water are CTAB micelles or DODAB BF. In (**c,d**), PMMA/QAC NPs were obtained by the emulsion polymerization of MMA in the presence of QACs. These NPs were obtained either using AIBN (○) or KPS (□) as the initiator. [MMA] and [QAC] used during particle synthesis were 0.56 M and 4.0 mM, respectively, for squares in (**c**), 0.4 M and 2.0 mM, respectively, for circles in (**c,d**), and 0.56 M and 10 mM, respectively, for squares in (**d**).

4. Conclusions

Over a range of MMA or QAC concentrations, 0.4 M MMA and 2 mM QAC yielded optimal physical properties for the PMMA/DODAB and PMMA/CTAB NPs in dispersion, such as nanometric size (Dz < 100 nm), low polydispersity (<0.05), high and positive zeta-potential (>20 mV), high yield (>70%), high particle number density (>10^{13} particles.mL^{-1}), and high colloidal stability (absence of aggregates and precipitates). Among two initiators (KPS or AIBN), AIBN was the best one to obtain optimal properties for the NPs synthesized at 2 mM QAC and 0.56 M MMA; the low sizes, high positive zeta-potentials, and low polydispersities occurred only using AIBN.

Inhibition halos by CTAB and PMMA/CTAB NPs against bacteria and yeast showed that PMMA/CTAB NPs behaved as reservoirs for the release of CTAB with time after dialysis; CTAB was able to move both through the dialysis membrane and the agar to inhibit microbial growth, highlighting hydrogels as good vehicles for CTAB. In contrast, DODAB preferred to remain incorporated in the PMMA polymeric matrix, did not move in the agar, and did not cross the dialysis bag membrane; for PMMA/DODAB NPs or DODAB BF, inhibition halos were not observed due to the lack of DODAB BF diffusion in the agar medium.

The incorporation of QACs in the PMMA/QAC NPs reduced antimicrobial activity in comparison to the QACs dispersions. CTAB was the most active microbicidal agent against the three microbes tested (*E. coli*, *S. aureus*, and *C. albicans*), reducing cell viability countings by 7 logs at submicellar concentrations. The controlled release of CTAB from PMMA/CTAB NPs, however, would be a promising strategy for CTAB delivery. CTAB mobility in hydrated medium favored its electrostatic interaction and penetration through the microbes' cell wall and membrane, imparting a lytic effect on the cells. DODAB BF revealed an important fungicidal activity against *C. albicans* not described before; similar to rod-like, cationic supramolecular assemblies, the disk-like cationic DODAB BF possibly entered the outer glycoproteins layer of the fungus penetrating the cell and causing a 5-logs reduction in yeast viability.

The real potency of QACs antimicrobials should not be evaluated in percentiles of initial CFU counting; potent agents often display reduction in microbial cell viability larger than the 2 logs of the initial counting of viable cells.

The PMMA/QAC NPs here described still require further evaluation regarding their cytotoxicity against mammalian cells before fulfilling their potential in drug and vaccine delivery. Due to their nanometric size, positive zeta-potential, narrow size distribution, and high colloidal stability, they are expected to combine well with oppositely charged antigens (proteins, peptides or DNA) for subunit vaccines' design, as many cationic adjuvants do. CTAB leakage and lytic property against eukaryotic cells, such yeast *C. albicans*, would not recommend the PMMA/CTAB NPs for vaccines. DODAB, on the other hand, remains embedded in the PMMA matrix, imparting a positive charge to the NPs without leaking to the outer medium. These considerations suggest that PMMA/DODAB NPs should be kept in perspective for further testing and prospective uses in drug and vaccine delivery.

Author Contributions: Conceptualization, A.M.C.-R.; Data curation, A.M.C.-R.; Formal analysis, B.I.M., A.M.C.-R.; Funding acquisition, A.M.C.-R.; Investigation, B.I.M., A.M.C.-R.; Project administration, A.M.C.-R.; Resources, A.M.C.-R.; Supervision, A.M.C.-R.; Writing—original draft, B.I.M., A.M.C.-R.; Writing—review & editing, A.M.C.-R. All authors have read and agreed to the published version of the manuscript.

Funding: This research and the APC were funded by Conselho Nacional de Desenvolvimento Científico e Tecnológico (CNPq), grants 302758/2019-4 and 302352/2014-7. B.I.M. was the recipient of undergraduate fellowships of the Programa Unificado de Bolsas da Universidade de São Paulo granted to the Project "Cationic Supramolecular Assemblies and their Films" by A.M.C.-R.

Acknowledgments: The technical support of Rodrigo Tadeu Ribeiro is gratefully acknowledged.

Conflicts of Interest: The authors declare no conflict of interest. The funders had no role in the design of the study; in the collection, analyses, or interpretation of data; in the writing of the manuscript, or in the decision to publish the results.

References

1. Arif, U.; Haider, S.; Haider, A.; Khan, N.; Alghyamah, A.A.; Jamila, N.; Khan, M.I.; Almasry, W.A.; Kang, I.-K. Biocompatible Polymers and their Potential Biomedical Applications: A Review. *Curr. Pharm. Des.* **2019**, *25*, 3608–3619. [CrossRef] [PubMed]
2. Shastri, V.P. Non-Degradable Biocompatible Polymers in Medicine: Past, Present and Future. *Curr. Pharm. Biotechnol.* **2003**, *4*, 331–337. [CrossRef] [PubMed]
3. Calzoni, E.; Cesaretti, A.; Polchi, A.; Di Michele, A.; Tancini, B.; Emiliani, C. Biocompatible Polymer Nanoparticles for Drug Delivery Applications in Cancer and Neurodegenerative Disorder Therapies. *J. Funct. Biomater.* **2019**, *10*, 4. [CrossRef] [PubMed]
4. Patra, C.N.; Priya, R.; Swain, S.; Kumar Jena, G.; Panigrahi, K.C.; Ghose, D. Pharmaceutical significance of Eudragit: A review. *Future J. Pharm. Sci.* **2017**, *3*, 33–45. [CrossRef]
5. Thakral, S.; Thakral, N.K.; Majumdar, D.K. Eudragit®: A technology evaluation. *Expert Opin. Drug Deliv.* **2013**, *10*, 131–149. [CrossRef]
6. Ali, U.; Karim, K.J.B.A.; Buang, N.A. A Review of the Properties and Applications of Poly (Methyl Methacrylate) (PMMA). *Polym. Rev.* **2015**, *55*, 678–705. [CrossRef]

7. Carmona-Ribeiro, A.M. Biomimetic Nanomaterials from the Assembly of Polymers, Lipids, and Surfactants. In *Surfactants and Detergents*; Dutta, A., Ed.; IntechOpen: London, UK, 2019; Volume 1, ISBN 978-1-78984-661-4.
8. Fournier, R.L. *Basic Transport Phenomena in Biomedical Engineering*, 3rd ed.; CRC Press: Boca Raton, FL, USA, 2011; ISBN 978-1-4398-2670-6.
9. Makadia, H.K.; Siegel, S.J. Poly Lactic-co-Glycolic Acid (PLGA) as Biodegradable Controlled Drug Delivery Carrier. *Polymers* **2011**, *3*, 1377–1397. [CrossRef]
10. Malikmammadov, E.; Tanir, T.E.; Kiziltay, A.; Hasirci, V.; Hasirci, N. PCL and PCL-based materials in biomedical applications. *J. Biomater. Sci. Polym. Ed.* **2018**, *29*, 863–893. [CrossRef]
11. Lasprilla, A.J.R.; Martinez, G.A.R.; Lunelli, B.H.; Jardini, A.L.; Filho, R.M. Poly-lactic acid synthesis for application in biomedical devices—A review. *Biotechnol. Adv.* **2012**, *30*, 321–328. [CrossRef]
12. Rivera-Briso, A.L.; Serrano-Aroca, Á. Poly (3-Hydroxybutyrate-co-3-Hydroxyvalerate): Enhancement Strategies for Advanced Applications. *Polymers* **2018**, *10*, 732. [CrossRef]
13. Guan, G.; Azad, M.A.K.; Lin, Y.; Kim, S.W.; Tian, Y.; Liu, G.; Wang, H. Biological Effects and Applications of Chitosan and Chito-Oligosaccharides. *Front. Physiol.* **2019**, *10*, 516. [CrossRef]
14. Younes, I.; Rinaudo, M. Chitin and Chitosan Preparation from Marine Sources. Structure, Properties and Applications. *Mar. Drugs* **2015**, *13*, 1133–1174. [CrossRef]
15. Moohan, J.; Stewart, S.A.; Espinosa, E.; Rosal, A.; Rodríguez, A.; Larrañeta, E.; Donnelly, R.F.; Domínguez-Robles, J. Cellulose Nanofibers and Other Biopolymers for Biomedical Applications. A Review. *Appl. Sci.* **2020**, *10*, 65. [CrossRef]
16. Cascone, S.; Lamberti, G. Hydrogel-based commercial products for biomedical applications: A review. *Int. J. Pharm.* **2020**, *573*, 118803. [CrossRef]
17. Yoshii, E. Cytotoxic effects of acrylates and methacrylates: Relationships of monomer structures and cytotoxicity. *J. Biomed. Mater. Res.* **1997**, *37*, 517–524. [CrossRef]
18. Hua, C.; Chen, K.; Wang, Z.; Guo, X. Preparation, stability and film properties of cationic polyacrylate latex particles with various substituents on the nitrogen atom. *Prog. Org. Coat.* **2020**, *143*, 105628. [CrossRef]
19. Pereira, E.M.A.; Kosaka, P.M.; Rosa, H.; Vieira, D.B.; Kawano, Y.; Petri, D.F.S.; Carmona-Ribeiro, A.M. Hybrid Materials from Intermolecular Associations between Cationic Lipid and Polymers. *J. Phys. Chem. B* **2008**, *112*, 9301–9310. [CrossRef]
20. Melo, L.D.; Palombo, R.R.; Petri, D.F.S.; Bruns, M.; Pereira, E.M.A.; Carmona-Ribeiro, A.M. Structure–Activity Relationship for Quaternary Ammonium Compounds Hybridized with Poly(methyl methacrylate). *ACS Appl. Mater. Interfaces* **2011**, *3*, 1933–1939. [CrossRef] [PubMed]
21. Sanches, L.M.; Petri, D.F.S.; de Melo Carrasco, L.D.; Carmona-Ribeiro, A.M. The antimicrobial activity of free and immobilized poly (diallyldimethylammonium) chloride in nanoparticles of poly (methylmethacrylate). *J. Nanobiotechnol.* **2015**, *13*, 58. [CrossRef]
22. Galvão, C.N.; Sanches, L.M.; Mathiazzi, B.I.; Ribeiro, R.T.; Petri, D.F.S.; Carmona-Ribeiro, A.M. Antimicrobial Coatings from Hybrid Nanoparticles of Biocompatible and Antimicrobial Polymers. *Int. J. Mol. Sci.* **2018**, *19*, 2965. [CrossRef]
23. Ribeiro, R.T.; Galvão, C.N.; Betancourt, Y.P.; Mathiazzi, B.I.; Carmona-Ribeiro, A.M. Microbicidal Dispersions and Coatings from Hybrid Nanoparticles of Poly (Methyl Methacrylate), Poly (Diallyl Dimethyl Ammonium) Chloride, Lipids, and Surfactants. *Int. J. Mol. Sci.* **2019**, *20*, 6150. [CrossRef] [PubMed]
24. Lincopan, N.; Espíndola, N.M.; Vaz, A.J.; Carmona-Ribeiro, A.M. Cationic supported lipid bilayers for antigen presentation. *Int. J. Pharm.* **2007**, *340*, 216–222. [CrossRef] [PubMed]
25. Pérez-Betancourt, Y.; Távora, B.D.C.L.F.; Colombini, M.; Faquim-Mauro, E.L.; Carmona-Ribeiro, A.M. Simple Nanoparticles from the Assembly of Cationic Polymer and Antigen as Immunoadjuvants. *Vaccines* **2020**, *8*, 105. [CrossRef] [PubMed]
26. Efron, N. *Contact Lens Practice E-Book*; Elsevier Health Sciences: Amsterdam, The Netherland, 2016; ISBN 978-0-7020-6661-0.
27. Naves, A.F.; Palombo, R.R.; Carrasco, L.D.M.; Carmona-Ribeiro, A.M. Antimicrobial Particles from Emulsion Polymerization of Methyl Methacrylate in the Presence of Quaternary Ammonium Surfactants. *Langmuir* **2013**, *29*, 9677–9684. [CrossRef]
28. Ahlström, B.; Chelminska-Bertilsson, M.; Thompson, R.A.; Edebo, L. Submicellar complexes may initiate the fungicidal effects of cationic amphiphilic compounds on *Candida albicans*. *Antimicrob. Agents Chemother.* **1997**, *41*, 544–550. [CrossRef]

29. Martins, L.M.S.; Mamizuka, E.M.; Carmona-Ribeiro, A.M. Cationic Vesicles as Bactericides. *Langmuir* **1997**, *13*, 5583–5587. [CrossRef]
30. Carmona-Ribeiro, A.M.; Vieira, D.B.; Lincopan, N. Cationic Surfactants and Lipids as Anti-Infective Agents. *Anti-Infect. Agents Med. Chem.* **2006**, *5*, 33–51. [CrossRef]
31. Vieira, D.B.; Carmona-Ribeiro, A.M. Cationic lipids and surfactants as antifungal agents: Mode of action. *J. Antimicrob. Chemother.* **2006**, *58*, 760–767. [CrossRef]
32. Israelachvili, J.N.; Mitchell, D.J.; Ninham, B.W. Theory of self-assembly of hydrocarbon amphiphiles into micelles and bilayers. *J. Chem. Soc. Faraday Trans. 2 Mol. Chem. Phys.* **1976**, *72*, 1525–1568. [CrossRef]
33. Israelachvili, J.N. *Intermolecular and Surface Forces*; Academic Press: Cambridge, MA, USA, 2015; ISBN 978-0-08-092363-5.
34. Carmona-Ribeiro, A.M. Synthetic amphiphile vesicles. *Chem. Soc. Rev.* **1992**, *21*, 209–214. [CrossRef]
35. Carmona-Ribeiro, A.M. Lipid Bilayer Fragments and Disks in Drug Delivery. *Curr. Med. Chem.* **2006**, *13*, 1359–1370. [CrossRef] [PubMed]
36. Carmona-Ribeiro, A.M. The Versatile Dioctadecyldimethylammonium Bromide. In *Application and Characterization of Surfactants*; Najjar, R., Ed.; IntechOpen: Rijeka, Croatia, 2017; Volume 1, pp. 157–181. ISBN 978-953-51-3325-4.
37. Tapias, G.N.; Sicchierolli, S.M.; Mamizuka, E.M.; Carmona-Ribeiro, A.M. Interactions between Cationic Vesicles and *Escherichia coli*. *Langmuir* **1994**, *10*, 3461–3465. [CrossRef]
38. Sicchierolli, S.M.; Mamizuka, E.M.; Carmona-Ribeiro, A.M. Bacteria Flocculation and Death by Cationic Vesicles. *Langmuir* **1995**, *11*, 2991–2995. [CrossRef]
39. Campanhã, M.T.N.; Mamizuka, E.M.; Carmona-Ribeiro, A.M. Interactions between cationic liposomes and bacteria: The physical-chemistry of the bactericidal action. *J. Lipid Res.* **1999**, *40*, 1495–1500. [PubMed]
40. Campanhã, M.T.N.; Mamizuka, E.M.; Carmona-Ribeiro, A.M. Interactions between Cationic Vesicles and *Candida albicans*. *J. Phys. Chem. B* **2001**, *105*, 8230–8236. [CrossRef]
41. Mamizuka, E.M.; Carmona-Ribeiro, A.M. Cationic Liposomes as Antimicrobial Agents. In *Communicating Current Research and Educational Topics and Trends in Applied Microbiology*; A. Méndez Vila: Badajoz, Spain, 2007; Volume 2, pp. 636–647, ISBN 13: 978-84-611-9423-0.
42. Vieira, D.B.; Carmona-Ribeiro, A.M. Cationic nanoparticles for delivery of amphotericin B: Preparation, characterization and activity in vitro. *J. Nanobiotechnol.* **2008**, *6*, 6. [CrossRef]
43. Carvalho, L.A.; Carmona-Ribeiro, A.M. Interactions between Cationic Vesicles and Serum Proteins. *Langmuir* **1998**, *14*, 6077–6081. [CrossRef]
44. Xavier, G.R.S.; Carmona-Ribeiro, A.M. Cationic Biomimetic Particles of Polystyrene/Cationic Bilayer/Gramicidin for Optimal Bactericidal Activity. *Nanomaterials* **2017**, *7*, 422. [CrossRef]
45. Ragioto, D.A.; Carrasco, L.D.; Carmona-Ribeiro, A.M. Novel gramicidin formulations in cationic lipid as broad-spectrum microbicidal agents. *Int. J. Nanomed.* **2014**, *9*, 3183–3192.
46. Kikuchi, I.S.; Carmona-Ribeiro, A.M. Interactions between DNA and Synthetic Cationic Liposomes. *J. Phys. Chem. B* **2000**, *104*, 2829–2835. [CrossRef]
47. Rosa, H.; Petri, D.F.S.; Carmona-Ribeiro, A.M. Interactions between Bacteriophage DNA and Cationic Biomimetic Particles. *J. Phys. Chem. B* **2008**, *112*, 16422–16430. [CrossRef]
48. Rozenfeld, J.H.K.; Silva, S.R.; Ranéia, P.A.; Faquim-Mauro, E.; Carmona-Ribeiro, A.M. Stable assemblies of cationic bilayer fragments and CpG oligonucleotide with enhanced immunoadjuvant activity in vivo. *J. Controll. Release* **2012**, *160*, 367–373. [CrossRef] [PubMed]
49. Carmona-Ribeiro, A.M. Bilayer-Forming Synthetic Lipids: Drugs or Carriers? *Curr. Med. Chem.* **2003**, *10*, 2425–2446. [CrossRef] [PubMed]
50. Vieira, D.B.; Carmona-Ribeiro, A.M. Synthetic Bilayer Fragments for Solubilization of Amphotericin B. *J. Colloid Interface Sci.* **2001**, *244*, 427–431. [CrossRef]
51. Carvalho, C.A.; Olivares-Ortega, C.; Soto-Arriaza, M.A.; Carmona-Ribeiro, A.M. Interaction of gramicidin with DPPC/DODAB bilayer fragments. *Biochim. Biophys. Acta BBA-Biomembr.* **2012**, *1818*, 3064–3071. [CrossRef]
52. Melo, L.D.; Mamizuka, E.M.; Carmona-Ribeiro, A.M. Antimicrobial Particles from Cationic Lipid and Polyelectrolytes. *Langmuir* **2010**, *26*, 12300–12306. [CrossRef]
53. Carmona-Ribeiro, A.M.; de Melo Carrasco, L.D. Novel Formulations for Antimicrobial Peptides. *Int. J. Mol. Sci.* **2014**, *15*, 18040–18083. [CrossRef]

54. Carmona-Ribeiro, A.M.; de Melo Carrasco, L.D. Cationic Antimicrobial Polymers and Their Assemblies. *Int. J. Mol. Sci.* **2013**, *14*, 9906–9946. [CrossRef]
55. Schales, O.; Schales, S. A simple and accurate method for the determination of chloride in biological fluids. *J. Biol. Chem.* **1941**, *140*, 879–884.
56. Carmona-Ribeiro, A.M. Preparation and Characterization of Biomimetic Nanoparticles for Drug Delivery. In *Nanoparticles in Biology and Medicine; Methods in Molecular Biology*; Humana Press: Totowa, NJ, USA, 2012; pp. 283–294. ISBN 978-1-61779-952-5.
57. Grabowski, E.; Morrison, I. Particle size distribution from analysis of quasi-elastic light scattering data. In *Measurement of Suspended Particles by Quasi-elastic Light Scattering*; John Wiley & Sons: New York, NY, USA, 1983; Volume 21, pp. 199–236.
58. Lincopan, N.; Santana, M.R.; Faquim-Mauro, E.; da Costa, M.H.B.; Carmona-Ribeiro, A.M. Silica-based cationic bilayers as immunoadjuvants. *BMC Biotechnol.* **2009**, *9*, 5. [CrossRef]
59. Carrasco, L.D.; de, M.; Bertolucci, R.J.; Ribeiro, R.T.; Sampaio, J.L.M.; Carmona-Ribeiro, A.M. Cationic Nanostructures against Foodborne Pathogens. *Front. Microbiol.* **2016**, *7*, 1804. [CrossRef] [PubMed]
60. Goyal, P.S.; Dasannacharya, B.A.; Kelkar, V.K.; Manohar, C.; Srinivasa Rao, K.; Valaulikar, B.S. Shapes and sizes of micelles in CTAB solutions. *Phys. B Condens. Matter* **1991**, *174*, 196–199. [CrossRef]
61. Carmona-Ribeiro, A.M.; Chaimovich, H. Preparation and characterization of large dioctadecyldimethylammonium chloride liposomes and comparison with small sonicated vesicles. *Biochim. Biophys. Acta BBA-Biomembr.* **1983**, *733*, 172–179. [CrossRef]
62. Carmona-Ribeiro, A.M.; Yoshida, L.S.; Chaimovich, H. Salt effects on the stability of dioctadecyldimethylammonium chloride and sodium dihexadecyl phosphate vesicles. *J. Phys. Chem.* **1985**, *89*, 2928–2933. [CrossRef]
63. Lo, C.T.; Van Tassel, P.R.; Saltzman, W.M. Simultaneous release of multiple molecules from poly(lactide-co-glycolide) nanoparticles assembled onto medical devices. *Biomaterials* **2009**, *30*, 4889–4897. [CrossRef] [PubMed]
64. Date, P.; Ottoor, D. pH Dependent Controlled Release of CTAB Incorporated Dipyridamole Drug from Agar-Based Hydrogel. *Polym.-Plast. Technol. Eng.* **2016**, *55*, 403–413. [CrossRef]
65. Buffet-Bataillon, S.; Tattevin, P.; Bonnaure-Mallet, M.; Jolivet-Gougeon, A. Emergence of resistance to antibacterial agents: The role of quaternary ammonium compounds—A critical review. *Int. J. Antimicrob. Agents* **2012**, *39*, 381–389. [CrossRef]
66. Sun, M.; Ding, Z.; Wang, H.; Yu, G.; Li, B.; Li, M.; Zhen, M. Antifungal effects of BiOBr nanosheets carrying surfactant cetyltrimethylammonium bromide. *J. Biomed. Res.* **2018**, *32*, 380–388.
67. Ramakrishna, S.; Mayer, J.; Wintermantel, E.; Leong, K.W. Biomedical applications of polymer-composite materials: A review. *Compos. Sci. Technol.* **2001**, *61*, 1189–1224. [CrossRef]
68. Cheng, C.J.; Tietjen, G.T.; Saucier-Sawyer, J.K.; Saltzman, W.M. A holistic approach to targeting disease with polymeric nanoparticles. *Nat. Rev. Drug Discov.* **2015**, *14*, 239–247. [CrossRef]
69. Otto, M. Staphylococcus epidermidis—The "accidental" pathogen. *Nat. Rev. Microbiol.* **2009**, *7*, 555–567. [CrossRef] [PubMed]
70. Fukushima, K.; Tan, J.P.K.; Korevaar, P.A.; Yang, Y.Y.; Pitera, J.; Nelson, A.; Maune, H.; Coady, D.J.; Frommer, J.E.; Engler, A.C.; et al. Broad-Spectrum Antimicrobial Supramolecular Assemblies with Distinctive Size and Shape. *ACS Nano* **2012**, *6*, 9191–9199. [CrossRef] [PubMed]
71. Carmona Ribeiro, A.M.; Carrasco, L.D.M. Fungicidal assemblies and their mode of action. *OA Biotechnol.* **2013**, *2*, 25. [CrossRef]

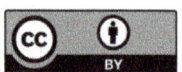

© 2020 by the authors. Licensee MDPI, Basel, Switzerland. This article is an open access article distributed under the terms and conditions of the Creative Commons Attribution (CC BY) license (http://creativecommons.org/licenses/by/4.0/).

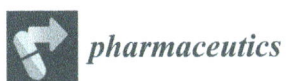

Article

Zein/MCM-41 Nanocomposite Film Incorporated with Cinnamon Essential Oil Loaded by Modified Supercritical CO_2 Impregnation for Long-Term Antibacterial Packaging

Xiaojing Liu [1,†], Jingfu Jia [2,*,†], Shulei Duan [1], Xue Zhou [2], Anya Xiang [2], Ziling Lian [2] and Fahuan Ge [1,2,*]

[1] School of Traditional Chinese Medicine, Guangdong Pharmaceutical University, Guangzhou 510006, China; LXJ_18826238139@163.com (X.L.); 17854223645@163.com (S.D.)
[2] School of Pharmaceutical Sciences, Sun Yat-sen University, Guangzhou 510006, China; zhouxue9@mail.sysu.edu.cn (X.Z.); xiangany@mail2.sysu.edu.cn (A.X.); lianzling@mail2.sysu.edu.cn (Z.L.)
* Correspondence: jiajingfu@mail.sysu.edu.cn (J.J.); gefahuan@mail.sysu.edu.cn (F.G.); Tel.: +86-20-39099722 (J.J.); +86-20-39099733 (F.G.)
† These authors contributed equally to this work.

Received: 3 January 2020; Accepted: 7 February 2020; Published: 18 February 2020

Abstract: Antimicrobial medicine and food packages based on bio-based film containing essential oils have attracted great attention worldwide. However, the controlled release of essential oils from these film nanocomposites is still a big challenge. In this study, a long-term antibacterial film nanocomposite composed of zein film and cinnamon essential oil (CEO) loaded MCM-41 silica nanoparticles was prepared. The CEO was loaded into MCM-41 particles via modified supercritical impregnation efficiently with a high drug load (>40 $wt\%$). The morphologies of the prepared nanoparticles and film nanocomposite were characterized by a scanning electron microscope. The release behaviors of CEO under different temperatures, high humidity, continuous illumination and in phosphate buffer solution (PBS) solution were investigated. The results showed that the film nanocomposite had an outstanding release-control effect. The addition of MCM-41 nanoparticles also improved the mechanical properties of zein films. The antibacterial effect of CEO was significantly prolonged by the film nanocomposite; indicating the CEO film nanocomposite fabricated via modified supercritical CO_2 impregnation was a potential long-term antibacterial medicine or food package material.

Keywords: film nanocomposite; essential oil; supercritical CO_2; long-term package

1. Introduction

With increasing concerns about the environment, ecology and safety in the last decade, biodegradable medicine and food packaging materials have gained more and more attention all over the world [1]. These film materials normally originated from regenerative resources such as proteins, lipids, cellulose, polysaccharides, lactic acid, and so on [2–4]. Furthermore, for the purpose of extending the shelf-life or avoiding microbial contamination, active packaging materials generated via the incorporation of bio-based films and antimicrobial components such as essential oils, were developed [5,6]. Several studies have shown that adding essential oils into polymeric films significantly enhanced the antibacterial properties of the package [7–9]. However, the components in essential oils generally have some inherent drawbacks such as high volatility and decomposing tendency. Therefore, the essential oil was lost rather fast from the polymeric films, and this short lifespan of active components could hardly meet the needs of long-term activity for package application [10]. Therefore, the development of controlled-release films was demanded.

Encapsulating essential oil into nanoparticles and incorporating these nanoparticles with bio-based film to fabricate film nanocomposite is an effective strategy to control the release of essential oils. It has been reported that chitosan or silicate nanoparticles could help essential oils release in a slow but sustained way, as well as improve their stability and long-term antimicrobial effect [11–13]. However, encapsulating or loading essential oils into nanoparticles is still a big challenge. In most of the process that was reported, large amounts of organic solvents or surfactants were used, and the drug loads were unsatisfactory (<10 $wt\%$) [11,14,15]. Thus, nanoparticles in some film nanocomposite containing essential oil only played the role of improving the film mechanical properties, but not as a drug carrier [16].

Supercritical CO_2 technology may be an alternative to loading essential oils into mesoporous nanoparticles with high efficiency [17,18]. Many natural active components including essential oils have considerable solubility in supercritical CO_2, making the supercritical CO_2 a good vehicle for transporting essential oil. Furthermore, supercritical CO_2 possesses strong permeability benefit from its gas-like viscosity, and its solvation stability will be deprived after the phase transformation of supercritical to gaseous state, which can be achieved readily by operation adjustment [19]. Therefore, supercritical CO_2 can be a good vehicle for essential oil to transport into nanoparticles and make no solvent residue after drug loading. In our previous study, essential oil was loaded into mesoporous silica nanoparticles with a high drug load (>35 $wt\%$) using a modified supercritical CO_2 impregnation method [20].

Cinnamon essential oil (CEO) has been reported to have good antimicrobial effects [21,22], and its leading component is cinnamaldehyde. The aim of this study was to develop a biodegradable long-term antibacterial film nanocomposite for medicine or food packaging, based on the combination of zein film and CEO loaded silica nanoparticles. To the best of our knowledge, this type of film nanocomposite having a long-term antibacterial effect for medicine or food package has not been reported. Supercritical CO_2 technology was used to load CEO into MCM-41 silicate nanoparticles. Furthermore, the mechanical properties and antibacterial effect of the prepared film nanocomposite were evaluated.

2. Materials and Methods

2.1. Materials

Zein powders extracted from corn germ were delivered by Sinopharm Chemical Reagent Co., Ltd. (Shanghai, China). CEO (Cinnamaldehyde content >95%) of pharmaceutical grade with quality inspection meeting the Chinese Pharmacopoeia standards was supplied by Jiangxi Anbang Pharmacy Co., Ltd. (Ji'an, China). Tetraethyl orthosilicate (TEOS, >99%), cetyltrimethyl ammonium bromide (CTAB, >99%), diethanol amine (DEA, >99%), glycerol (>99.7%, GC), and standard substance of cinnamyl aldehyde (>99.5%, GC) were purchased from Aladdin (Shanghai, China). Carbon dioxide (99.99%) was obtained from Guangzhou Gas Factory Co., Ltd. (Guangzhou, China). Tryptone agar and yeast extract were from Coolaber Science & Technology Co. Ltd. (Beijing, China). Stock culture of *Staphylococcus aureus* (ATCC 27217) was obtained from Solarbio Science & Technology Co., Ltd. (Beijing, China). Deionized water was produced by a Milli-Q system and acetonitrile was chromatographically pure. Other reagents were analytical grade and used directly.

2.2. Preparation of CEO Loaded Silica Nanoparticles (CEO@MCM-41)

The mesoporous silica nanoparticles MCM-41 were prepared using the method described previously [23]. Typically, 0.4 mol CTAB and 0.062 mol DEA was mixed in 165 mL water and stirred at 350 r/min under 95 °C, then 1 mol TEOS was dropwise added within 45 min. After reacting for another 1 h, the white emulsion was centrifuged and washed with water and methanol several times. Finally, the obtained particles were soaked in ethanol/HCl (8/1, v/v) at 60 °C for 24 h to remove the surfactant template, resulting in CTAB free MCM-41.

CEO was loaded into MCM-41 by modified supercritical CO_2 impregnation and the equipment was described in a previous study [20]. In this step, 200 mg MCM-41 particles were firstly put in a stainless basket with an air-permeable bottom and sealed in a high-pressure drug loading kettle, where a magnetic stirring apparatus was loaded at the kettle base. Next, 2 mL CEO was injected into the kettle to make the MCM-41 particles soaked for 15 min. Afterwards, CO_2 was delivered into the kettle continuously until the pressure rose to 15 MPa, and the kettle was heated to 40 °C at the same time. This supercritical state was kept for 1 h to load CEO into MCM-41 particles, then the kettle temperature was cooled below 20 °C followed by depressurization. The procedure of "CEO injection, soak, CEO loading under supercritical state and depressurization" was cycled five times to make an almost saturated drug load. The final obtained CEO@MCM-41 particles were stored at 4 °C.

2.3. Film Nanocomposite Fabrication

Zein-based filmed nanocomposite was prepared by a casting method. Firstly, 2 g zein and 0.5 g glycerol were dissolved in 97% ethanol solution (10 mL) at 70 °C and stirred for 1 h at 300 rpm through magnetic stirring. Then, a certain amount of CEO@MCM-41 particles were added into the zein solution, and stirred for another 30 min. Finally, the solution was casted in Teflon molds and dried at 40 °C for 8 h. Thus, the CEO@MCM-41/zein film nanocomposite was obtained and peeled off for later use.

By the same methods, zein-based film containing blank MCM-41 (blank film nanocomposite) or CEO alone (CEO/zein film) were prepared, where the amounts of MCM-41 and CEO used were equal to those in the film nanocomposite.

2.4. MCM-41 Particles Characterization

Brunner–Emmet–Teller (BET) and Barrett-Joyner-Halenda (BJH) measurements were carried out to examine the internal pore structures of MCM-41 and nitrogen-adsorption-desorption isotherms were plotted using a specific surface meter (JW-BK200C, JWGB Sci. & Tech. Co., Ltd., Beijing, China). The morphology of MCM-41 particles were observed by a high-resolution scanning electron microscope (SEM, Gemini500, Zeiss/Bruker, Karlsruhe, Germany).

2.5. Film Nanocomposite Characterization

2.5.1. Morphology

The morphology of the film nanocomposite was observed by a scanning electron microscope (SEM, JSM-6330F, JEOL Ltd., Tokyo, Japan) of both surface and cross section. The samples were attached on an electrically conductive adhesive stuck to an aluminum stub and then coated with platinum using a sputter coater (1.2 kW, E-1045, Hitachi, Tokyo, Japan) for 120 s.

2.5.2. Film Thickness and Mechanical Properties

The film thickness was determined using a professional digital display thickness gauge (EXPLOIT, Jinhua, China), which had a sensitivity of 0.001 mm. Different locations (>6) of the film were picked randomly to be measured, and an average value was considered the final thickness value.

For tensile strength (TS) and elongation at break (EAB%) determination, the film was firstly stored under 50% humidity for 60 h before being cut into 5 × 25 mm rectangular strips. The strips were then determined by a fastener tension tester (QJ212, Qingji, Shanghai, China). Parallel determinations of ten times for each sample were carried out.

2.6. Contents and Release Behavior of CEO

As only one effective peak referring to cinnamaldehyde was displayed in the chromatogram (see Figure S1 in the Supporting Materials), the amount of CEO was calculated based on the determination of cinnamaldehyde (96.8% in the CEO used) using a high-performance liquid chromatography system (HPLC, UltiMate 300, Thermo Fisher Scientific Ltd., Waltham, MA, USA).

During the determination, a Sharpsil-HC18 chromatography column (250 L × 4.6 mm I.D., S-5 μm 100A) was used, with a gradient acetonitrile/water mobile phase, in which the acetonitrile ratio increased gradually from 35% to 38% within 0–10 min, and continued to rise to 50% within 10–15 min. The samples were detected by UV at 290 nm, the temperature was 30 °C, and the flow rate was 1 mL/min.

The release behaviors of CEO from CEO/zein film, CEO@MCM-41 and film nanocomposite under high temperature (40, 60 and 80 °C, humidity of 40%), high humidity (80%, 25 °C), continuous illumination, and in phosphate buffer solution (PBS, pH 7.0) were investigated. For temperature and humidity tests, several precisely weighed samples were put into a constant temperature and humidity chamber (LHS-80HC-I, Yiheng, Shanghai, China), and one of them was taken out at preset time intervals. The fetched samples were immediately dissolved in 90% ethanol solutions for HPLC determination.

For the illumination test, the samples were put in a clean fuming cupboard with the light open, but the window of the cupboard was shielded by a thick black curtain from external light. The sampling and determination methods were the same as the temperature and humidity tests.

For the release test in PBS, 50 mg CEO@MCM-41 nanoparticles or 100 × 100 mm film samples (precisely weighed) were directly put into 120 mL PBS solution with 180 rpm magnetic stirring. At each time interval, 1 mL solution was withdrawn from the same water level for HPCL determination, and 1 mL PBS solution was replenished immediately.

2.7. Antibacterial Activity

The antibacterial activity of the CEO/zein film (1.0 wt%) and CEO film nanocomposite (1.0% CEO@MCM-41 nanoparticles) were tested against *Staphylococcus aureus* (*S. aureus*, LA9190, Solarbio, Beijing, China) using the plate diffusion method, as well as the CEO solution (2 mg/mL in ethanol) and blank film nanocomposite for the control. 25 mL culture medium (Macklin, Shanghai, China) was firstly put in a 100 mm diameter plate, and 0.4 mL inoculum containing 4×10^4 CFU/mL bacteria was spread after the medium cooled. Then an oxford cup was set in the center, and 250 μL CEO solution or 340 mg film sample was put together with 1 mL ethanol into the oxford cup carefully. Finally, the plates were incubated at 36 °C for 20 h before observing the inhibitory zone surrounding the oxford cup.

3. Results and Discussion

3.1. Morphology and Structures of MCM-41 and CEO@MCM-41

The morphology of the prepared silica MCM-41 and CEO@MCM-41 particles were observed by SEM, and the images are shown in Figure 1A,B, separately. Both powders had spherical particles with uniform diameters around 50 nm, indicating that loading CEO into MCM-41 by supercritical impregnation brought no change to the particle morphology. The nitrogen-adsorption-desorption isotherms of MCM-41 displayed in Figure 1C demonstrated that uniform mesoporous channels were formed in the particles, as well as CEO@MCM-41 in Figure 1D. Furthermore, it could be seen that the adsorption/desorption volume of CEO@MCM-41was decreased compared to that of MCM-41, indicating that CEO was loaded into the inner pore channels. The BET and BJH determination results including specific surface area, pore volume and pore size are listed in Table 1. It can be seen that MCM-41 had a high BET specific surface area value of 596.36 m^2/g, and the BJH adsorption and desorption values were close. However, BET surface area decreased to 264.47 m^2/g for CEO@MCM-41, indicating that CEO was successfully loaded into the mesoporous channels, which was also supported by the obvious differences between the BJH adsorption and desorption values.

Table 1. Results of BET and BJH determination for MCM-41 and CEO@ MCM-41.

Name	MCM-41	CEO@MCM-41
BET surface area	596.36 m^2/g	264.47 m^2/g
BJH adsorption surface area	857.53 m^2/g	407.73 m^2/g
BJH desorption surface area	868.25 m^2/g	455.03 m^2/g
BJH adsorption pore volume	1.56 cm^3/g	0.46 cm^3/g
BJH desorption pore volume	1.56 cm^3/g	0.82 cm^3/g
BJH adsorption pore width	7.28 nm	4.54 nm
BJH desorption pore width	7.19 nm	7.19 nm

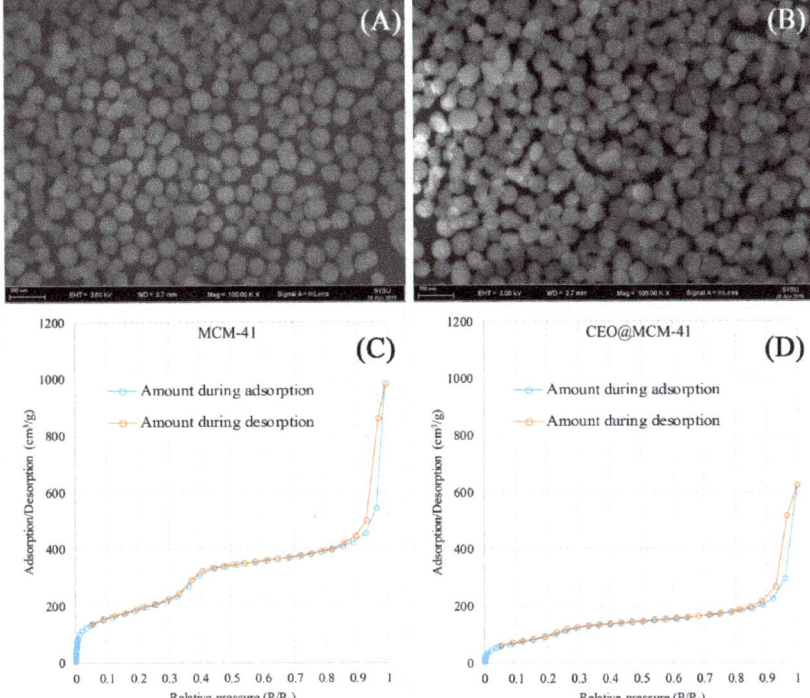

Figure 1. Scanning electron microscope images of (**A**) MCM-41 and (**B**) CEO@MCM-41 particles, and nitrogen-adsorption–desorption isotherms of (**C**) MCM-41 and (**D**) CEO@MCM-41 particles.

3.2. Drug Load of CEO in CEO@MCM-41

CEO was loaded into MCM-41 via modified supercritical impregnation and the circle time was a crucial factor for the drug load of CEO@MCM-41. In this study, with the circle time increased, the drug load increased rapidly to 44.5 ± 0.6% at the first stage (before five times, Figure 2). However, the growth stopped when the circle time went over five, indicating a saturated drug load was achieved. Multiple circle operations were necessary for getting the maximum drug load and the reason has been discussed in our early study [20]. Simply, partial CEO loaded in the MCM-41 particles during the previous circle could hardly dissolve in supercritical CO_2 again (or the dissolution rate decreased seriously) in the following circle, due to the strong absorption caused by the silanol groups of MCM-41.

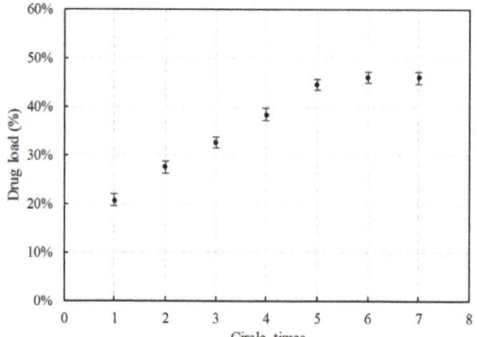

Figure 2. Drug load of CEO@MCM-41 prepared under different circle times by modified supercritical impregnation.

3.3. Morphology of the Film Nanocomposite

The morphology of the zein-based film containing CEO@MCM-41 nanoparticles, that is film nanocomposite, is shown in Figure 3. It can be seen that lots of pore channels existed in the film nanocomposite, enabling the CEO@MCM-41 nanoparticles to become well dispersed, which impacted the uniformity of film quality such as the mechanical properties and the local release behavior of the loaded CEO. These channels could also help the CEO loaded in the nanoparticles release out from the film. It was interesting to note, that the pore size on the film surface was much smaller than the size of the inner channel, which might be able to slow the CEO release to some extent.

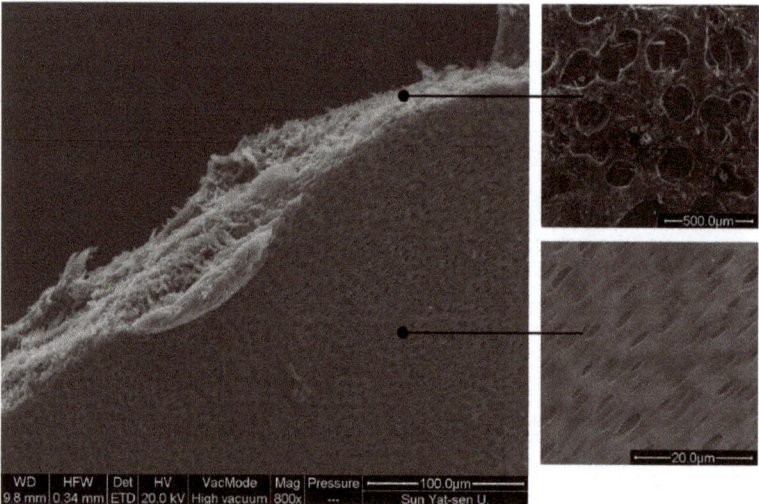

Figure 3. Scanning electron microscope images of the crack edge for the film nanocomposite.

3.4. Physical and Mechanical Properties of Zein-Based Films

The physical and mechanical properties of the prepared film nanocomposite is very important for its use in medicine or food packaging, and the film thickness should be considered at first. Shown in Table 2, compared to the blank zein film, adding MCM-41 particles made a thicker film nanocomposite, and the thickness grew slowly with MCM-41 content increase. In comparison, the thickness had no significant change with the addition of 1% CEO. The thickness turned higher when MCM-41 existed, probably attributed to the nanoparticle movement that caused an amplified cavity in the film.

Table 2. Film thickness of the zein-based film.

Samples	MCM-41 Contents (%)	Thickness (μm)
Zein film (blank)	0	186.0 ± 16.2
CEO/zein film	-	183.3 ± 16.4
Film nanocomposite	0.5%	218.1 ± 21.6
Film nanocomposite	1.0%	216.5 ± 16.7
Film nanocomposite	2.0%	223.5 ± 11.1
Film nanocomposite	3.0%	227.2 ± 15.2
Film nanocomposite	4.0%	235.6 ± 23.9
Film nanocomposite	5.0%	243.1 ± 19.8

Tensile strength (TS) and elongation at break (EAB%) are also crucial parameters for the package-use film nanocomposite. Figure 4 represents TS and EAB% of film nanocomposite with different MCM-41 contents. The TS of the film nanocomposite could be seen without the CEO in MCM-41, which increased gradually with the MCM-41 content from 0.6 ± 0.1 MPa (blank zein film) to 3.2 ± 0.1 MPa (5% MCM-41), while EAB% decreased from 85.9 ± 2.7% to 22.0 ± 3.1%, where a sharp decrease occurred when the MCM-41 particle content increased from 1.0% to 2.0%. The TS reinforced the film nanocomposite by MCM-41 addition, which may have been because of the netted internal hydrogen bonds formed between the nanoparticles and the zein matrix, which enabled the MCM-41 particles to share the drawing force. Similar results were also reported in other studies on film nanocomposite of different types [16]. Meanwhile, although adding lipid substances might modify the mechanical properties of protein-based films via crosslinking effect [24,25], the TS and EAB% had no significant change for the film nanocomposite with or without CEO in this study, as the essential oil was loaded inside the nanoparticles. According to the results, 1.0 *wt*% of MCM-41 nanoparticles in zein film was selected for the following studies.

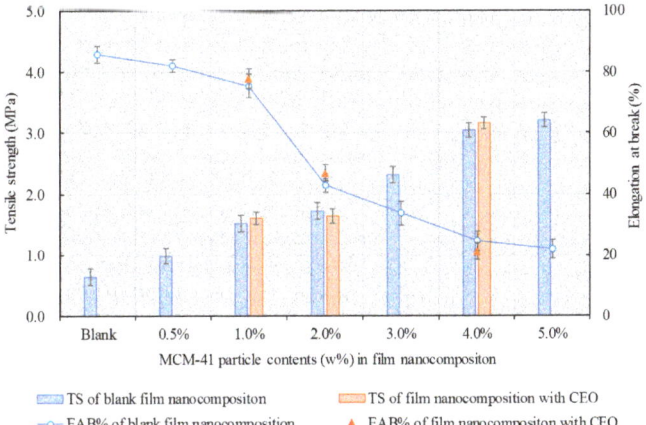

Figure 4. Tensile strength (TS, bars) and elongation at break (EAB%, dots and line) of the film nanocomposite with different MCM-41 particle contents.

3.5. Release Behavior of CEO from the Film Nanocomposite

The stability and shelf life of CEO in the film nanocomposite was crucial for the duration of the antibacterial effect. In this study, the CEO losses from the CEO/zein film, CEO@MCM-41 and film nanocomposite over time were investigated under different conditions including high temperatures, continuous illumination, high humidity and in PBS solutions. Under all conditions, no newly generated component except for cinnamaldehyde was detected by HPCL, indicating the loss of CEO was mostly caused by the release of cinnamaldehyde or its escape after decomposition.

Shown in Figure 5A–C, the release rates of CEO exposed to air, as well as in all three carries were accelerated with the temperature increase. The CEO released very fast when exposed to air. For example, it released 37.2% at 40 °C (Figure 5A) and was nearly exhausted at 60 °C (Figure 5B) after a 84 h test. However, the accumulated release amounts of CEO from the CEO/zein film after 84 h at 40 °C and 60 °C dropped to 16.0% (Figure 5A) and 74.56% (Figure 5B), while full release at 80 °C needed 60 h (Figure 5C). Furthermore, the CEO release rate dropped drastically in the order of CEO/zein film, CEO@MCM-41 and film nanocomposite. After 120 h temperature acceleration tests at 40 °C, CEO released only 4.0% and 1.2% from CEO@MCM-41 and film nanocomposite (Figure 5A), respectively. Their accumulated release amounts at 80 °C after 60 h also decreased to 69.1% and 38.2%, compared to CEO/zein film. It could be concluded that both the matrix structure of the zein film and the mesoporous structure helped prolong the life-span of CEO, probably attributed to the hydrogen-bond interaction of CEO molecules provided by the silica hydroxyl inside the MCM-41 particles and the polar groups in the protein matrix.

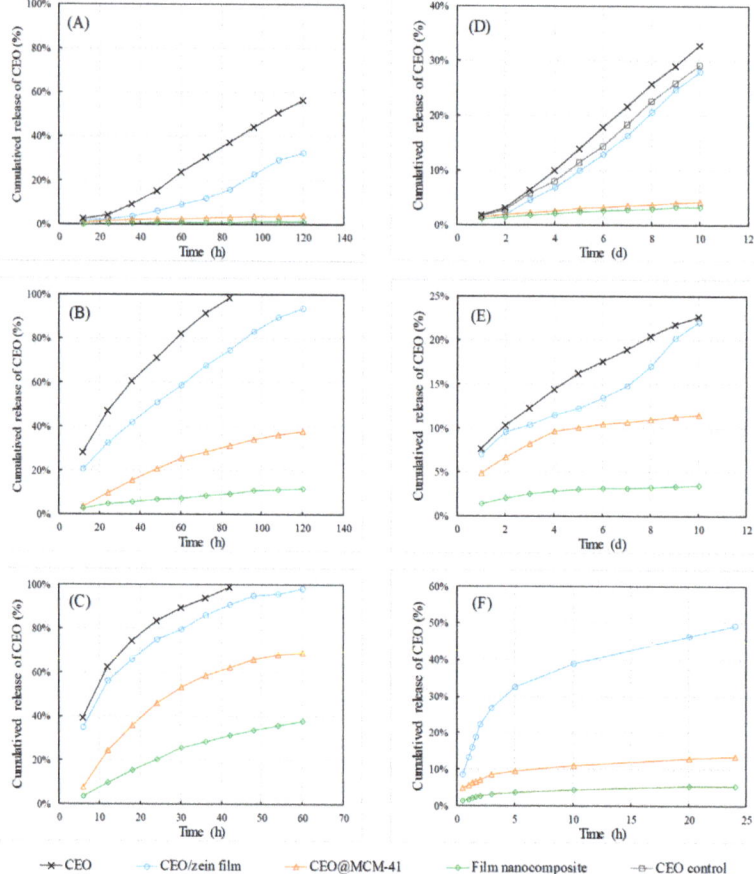

Figure 5. Release behavior of CEO from CEO/zein film, CEO@MCM-41 and film nanocomposite at different conditions. Including: at a high temperature of (**A**) 40 °C, (**B**) 60 °C and (**C**) 80 °C, (**D**) under continuous illumination at room temperature (the control CEO sample without illumination), (**E**) under high humidity of 80% and room temperature, and (**F**) in neutral PBS solution.

According to the comparison of CEO release behavior with or without illumination (Figure 5D), it could be seen that illumination was able to accelerate the loss of CEO, which might be attributed to the intensified decomposition and escaping of cinnamaldehyde under light. The release rate from CEO/zein film had a slight decrease. After a 10-day test, CEO released 28.1% from the CEO/zein film, while 32.8% CEO exposed to the air was lost. It was quite different for CEO@MCM-41 and film nanocomposite that CEO gained very low release rate, as the cumulative release amounts of CEO after 10 days were only 4.2% and 3.3%, separately. This was because unlike the transparent zein film, the wall of MCM-41 nanoparticles could prevent CEO molecules from contacting the light.

High humidity could also affect the release behavior of CEO (Figure 5E). After a 10-day test, the cumulative release amounts of CEO exposed to air was 22.7%, which decreased to 22.1% from CEO/zein, 11.6% from CEO@MCM-41, and only 3.5% from film/nanocomposite, respectively. The interesting thing was the released amount from CEO/zein film was less than that of CEO exposed at the beginning, but gradually rose close to the latter. This result indicated that the zein film would loose its protective effect for CEO when it was wetted, because the internal hydrogen bonds were weakened with a water increase. The water-isolation effect of MCM-41 nanoparticles was stronger than that of zein film, since it was more difficult for water to permeate into the nanosized mesoporous channel in the particle. However, high humidity had little effect under the combined use of a zein film and MCM-41, because the matrix structure of the zein film had strong absorption to the permeated water molecules, making the channels of MCM-41 dry.

Compared to the release behaviors in air, CEO released much faster in a PBS solution of pH 7.0 (Figure 5F). CEO/zein film had an initial burst release (22.3%) in the first 2 h, and then released gradually to 49.3% after 24 h. The release rate dropped significantly for CEO@MCM-41 and the film nanocomposite, and the cumulative released amounts were 13.6% and 5.5% at 24 h, respectively. The results demonstrated that the film nanocomposite had an outstanding control-release effect for CEO even in an aqueous solution. This unique property made the CEO film nanocomposite a potential long-acting antibacterial package material for medicine or food.

3.6. Antibacterial Properties

Figure 6 shows the antibacterial effects of a CEO/zein film (1 w/w% CEO) and CEO film nanocomposite (1 w/w% CEO@MCM-41) against *S. aureus*, as well as a CEO solution (2 mg/mL in ethanol) and blank film nanocomposite (1 w/w% MCM-41 nanoparticles) for the control. The large inhibition zone in Figure 6A demonstrated the significant antibacterial effect of CEO against *S. aureus*, while the blank film nanocomposite had no such effect according to Figure 6B. Shown in Figure 6C,D, it can be seen that the fresh CEO/zein film had a stronger antibacterial effect than that of the fresh CEO film nanocomposite, attributing to more CEO being released in the same period from the CEO/zein film. However, after being soaked in PBS solution for 4 days, the CEO/zein film lost its antibacterial effect (Figure 6E), while the film nanocomposite remained with a similar antibacterial effect as in the beginning (Figure 6F). The sustained but much slower release of CEO from the film nanocomposite was the crucial factor for this long-term antibacterial effect, which is very important for a medicine/food package.

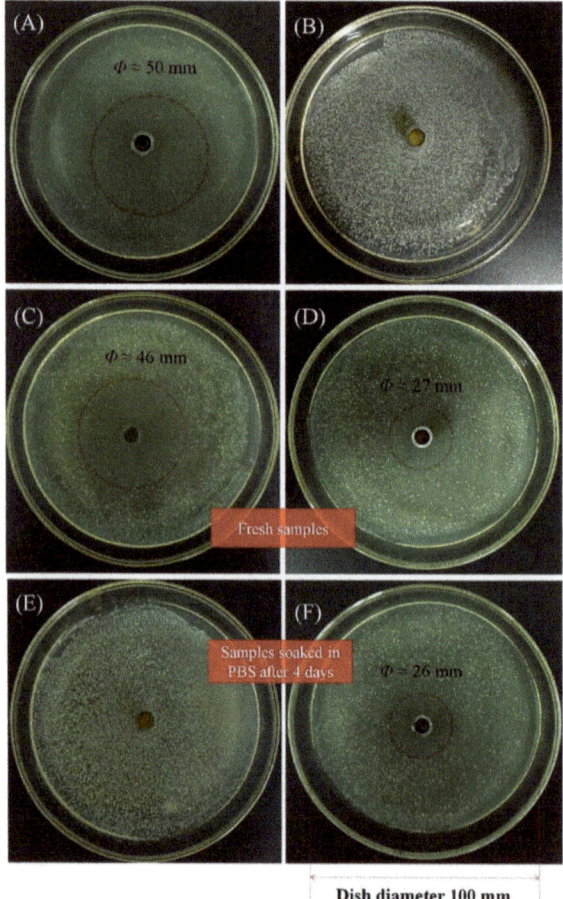

Figure 6. Antibacterial properties of different samples against *S. aureus*. (**A**) CEO solution (2 mg/mL) in ethanol, (**B**) zein film containing blank MCM-41, (**C**) fresh CEO/zein film, (**D**) fresh film nanocomposite, (**E**) CEO/zein film soaked in neutral PBS solution for four days and a (**F**) film nanocomposite soaked in neutral PBS solution for four days.

4. Conclusions

A long-term antibacterial film nanocomposite containing CEO for medicine or food packaging applications was prepared in this study. The method of modified supercritical CO_2 impregnation was used to load CEO into MCM-41 silica nanoparticles, and the drug load of CEO@MCM-41 was up to 44.5 ± 0.6 wt%. According to the SEM observation, MCM-41 particles around 50 nm were dispersed uniformly in the polyporous matrix of the zein film. The TS of the zein film was reinforced with the addition of MCM-41 particles, while the EAB% decreased sharply when the content of MCM-41 was higher than 1.0 wt%. The release of CEO from the film nanocomposite was controlled under all extreme test conditions. Whatever was under high humidity (80%) or continuous illumination conditions in air, the cumulative release amounts of CEO were below 5% after 10 days, while CEO only released 5.5% after 24 h in PBS solution. After being soaked in PBS solution for 4 days, the CEO film nanocomposite still had a strong antibacterial effect against *S. aureus*, the same as the fresh one. It can be concluded that the CEO film nanocomposite can be proposed as a promising long-term antibacterial natural packaging material for medicine and food.

Supplementary Materials: The following are available online at http://www.mdpi.com/1999-4923/12/2/169/s1, Figure S1: HPLC profile of CEO.

Author Contributions: Data curation, X.L. and S.D.; funding acquisition, F.G.; investigation, X.L., A.X. and Z.L.; methodology, X.Z.; project administration, J.J.; supervision, J.J.; validation, F.G.; writing—original draft, X.L.; writing—review and editing, J.J. All authors have read and agreed to the published version of the manuscript.

Funding: This work was supported by the financial support of the Nature Science Foundation of Guangdong Province (2017A030313650) and the National Key R&D Program of China (2017YFC1703102).

Acknowledgments: This work was supported by the financial support of the Nature Science Foundation of Guangdong Province (2017A030313650) and the National Key R&D Program of China (2017YFC1703102).

Conflicts of Interest: The authors declare no conflict of interest.

References

1. Garavand, F.; Rouhi, M.; Razavi, S.H.; Cacciotti, I.; Mohammadi, R. Improving the integrity of natural biopolymer films used in food packaging by crosslinking approach: A review. *Int. J. Biol. Macromol.* **2017**, *104*, 687–707. [CrossRef] [PubMed]
2. Wang, H.; Qian, J.; Ding, F. Emerging Chitosan-Based Films for Food Packaging Applications. *J. Agric. Food Chem.* **2018**, *66*, 395–413. [CrossRef] [PubMed]
3. Youssef, A.; El-Sayed, S. Bionanocomposites materials for food packaging applications: Concepts and future outlook. *Carbohydr. Polym.* **2018**, *193*, 19–27. [CrossRef] [PubMed]
4. Muller, J.; González-Martínez, C.; Chiralt, A. Combination of poly(lactic) acid and starch for biodegradable food packaging. *Materials* **2017**, *10*, 952. [CrossRef]
5. Atarés, L.; Chiralt, A. Essential oils as additives in biodegradable films and coatings for active food packaging. *Trends Food Sci. Technol.* **2016**, *48*, 51–62. [CrossRef]
6. Ribeiro-Santos, R.; Andrade, M.; Melo, N.R.D.; Sanches-Silva, A. Use of essential oils in active food packaging: Recent advances and future trends. *Trends Food Sci. Technol.* **2017**, *61*, 132–140. [CrossRef]
7. Acevedo-Fani, A.; Salvia-Trujillo, L.; Rojas-Graü, M.A.; Martín-Belloso, O. Edible films from essential-oil-loaded nanoemulsions: Physicochemical characterization and antimicrobial properties. *Food Hydrocoll.* **2015**, *47*, 168–177. [CrossRef]
8. Yuan, G.; Chen, X.; Li, D. Chitosan films and coatings containing essential oils: The antioxidant and antimicrobial activity, and application in food systems. *Food Res. Int.* **2016**, *89*, 117–128. [CrossRef]
9. Hafsa, J.; Smach, M.A.; Ben Khedher, M.R.; Charfeddine, B.; Limem, K.; Majdoub, H.; Rouatbi, S. Physical, antioxidant and antimicrobial properties of chitosan films containing Eucalyptus globulus essential oil. *LWT Food Sci. Technol.* **2016**, *68*, 356–364. [CrossRef]
10. Khaneghah, A.M.; Hashemi, S.M.B.; Limbo, S. Antimicrobial agents and packaging systems in antimicrobial active food packaging: An overview of approaches and interactions. *Food Bioprod. Process.* **2018**, *111*, 1–19. [CrossRef]
11. Cadena, M.B.; Preston, G.M.; Van der Hoorn, R.A.L.; Flanagan, N.A.; Townley, H.E.; Thompson, I.P. Enhancing cinnamon essential oil activity by nanoparticle encapsulation to control seed pathogens. *Ind. Crops Prod.* **2018**, *124*, 755–764. [CrossRef]
12. Liu, F.; Avena-Bustillos, R.J.; Chiou, B.S.; Li, Y.; Ma, Y.; Williams, T.G.; Wood, D.F.; McHugh, T.H.; Zhong, F. Controlled-release of tea polyphenol from gelatin films incorporated with different ratios of free/nanoencapsulated tea polyphenols into fatty food simulants. *Food Hydrocoll.* **2017**, *62*, 212–221. [CrossRef]
13. Ghaderi-Ghahfarokhi, M.; Barzegar, M.; Sahari, M.A.; Ahmadi Gavlighi, H.; Gardini, F. Chitosan-cinnamon essential oil nano-formulation: Application as a novel additive for controlled release and shelf life extension of beef patties. *Int. J. Biol. Macromol.* **2017**, *102*, 19–28. [CrossRef] [PubMed]
14. Bernardos, A.; Marina, T.; Žáček, P.; Pérez-Esteve, E.; Martínez-Mañez, R.; Lhotka, M.; Kouřimská, L.; Pulkrábek, J.; Klouček, P. Antifungal effect of essential oil components against Aspergillus niger when loaded into silica mesoporous supports. *J. Sci. Food Agric.* **2015**, *95*, 2824–2831. [CrossRef] [PubMed]

15. Chan, A.C.; Cadena, M.B.; Townley, H.E.; Fricker, M.D.; Thompson, I.P. Effective delivery of volatile biocides employing mesoporous silicates for treating biofilms. *J. R. Soc. Interface* **2017**, *14*, 20160650. [CrossRef] [PubMed]
16. Vahedikia, N.; Garavand, F.; Tajeddin, B.; Cacciotti, I.; Jafari, S.M.; Omidi, T.; Zahedi, Z. Biodegradable zein film composites reinforced with chitosan nanoparticles and cinnamon essential oil: Physical, mechanical, structural and antimicrobial attributes. *Colloids Surf. B Biointerfaces* **2019**, *177*, 25–32. [CrossRef] [PubMed]
17. Champeau, M.; Thomassin, J.M.; Tassaing, T.; Jérôme, C. Drug loading of polymer implants by supercritical CO_2 assisted impregnation: A review. *J. Control. Release* **2015**, *209*, 248–259. [CrossRef]
18. Sovova, H.; Sajfrtova, M.; Topiar, M. Supercritical CO_2 extraction of volatile thymoquinone from Monarda didyma and *M. fistulosa* herbs. *J. Supercrit. Fluid* **2017**, *105*, 29–34. [CrossRef]
19. Da Silva, R.P.F.F.; Rocha-Santos, T.A.P.; Duarte, A.C. Supercritical fluid extraction of bioactive compounds. *Trac Trends Anal. Chem.* **2016**, *76*, 40–51. [CrossRef]
20. Jia, J.; Liu, X.; Wu, K.; Zhou, X.; Ge, F. Loading zedoary oil into pH-sensitive chitosan grafted mesoporous silica nanoparticles via gate-penetration by supercritical CO_2 (GPS). *J. CO2 Util.* **2019**, *33*, 12–20. [CrossRef]
21. Ahmed, J.; Mulla, M.Z.; Arfat, Y.A. Thermo-mechanical, structural characterization and antibacterial performance of solvent casted polylactide/cinnamon oil composite films. *Food Control.* **2016**, *69*, 196–204. [CrossRef]
22. Xu, T.; Gao, C.; Yang, Y.; Shen, X.; Huang, M.; Liu, S.; Tang, X. Retention and release properties of cinnamon essential oil in antimicrobial films based on chitosan and gum Arabic. *Food Hydrocoll.* **2018**, *84*, 84–92. [CrossRef]
23. Niedermayer, S.; Weiss, V.; Herrmann, A.; Schmidt, A.; Datz, S.; Müller, K.; Wagner, E.; Bein, T.; Bräuchle, C. Multifunctional polymer-capped mesoporous silica nanoparticles for pH-responsive targeted drug delivery. *Nanoscale* **2015**, *7*, 7953–7964. [CrossRef] [PubMed]
24. Noshirvani, N.; Ghanbarzadeh, B.; Gardrat, C.; Rezaei, M.R.; Hashemi, M.; Coz, C.L.; Coma, V. Cinnamon and ginger essential oils to improve antifungal, physical and mechanical properties of chitosan-carboxymethyl cellulose films. *Food Hydrocoll.* **2017**, *70*, 36–45. [CrossRef]
25. Atef, M.; Rezaei, M.; Behrooz, R. Characterization of physical, mechanical, and antibacterial properties of agar-cellulose bionanocomposite films incorporated with savory essential oil. *Food Hydrocoll.* **2015**, *45*, 150–157. [CrossRef]

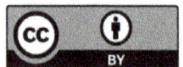

© 2020 by the authors. Licensee MDPI, Basel, Switzerland. This article is an open access article distributed under the terms and conditions of the Creative Commons Attribution (CC BY) license (http://creativecommons.org/licenses/by/4.0/).

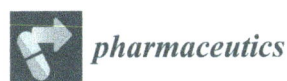

Article

Sustained Release of Linezolid from Prepared Hydrogels with Polyvinyl Alcohol and Aliphatic Dicarboxylic Acids of Variable Chain Lengths

Gustavo Carreño [1,2], Adolfo Marican [1,2], Sekar Vijayakumar [3], Oscar Valdés [4], Gustavo Cabrera-Barjas [5], Johanna Castaño [6] and Esteban F. Durán-Lara [2,7,*]

[1] Instituto de Química de Recursos Naturales, Universidad de Talca, Talca 3460000, Maule, Chile; gcarreno@utalca.cl (G.C.); amarican@utalca.cl (A.M.)
[2] Bio and NanoMaterials Lab, Drug Delivery and Controlled Release, Universidad de Talca, Talca 3460000, Maule, Chile
[3] Marine College, Shandong University, Weihai 264209, China; vijaysekar05@gmail.com
[4] Vicerrectoría de Investigación y Postgrado, Universidad Católica del Maule, Talca 3460000, Maule, Chile; ovaldes@ucm.cl
[5] Unidad de Desarrollo Tecnológico, Universidad de Concepción, Av. Cordillera 2634, Parque Industrial Coronel, Coronel 4191996, Biobío, Chile; g.cabrera@udt.cl
[6] Facultad de Ingeniería y Tecnología, Universidad San Sebastián, Lientur 1457, Concepción 4080871, Chile; johanna.casta@gmail.com
[7] Departamento de Microbiología, Facultad de Ciencias de la Salud, Universidad de Talca, Talca 3460000, Maule, Chile
* Correspondence: eduran@utalca.cl; Tel.: +56-71-220-0363

Received: 10 September 2020; Accepted: 15 October 2020; Published: 17 October 2020

Abstract: A series of hydrogels with a specific release profile of linezolid was successfully synthesized. The hydrogels were synthesized by cross-linking polyvinyl alcohol (PVA) and aliphatic dicarboxylic acids, which include succinic acid (SA), glutaric acid (GA), and adipic acid (AA). The three crosslinked hydrogels were prepared by esterification and characterized by equilibrium swelling ratio, infrared spectroscopy, thermogravimetric analysis, mechanical properties, and scanning electron microscopy. The release kinetics studies of the linezolid from prepared hydrogels were investigated by cumulative drug release and quantified by chromatographic techniques. Mathematical models were carried out to understand the behavior of the linezolid release. These data revealed that the sustained release of linezolid depends on the aliphatic dicarboxylic acid chain length, their polarity, as well as the hydrogel crosslinking degree and mechanical properties. The in vitro antibacterial assay of hydrogel formulations was assessed in an *Enterococcus faecium* bacterial strain, showing a significant activity over time. The antibacterial results were consistent with cumulative release assays. Thus, these results demonstrated that the aliphatic dicarboxylic acids used as crosslinkers in the PVA hydrogels were a determining factor in the antibiotic release profile.

Keywords: hydrogel; polyvinyl alcohol; aliphatic dicarboxylic acids; sustained release; linezolid; equilibrium swelling ratio; accumulative release; thermogravimetric analysis

---

1. Introduction

Multidrug-resistant (MDR) bacteria or "superbugs" represent one of the most important challenges to public health and pose a huge economic burden on global health care [1,2]. Indeed, antibacterial resistance causes 700,000 deaths per year worldwide [3]. The World Health Organization (WHO) has classified *Enterococcus faecium* as one of the primary drug-resistant pathogens posing the most significant risk to public health. This bacterium causes urinary tract infections, hospital-acquired bloodstream infections, abdominal and pelvic abscesses, endocarditis, and chronic periodontitis. The importance of this pathogen in these types of infection is reinforced by their intrinsic and acquired resistance to various antimicrobial agents, which renders them challenging to treat [4]. Linezolid is among the few available antibiotics that can treat bacterial resistance. This antibiotic is the first clinically useful oxazolidinone antibacterial agent [5]. This chemotherapeutic agent has been approved for the treatment of complicated skin and skin-structure tissue infections principally caused by vancomycin-resistant *E. faecium* [6]. Recent studies indicate that the effectiveness of antibacterial agents is better when they are released through drug delivery systems. Furthermore, these systems could slow down the progression of bacterial resistance to antibiotics [7,8]. In this context, hydrogels appear to be excellent candidates as antibiotic delivery platforms [9]. Hydrogels are a form of 3D porous material; these biomaterials consist of polymer chains with physical or chemical crosslinking [10]. Hydrogels can be of natural and/or synthetic origin [11]. Polyvinyl alcohol (PVA) hydrogels have been deeply explored due to their excellent biocompatibility properties and have been FDA (Food and Drug Administration) approved [12]. Hydrogels have received growing attention as drug delivery systems over the last decade due to their exclusive properties, such as high biocompatibility, tunable release rate, and versatility to be loaded with different molecules [13,14]. The most relevant characteristics of hydrogels are their porosity, pore size, and physicochemical environment of the matrix, which is tunable by modifying the crosslink density and/or varying the crosslinker type in their network. Therefore, the crosslinking agents such as aliphatic dicarboxylic acids (ADAs) could play a key role in the drug release profile from the hydrogel. In the hydrogel network, the pore size, swelling capacity, affinity with the drug, and subsequent sustained release have a very close relationship with the chemical structure and length of ADAs [14,15]. New antibacterial therapy strategies based on the sustained or prolonged release of linezolid could be an effective solution to fight pathogens. Thus, the purpose of this study was to develop hydrogels with ADAs of variable chain lengths as crosslinker agents featuring the tunable sustained release of linezolid.

2. Materials and Methods

2.1. Materials

Polyvinyl alcohol (PVA) 30–60 KDa, succinic acid (SA), glutaric acid (GA) adipic acid (AA), $NaHCO_3$, acetonitrile (HPLC grade), and linezolid analytical standards were purchased from Sigma-Aldrich (St. Louis, MO, USA). HCl, methanol (HPLC grade), K_2HPO_4, and H_3PO_4 were purchased from Merck (Darmstadt, Germany). All solutions were prepared using MilliQ water. *Enterococcus faecium* ATCC® 19434 bacterial strain, brain heart infusion (BHI) agar, Luria–Bertani (LB), and peptone water were purchased from Merck (Darmstadt, Germany). Distilled water was utilized for the preparation of all the solutions in the antibacterial study. The mouse fibroblast cell line L929 (ATCC® CCL-1™) was purchased from ATCC (Manassas, VA, USA). The cells were cultured in Dulbecco's modified Eagle's medium (DMEM, Gibco®, Grand Island, NY, USA) containing 10% fetal bovine serum (FBS, Gibco®, Grand Island, NY, USA) and antibiotics (100 U penicillin and 100 U/mL streptomycin, Gibco®, Grand Island, NY, USA) under 5% CO_2 at 37 °C. Cells were harvested after reaching confluence by using 0.05% trypsin–EDTA (Gibco®, Grand Island, NY, USA).

2.2. Synthesis of Hydrogels Based on PVA, ADAs, and Linezolid Loading

For this study, three hydrogels based on PVA and ADAs were synthetized. The methodology for preparing the hydrogels was performed through the esterification of PVA with ADAs according to the method from Rodríguez Nuñez et al. with minor modifications [16]. Briefly, the esterification reactions were performed by mixing an aqueous solution of PVA with an aqueous solution of a specific ADA (20 wt%) using HCl (1×10^{-1} mol·L^{-1}) and temperature as catalysts of crosslinking. Then, each reaction was performed under reflux at ~90 °C in a necked flask with magnetic agitation in the presence of air. After 3 h, each pre-hydrogel solution was poured into a new flask, and 8 mg of linezolid was added for its encapsulation, as depicted in Table 1. Then, each solution was vigorously stirred for 1 h and then sonicated for another hour until a homogenized solution was reached. After that, each pre-hydrogel-linezolid solution was put in an oven at 45 °C overnight until the crosslinking was complete. The hydrogel of PVA cross-linked with SA is named PSAH, the hydrogel of PVA cross-linked with GA named PGAH, and the hydrogel of PVA cross-linked with AA named PAAH. Afterward, the PSAH, PGAH, and PAAH hydrogels with the encapsulated linezolid were partially neutralized with $NaHCO_3$ to remove the excess acid and increase water uptake [17]. Then, the linezolid-loaded hydrogels were lyophilized to obtain the xerogel. The linezolid-loaded PSAH, linezolid-loaded PGAH, and linezolid-loaded PAAH were termed PSAH-Li, PGAH-Li, PAAH-Li, respectively. At the same time, three hydrogels were prepared without linezolid to perform the following characterizations: ESR, FT-IR, TGA, mechanical analysis, and SEM.

Table 1. Specifications of prepared hydrogels and the amount of linezolid loading.

Hydrogel	Crosslinker	Crosslinker Ratio (%) *	Linezolid (%) *
PVA-Succinic Acid (PSAH)	SA	20	2
PVA-Glutaric Acid (PGAH)	GA	20	2
PVA-Adipic Acid (PAAH)	AA	20	2

* % w/w respect to hydrogel; succinic acid (SA); glutaric acid (GA), and adipic acid (AA).

2.3. Swelling Behavior

The swelling behavior was calculated by the equilibrium swelling ratio (% ESR) at desired time intervals. Each xerogel film was immersed in phosphate buffer saline (PBS) [18] and acetate buffer (pH 3.0) at 25 °C for 21 h until swelling equilibrium was attained. The weight of the wet sample (W_w (g)) was obtained after carefully eliminating moisture on the surface with an absorbent paper. The weight of the dried sample (W_d (g)) was acquired after freeze-drying the hydrogel sample. The ESR of the hydrogel samples was obtained as follows:

$$\text{ESR } (\%) = \frac{W_w - W_d}{W_d} \times 100\% \tag{1}$$

2.4. FT-IR Analysis

The freeze-dried samples were ground into small fragments. After that, the PSAH, PGAH, and PAAH were analyzed in KBr (potassium bromide) disks by Fourier transform infrared spectroscopy (Nicolet Nexus 470 spectrometer, Thermo Scientific, Waltham, MA, USA). The wavenumber range scanned was 4000–500 cm^{-1}; 32 scans of 2 cm^{-1} resolution were signal-averaged and stored. The films utilized in this analysis were sufficiently thin to obey the Beer–Lambert law.

2.5. Thermogravimetric Analysis

The thermal stability of PVA crosslinked films was evaluated using a thermobalance Cahn-2000 (Ventron Corp., CA, USA). Thermal analysis was carried out by heating samples (10 mg) from 25 to 600 °C at a heating rate of 10 °C/min under a nitrogen atmosphere (50 mL/min). The sample weight loss was recorded as a function of temperature.

2.6. Mechanical Properties

The tensile strength (TS), tensile modulus (E), and elongation at break (eB) of the hydrogels were measured according to American Society for Testing Materials (ASTM) D 882 test methods using an Autograph AGS-X Universal Tester (Shimadzu, Kyoto, Japan). The tensile samples were cut into rectangular shapes with dimensions of 100 mm in length and 10 mm in width. The gauge length was fixed at 50 mm, and the speed of the moving clamp was 5 mm·min^{-1}. Three samples were tested, and the average values were taken as the reported results.

2.7. Scanning Electron Microscopy Analysis

Scanning Electron Microscopy (SEM) studies were carried out for all three formulations. The formulations morphology was evaluated using a scanning electron microscope (JEOL-JSM 6380, JEOL, Tokyo, Japan) operated at 15 kV. Surface views of cryogenically fracture films were examined. All samples were sputtered with a gold layer around 40 nm in thickness prior to the examination.

2.8. Release Kinetics Studies

The conformation of each proposed hydrogel is described in Table 1. Each linezolid-loaded hydrogel with a weight of 400 mg was placed into a 10 mL tube, and 5 mL of PBS [18] was poured over the formulation as a release medium. The tubes were transferred to an orbital shaking water bath (Faraz teb, Tehran, Iran) at 33.5 ± 0.1 °C [19] and shaken at 35 ± 2 rpm. At specific time intervals, the PBS was removed and replaced with an equal volume of PBS to maintain sink conditions throughout the study. For the quantification of linezolid, a stock solution (3 mg/mL) was prepared in methanol and stored at −18 °C. Standard solutions of the antibiotic were prepared with PBS (pH 7.4) in the range of 0.01–50 mg L^{-1}. The chromatographic system consisted of a Perkin Elmer series 200 HPLC system (Norwalk, CT, USA) with a UV–vis detector and a C-18 Kromasil 100-5-C18 (250 mm × 4.6 mm i.d. × 5 µm) column. Fifty microliters of the sample were injected into the HPLC apparatus. Isocratic elution with methanol/water (50:50, *v/v*) at a constant flow rate of 1.0 mL min^{-1} was utilized as the mobile phase. The analytical wavelength was 254 nm at room temperature The release rate of linezolid-loaded hydrogels was acquired by applying the concentration of released linezolid to the following correlation (Equation (2)):

$$\text{Cumulative Li release (\%)} = \text{Cumulative amount of Li released} \times \frac{100}{\text{Inicial amount of Li}} \quad (2)$$

Linezolid release kinetics were performed by employing different mathematical models of drug release equations, such as zero-order (Equation (3)), first-order (Equation (4)), Hixson–Crowell (Equation (5)), Higuchi (Equation (6)), Korsmeyer–Peppas (Equation (7)), and Peppas–Sahlin (Equation (8)) [20,21]:

$$Q_t/Q_0 = K_0 t \quad (3)$$

$$\ln Q_t/Q_0 = K_1 t \quad (4)$$

where Q_t is the amount of linezolid released at time t, and Q_0 is the original linezolid concentration in the formulation.

$$C_0^{1/3} - C_t^{1/3} = Kt \quad (5)$$

where C_t is the amount of drug released in time t, C_0 is the initial amount of linezolid in the formulation, and K is the rate constant.

$$Q = Kt^{1/2} \quad (6)$$

where Q is the cumulative linezolid release, K is the Higuchi release constant, and t is the time.

$$\frac{M_t}{M} = Kt^n \quad (7)$$

where M_t/M is the cumulative linezolid release, K is the release constant, t is the time, and n is the release exponent.

$$\frac{M_t}{M\infty} = K_d t^n + K_r t^{2n} \quad (8)$$

where M_t and M_∞ are the absolute cumulative amounts of linezolid release at time t and at infinite time, respectively.

2.9. Antibacterial Activity

The studies were performed according to Oscar Forero-Doria et al. [8]. First, 50 mg of each linezolid-loaded hydrogel was placed into a tube with 5 mL of PBS [18] as "release medium". Concurrently, a tube with 5 mL of PBS loaded with 1 mg of linezolid was prepared and utilized as a control. After that, the tubes were placed into an orbital shaking water bath (Farazteb, Iran) at 37 ± 0.1 °C. Depending on the assay, at certain time intervals (1, 3, 6, 24, and 48 h) 200 µL of release medium was taken and replaced with an equal volume of PBS to maintain sink conditions throughout the study. Lastly, the samples of each tube were evaluated by screening the antimicrobial activity and quantitatively testing the antibacterial activity utilizing the following protocols.

2.10. Assessment of Antimicrobial Activity of Proposed Hydrogels against E. faecium

To estimate the inhibitory activity against *E. faecium*, a qualitative test with a ring-diffusion method was implemented. With the aim of assessing the antibacterial activity of the prepared hydrogels, the Gram-positive strain *E. faecium* ATCC® 19434 was used as a model pathogen. The bacteria were grown overnight in MRS (de Man Rogosa Sharpe) broth at 37 °C. The inoculum (100 µL) containing *E. faecium* (adjusted to ~1.0×10^6 CFU·mL^{-1}) was seeded previously on the agar. Next, wells (8 mm in diameter) were made on an agar plate and filled with 100 µL of release medium for the specific interval times from Section 2.9. Additionally, two internal controls were treated with linezolid (10 and 15 µg·mL^{-1}, respectively). The plates were incubated at 37 °C for 24 h, and the antibacterial activity was calculated by the formation of bacterial inhibition zones surrounding the film disks. All tests were performed in duplicate.

2.11. Quantitative Assay of the Antibacterial Activity of Proposed Hydrogels against E. faecium

In this analysis, *E. faecium* ATCC® 19434 (concentration range of 1.0×10^6 CFU·mL^{-1}) was inoculated in 1 mL of LB broth at 37 °C until reaching turbidity equivalent to a 0.5 McFarland standard. Afterward, 150 µL of release medium from the samples and controls of Section 2.8 was added to 2 mL of the previous inoculation solution and then shaken at 200 rpm for 24 h at 37 °C. Afterward, each culture was tested; serial dilutions were made in 0.1% sterile peptone water. From each of these dilutions, 100 µL aliquots were collected, which were placed in plate count agar and incubated at 37 °C for 24 h. Then, viable cell counts were performed. All trials were performed in triplicate.

2.12. Cytotoxicity and Cell Viability

The cytotoxicity of the proposed hydrogels was evaluated on fibroblast cells. For this goal, the viability of the cells was assessed using the MTT technique according to the protocol of Mossman et al. [22]. Briefly, the cells were seeded in 24-well plates (5 µL, 1.6×10^4 cells per well) and 150 µL of Dulbecco's Modified Eagle Medium (DMEM)-High medium was added and incubated for 24 h at 37 °C in 5% CO_2. Afterward, the medium was replaced by 100 µL of fresh DMEM-High per well, which containing three diverse concentrations of PSAH, PGAH, and PAAH (500 µg·mL^{-1}, 1500 µg·mL^{-1}, and 2500 µg·mL^{-1} per hydrogel). Fresh medium without a sample was utilized as a control. Cell viability was assessed after 24 h by the MTT technique. Briefly, 5 µL of MTT solution (3 mg·mL^{-1} in PBS) and 50 µL of fresh medium were added to the respective sample and incubated for 4 h in the dark at 37 °C; formazan crystals were then dissolved in 100 µL of DMSO and incubated for 18 h. Supernatant optical density (o.d.) was analyzed at 570 nm (Spectrophotometer, Packard Bell, Meriden, CT, USA). Unprocessed fibroblast cells were taken as control with 100% viability. The hydrogels cytotoxicity was depicted as the relative viability (%), which correlates with the number of viable cells compared with the negative cell control (100%).

2.13. Statistical Analysis

In this work, all experiments were performed in triplicate. The SPSS 9.0 statistical software (IBM, Chicago, IL, USA, 1999) was used to perform the ANOVA analysis and Tukey's test ($p < 0.05$) to determine the statistical significance in some experiments such as the mechanical properties, ESR analysis, cumulative release test, quantitative test of antibacterial activity, and MTT assay. Graphs of the study results were designed by utilizing GraphPad Prism 6. Statistical significance was set at $p < 0.05$.

3. Results and Discussion

3.1. Synthesis and Load of Hydrogels

In Figure 1 the preparation of the hydrogels is depicted. Each hydrogel was prepared by esterification between PVA with a specific ADA (SA, GA, and AA). Once the pre-hydrogel was formed, the linezolid was added for its encapsulation (see Table 1). By this simple methodology, it is possible to achieve over 99% retention of the drug. Considering previous studies, a crosslinking degree of 10:2 of PVA:ADA was prepared, which was kept constant due to its good characteristics, such as porosity, mechanical properties, among others [14,16,23].

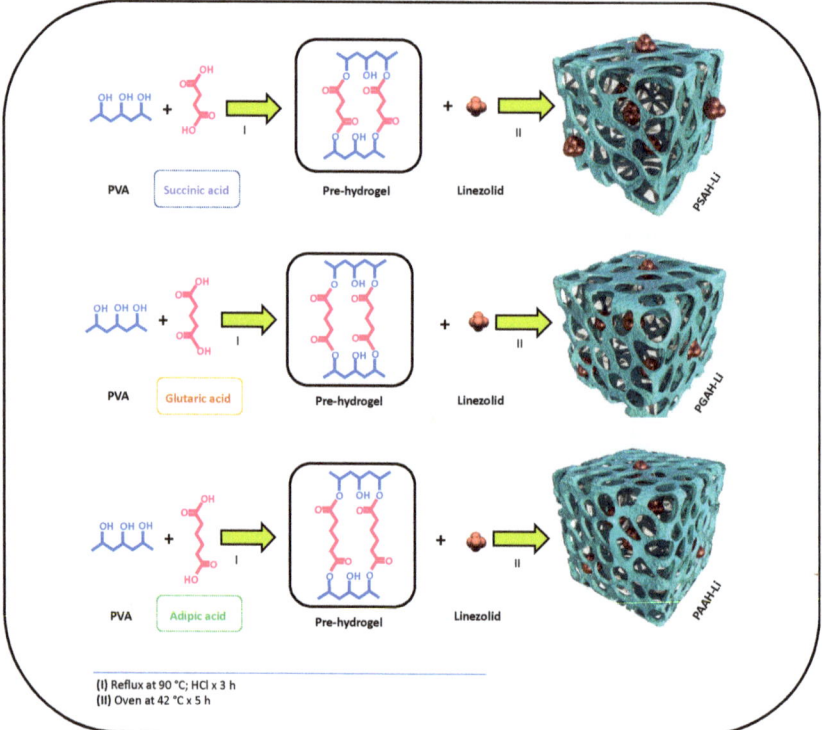

Figure 1. Synthesis and proposed structures of the linezolid-loaded hydrogels.

3.2. Swelling Behavior

This analysis allowed the confirmation of network formation in the three hydrogels. Since it is desirable to study the release of the antibiotic under physiological pH conditions, the ESR was evaluated at pH 7.4. Moreover, as a comparative analysis of swelling behavior, this analysis was also assessed at pH 4.0. Figure 2 shows the ESR for all formulations. An increase in the swelling index rate of the three hydrogels over time was observed at both pH values. In the beginning, the hydrogel swelling ratio increased fast and then slowed down to reach an equilibrium. This swelling behavior is characteristic of the hydrogel matrix obtaining the maximum swelling capacity. Specifically, PSAH, PGAH, and PAAH reached swelling equilibrium (zero-order) at approximately 3–4 h. On the other hand, a significant difference ($p < 0.05$) in all the cases was observed between the two pH models. For example, PSAH showed a better swelling degree at pH 7.4 with a value of approximately 600%, while at pH 4.0 the swelling degree was about 500%. For the other samples, PGAH and PAAH showed a swelling degree at pH 7.4 around 440% and 230%, and at pH 4.0 about 210% and 180%, respectively. The ESR difference at both pH values is due to the protonation degree of the free aliphatic carboxylic acids into the hydrogel network, which has different types of pKa [24]. Particularly, PGAH showed a higher difference in swelling behavior between pH values; such behavior can be attributed to the dissociation degree and ionization process of free COO- groups. These results are coherent, considering that the glutaric acid has the lowest pKa2 (5.22) compared to that of succinic and adipic acid (pKa2: 5.64 and 5.41), respectively. Therefore, in the network of PSAH more free carboxylic acid groups are susceptible to ionization by pH change.

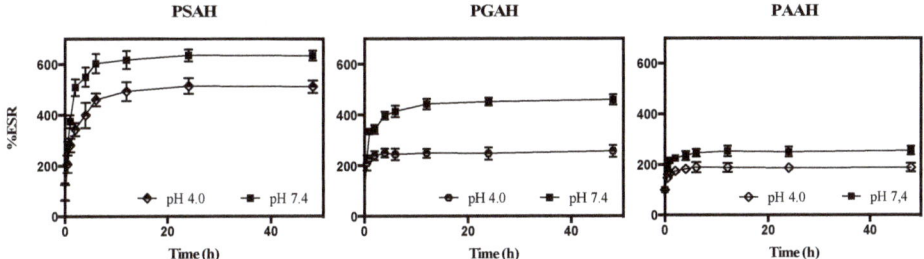

Figure 2. The swelling ratio of the hydrogels at 24–25 °C as a function of time, pH, and crosslinker nature. Data are shown as mean ± SD ($n = 3$).

When correlating the pH and Time variables for each formulation, it was found that for PSAH, the p-value < 0.05 (0.0140) in the ANOVA, therefore, there is a statistically significant relationship between the variables at the 95% confidence level. The highest p-value on the independent variables is 0.1175, belonging to pH. Thus, since the p-value > 0.05, pH is not statistically significant at the 95% or higher confidence level. In the case of PGAH, the p-value < 0.05 (0.0045) in the ANOVA, there is a statistically significant relationship between the variables at the 95% confidence level. On the other hand, the highest P-value on the independent variables is 0.0415 (p-value < 0.05), belonging to Time. In this context, Time is statistically significant at the 95% confidence level. Finally, in the case of PAAH, given that the p-value > 0.05 (0.1243) in the ANOVA, there is not a statistically significant relationship between the variables at the 95% or higher confidence level. The highest p-value on the independent variables is 0.9926 (p-value > 0.05), belonging to pH. Because of this, pH is not statistically significant at the 95% or higher confidence level. The correlation models are presented below:

PSAH correlation model:
$$\% \text{ ESR} = 167.86 + 6.5042t \; (R^2 = 35.85) \tag{9}$$

PGAH correlation model:
$$\% \text{ ESR} = 44.5875 + 37.3718 \text{pH} + 2.867t \; (R^2 = 44.84) \tag{10}$$

PAAH correlation model:
$$\% \text{ ESR} = 202.421 + 1.54335t \; (R^2 = 14.17) \tag{11}$$

3.3. FT-IR Analysis

The FT-IR analysis was conducted in the range from 4000 to 500 cm^{-1} to confirm the effectiveness of the crosslinking reaction between the PVA and different ADAs (SA, GA, and AA). Figure 3 shows the FT-IR spectra of hydrogel films (PSAH, PGAH, and PAAH). For PVA, all FT-IR spectra showed most of the characteristic infrared absorption bands (spectra not shown). The spectrum showed a broad band at around 3270 cm^{-1}, which was attributed to inter- and intramolecular hydrogen bonds of -OH groups in PVA [25]. After crosslinking, this band showed a significant shift to 3400 cm^{-1} caused by the chemical reaction, demonstrating a polymer structural change. Other FT-IR bands appeared between 2840 and 3000 cm^{-1}, around 1688 cm^{-1}, and between 1150 and 1085 cm^{-1}, corresponding to the vibrations of the -CH$_2$, C=O, and C-O-C groups, respectively [26]. In addition, the evidence of ester formation between the PVA hydroxyl groups and diacids carboxylic groups is the shifting of the ADA's -C=O absorption peak from 1691 to 1704 cm^{-1}. This result was in agreement with that previously reported in [27]. It the intensity difference for the -CH stretching vibration (between 2840 and 3000 cm^{-1}) between crosslinked films could also be noticed. The band intensity increased along with the crosslinker agent carbon numbers, as shown in Figure 1. It is important to note that other significant absorption bands recorded for PSAH, PGAH, and PAAH samples demonstrated the acid compounds in the hydrogel structure [14]. Table 2 summarizes the leading characteristics bands and their assignment for neat PVA and hydrogel samples. Finally, the spectral changes obtained in FT-IR analysis demonstrated the success of the crosslinking reaction between the hydroxyl group of PVA and the carboxylic groups from ADAs.

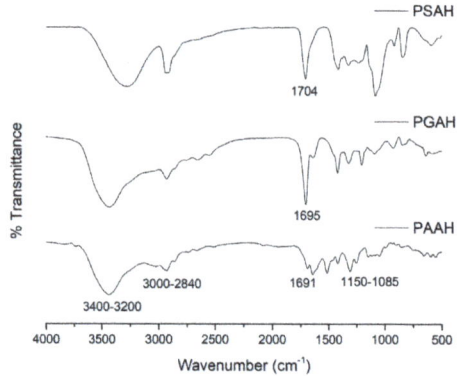

Figure 3. FT-IR spectra of PSAH, PGAH, and PAAH.

Table 2. Vibration modes and band frequencies in polyvinyl alcohol (PVA) and PVA crosslinked with SA, GA, and AA.

Sample	Chemical Group	Wave Numbers (cm^{-1})
PVA PSAH PGAH PAAH	O-H from the intermolecular and intramolecular hydrogen bonds	ν ~3400
PVA PSAH PGAH PAAH	C-H from alkyl groups	ν 2840–3000
PSAH PGAH PAAH	C=O	ν 1704 ν 1695 ν 1691
PVA	-C=C	ν 1640

Table 2. *Cont.*

Sample	Chemical Group	Wave Numbers (cm^{-1})
PVA	CO (crystallinity)	ν 1100
PVA PSAH PGAH PAAH	C-O-C	ν 1150–1085
PVA PSAH PGAH PAAH	CH$_2$	δ 1461–1417

3.4. Thermogravimetric Analysis

Thermogravimetric (TG) analysis has become a frequently used technique for studying the thermal stability of complex materials. In this work, the thermal properties of the prepared hydrogels based on PVA crosslinked with different ADAs are investigated using TG. The TG and Derivative thermogravimetry (DTG) curves of hydrogel samples are presented in Figure 4, and the analysis results are summarized in Table 3.

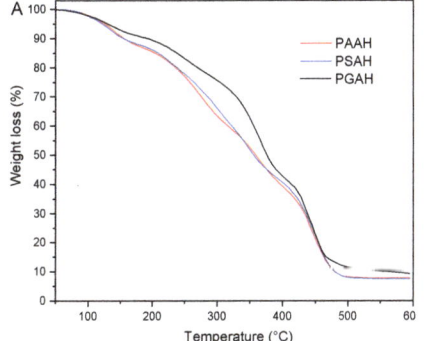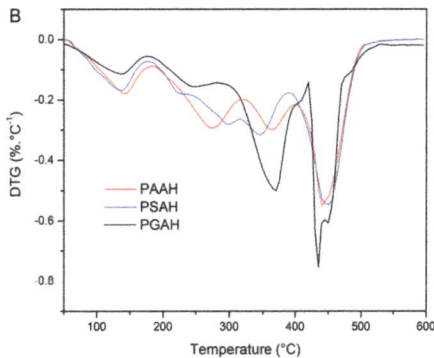

Figure 4. TG (**A**) and DTG (**B**) curves of the PSAH, PGAH, and PAAH recorded at 10 °C/min in the N$_2$ atmosphere.

Table 3. Thermogravimetric analysis results from hydrogels.

Sample	Temperature (°C)			Weight Loss (%)	Char (%)
	Onset	Peak	End		
PSAH	36.5	137.6	175.1	11.8	7.4
	177.5	224.2	240.9	8.5	
	241.0	297.2	316.9	17.8	
	317.0	345.8	390.6	19.5	
	391.0	449.9	528.9	34.8	
PGAH	36.1	138.7	174.8	8.8	9.3
	175.0	245.4	281.9	12.5	
	289.5	369.4	420.3	39.7	
	420.7	435.4	528.1	27.8	
PAAH	35.4	142.8	181.6	12.7	7.6
	182.4	273.6	319.1	27.9	
	319.2	363.5	399.7	20.1	
	400.0	440.9	530.9	31.3	

It is known the degradation of neat PVA is observed over three temperature regions, which are 80–250 °C, 275–450 °C, and 475–525 °C peaking at 142, 287, and 440 °C, respectively [27]. For all formulations, a first thermal effect with a maximum decomposition rate from 137 to 142 °C and an associated mass loss from 8.8% to 12.7% were observed. This effect is related to the evaporation of the bound and unbound water of the films [25]. The thermal degradation of crosslinked films occurred in three temperature regions for PGAH and PAAH, but in four regions for PSAH. The second degradation step showed two stages for PSAH; the first T_{Peak} appeared at 224 °C, and the second at 297 °C. The first process could be due to the thermal degradation of the free SA remaining in the hydrogel and showed a weight loss of 8.8%, whereas the second loss was 17.8%. In the case of PGAH and PAAH, the second effect was peaking at 245 and 273 °C with associated weight losses of 12.5% and 27.9%, respectively. All those peaks could correspond to a shift in PVA decomposition temperature (287 °C) (data not shown). In this thermal effect, the scission of partially esterified but still uncrosslinked PVA chains were co-occurring with polymer cyclization [27]. The third decomposition stage belonged to crosslinked PVA chain decomposition. The maximum decomposition rate appeared from 345 to 369 °C, demonstrating an increase in the thermal stability of formed hydrogels. Due to the formation of multiple inter- and intrachain ester bonds, an interpolymeric network that modifies the PVA structure was created. After crosslinking, an increase in the number of covalent bonds and hydrogen bonding between the polymer chains occurred, making them more thermally stable. This finding agrees with results from other authors that crosslinked PVA with AA and GA [28]. This thermal effect was more relevant for the PGAH sample, showing 39.7% of weight loss. The last thermal effect showed a maximum decomposition rate in the temperature interval of 435–449 °C and mass loss associated from 27.8% to 34.8%. Several authors reported that in this process the complete degradation of the PVA backbone occurs and cyclized chains turn them into charring residue [25,27].

3.5. Mechanical Properties

The influence of the ADA's chain length on the mechanical properties of crosslinked PVA hydrogel films is summarized in Table 4. Tensile strength (TS), tensile modulus (E), and elongation at break (eB) were included in the evaluated tensile properties.

Table 4. Mechanical properties of PVA crosslinked films *.

Formulation	Tensile Modulus (E) (MPa)	Tensile Strength (TS) (MPa)	Elongation at Break (eB) (%)
PSAH	80 ± 10 a	14 ± 1 a	88 ± 9 a
PGAH	70 ± 7 a	25 ± 5 b	126 ± 26 b
PAAH	104 ± 4 b	17 ± 4 b	66 ± 13 a

* Different letters next to the standard deviation, in each column, indicate statistically significant differences using Tukey HSD (honestly significant difference), at 95% confidence.

The results showed interesting mechanical properties of the hydrogel films prepared with ADAs. We hypothesized that the formation of the ester bond between the ADAs and the PVA matrix would play an important role in the mechanical properties, dependent on the chain length of the ADAs used. Thus, the PGAH hydrogel exhibits better mechanical properties (TS: 25 MPa; eB: 126%) than the PSAH and PAAH hydrogels. It was significantly different in TS values with the PSAH hydrogel and for eB values with the PSAH and PAAH samples, respectively. On the other hand, the PAAH hydrogel showed a significant difference in E values compared to the other ones, which means it is the stiffer sample. This result could be due to the degree of crosslinking obtained between the PVA matrix and glutaric acid chains during the formation of the hydrogel network. This fact agrees with the SEM analysis (Figure 5) of this sample, which showed a rough and homogeneous surface that improves mechanical strength. The mechanical properties of the materials are associated with their chemical nature and the interactions among the forming components [29]. The results reveal that crosslinking agents with intermediate chain lengths (GA) favor a higher chemical interaction with the PVA matrix.

Moreover, thermal analysis results confirm this finding because a higher crosslinking degree was found in this sample. Furthermore, previous hydrogels based on PVA found a linear relationship between mechanical strength and the crosslinking degree [30]. These results are in agreement with the FT-IR analysis regarding the ester band appearance around 1704 cm^{-1}. On the other hand, the PAAH hydrogel showed mechanical properties similar to the stiff and brittle materials with high tensile modulus and low elongation at break. This behavior could be associated with the porosity and the highly compact structure found in the fractured surface of hydrogel films observed by the SEM (Figure 5). The lower mechanical behavior of the hydrogel films prepared with PAAH was associated with the crosslinker characteristics, consisting of a larger molecule that restricts the formation of crosslinking density in the hydrogel [31]. The tensile strength and tensile modulus indicate the toughness, and the elongation at break indicates the elasticity of the materials, suggesting their possible applications. The hydrogels of this study can be used for drug delivery applications such as antibiotic release because they have adequate (strong and flexible) mechanical properties [32,33]. Thus, several authors [34,35] reported the following values for the mechanical properties of wound dressing hydrogel films (TS = 18 MPa; E = 98; eB = 200%) and drug delivery films (TS = 13–35; eB = 44–112%), respectively.

3.6. SEM Analysis

The hydrogel formulations with different crosslinkers were observed using Scanning Electron Microscopy (SEM) to understand surface properties. As depicted in Figure 5, for all samples, a rough surface is observed. In the case of PGAH (Figure 5B), a more uniform structure than those in the PSAH sample could be observed (Figure 5B). Finally, the PAAH micrograph (Figure 5C) revealed a different and more compact morphology with hollows fractures on the surface. It seems that in hydrogel formulations, the surface morphology was highly influenced by the crosslinker chemical structure, being stiff and dense when the ADA's chain length is longer. Then the hydrogel supramolecular structure could affect the drug release behavior.

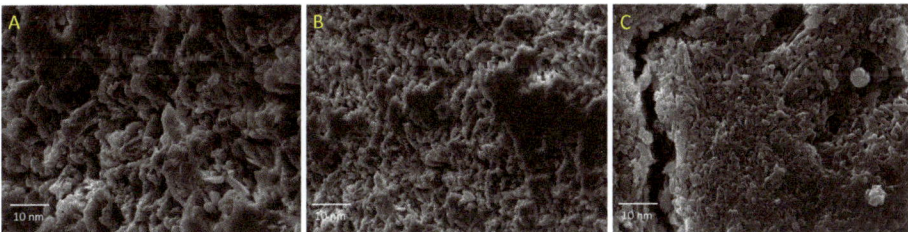

Figure 5. SEM micrographics of PSAH (**A**), PGAH (**B**), and PAAH (**C**).

3.7. Release Kinetics Studies

The linezolid release profile analysis was carried out by HPLC with a 400 mg hydrogel charged with linezolid. In vitro release kinetics of linezolid from each hydrogel were obtained under physiological conditions (37 °C, PBS at pH 7.4). The cumulative percent released of the antibiotic was monitored over time and results are shown in Figure 6.

For all loaded hydrogels (PSAH-Li, PGAH-Li, and PAAH-Li) a rapid antibiotic release into the medium was observed. The cumulative release of PSAH was significantly higher than the other samples from 2 h. From 6 h onward, all hydrogels showed a significantly different drug release profile. At this time, 51%, 40%, and 29% of the linezolid had been released from PSAH-Li, PGAH-Li, and PAAH-Li, respectively. The PAAH-Li revealed a slower release profile than the other two formulations, and PSAH-Li a higher one. After 6 h, the formulations exhibited a significantly lower and continuous antibiotic release into the medium. For PSAH-Li, PGAH-Li and PAAH-Li, the average rapid-release phase was 0.68, 0.53, and 0.39 mg/h of linezolid, respectively. This rate changed after 6 h for all cases, and the average of the slow-release phase was 0.06, 0.05, 0.04 mg/h of linezolid, respectively. In Table 5, all the average release values of the antibiotic are shown. According to these results and the graph depicted in Figure 6, the linezolid release profile follows the next order: PSAH-Li > PGAH-Li > PAAH-Li.

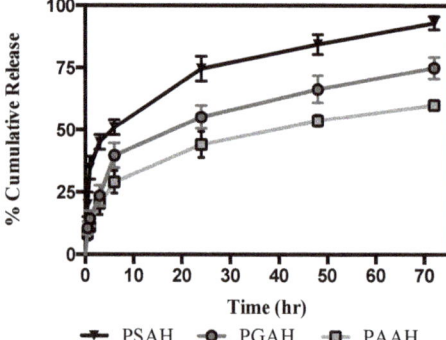

Figure 6. Release profile of linezolid from prepared hydrogels in phosphate buffer saline (PBS) at 33.4 °C; mean Scanning Electron Microscopy (SEM) (n = 3). Different letters next to the standard deviation on each point indicate statistically significant differences using Tukey HSD, at 95% confidence.

Table 5. Release profile of linezolid-loaded hydrogels.

	Formulation		PSAH-Li	PGAH-Li	PAAH-Li
Release phase	Rapid *	% Released	51 ± 3 c	40 ± 5 b	29 ± 4.6 a
		Release rate (mg/h)	0.68 ± 0.04 b	0.53 ± 0.07 a	0.39 ± 0.06 a
	Slow **	% Released	42 ± 3.6 b	35.3 ± 3.5 ab	30.3 ± 3.5 a
		Release rate (mg/h)	0.06 ± 0.005 b	0.05 ± 0.005 ab	0.04 ± 0.005 a

* The rapid phase occurred over 6 h. ** The release rate was calculated in a specific time frame because, until 72 h, the formulation still released antibiotic. Different letters next to the standard deviation, in each row, indicate statistically significant differences using Tukey HSD, at 95% confidence.

The release patterns of each formulation depend on the structure of the crosslinker agent, the intermolecular interactions between the linezolid drug and hydrogel network [12], and mostly on the swelling degree. Therefore, in light of the obtained outcomes, it could be deduced that the release rate of PAAH-Li was slower because the expansion of the compact network was minimal, as revealed by the water uptake process (% ESR). One of the reasons for this result is that the size of AA aliphatic chain is larger than SA and GA, respectively, which could contribute to a more apolar environment. Moreover, in concordance with the mechanical studies, PAAH showed a stiffer structure with high tensile modulus and low elongation at break. This performance has a direct relation with its highly compact morphology observed by SEM. The lower mechanical behavior of PAAH could be associated with the larger crosslinker agent that limits the formation of crosslinking density in the hydrogel. With a lesser crosslinking degree, there are less carboxylic groups potentially ionizable. Therefore, there are fewer charges of the electrostatic repulsion between chains from networks and, consequently, less capacity to generate an uptake of solvent into the matrix. This result is consistent with swelling behavior. On the contrary, for the case of PSAH and PGAH with a higher crosslinking degree, the increased swelling ability of the hydrogels contributes to the destruction of hydrogen bonding between the polymer molecules, resulting in an increase in chain mobility and network expansion [21]. The above mentioned results can explain the faster release of linezolid from PSAH-Li. In contrast, in a lesser expanded, more compacted, and stiff hydrogel (PAAH-Li), the encapsulated drug is released slower.

The average release profiles of samples were fitted through several mathematical models to elucidate the mechanism of linezolid release. The coefficients of correlation (R) and release exponents (n) are shown in Table 6. According to R^2 value obtained, among all the studied models, the Korsmeyer–Peppas model was the best fit for PSAH-Li and PGAH-Li with R^2 values of 0.9967 and 0.9845, respectively. In contrast, an with R^2 value of 0.9013, the Higushi model is the best fitted to PAAH-Li. On the other hand, for the case of PSAH-Li and PGAH-Li the release mechanism for linezolid was Fickian diffusion. For the case of PAAH-Li the mechanism for linezolid release was pseudo-Fickian.

Table 6. Linezolid release kinetics and correlation coefficient values from Fick, Hixon–Crowell, Higushi and Korsmeyer–Peppas models.

Hydrogel	Mathematical Model										
	Zero Order		First Order		Hixon-Crowell		Higushi		Korsmeyer-Peppas		
	R^2	K	R^2	K	R^2	K	R^2	K	R^2	K	n
PSAH-Li	0.8382	1.0054	0.6736	0.0227	0.4724	−0.0324	0.9632	3.4568	0.9967	5.7570	0.5112
PGAH-Li	0.8326	1.2624	0.6678	0.0225	0.4671	−0.0348	0.9529	4.3222	0.9845	7.3148	0.5167
PAAH-Li	0.7585	1.6056	0.6558	0.0159	0.3590	−0.0324	0.9013	4.8923	0.8938	14.6218	0.3539

3.8. Antibacterial Studies

Some studies indicate that the effectivity of antibacterial agents is better when they are applied through sustained release. Furthermore, this approach could lower bacterial resistance incidence [7,8,36]. Regarding the limitations presented by PSAH (faster release) and PAAH (reduced mechanical properties), PGAH was selected to carry out the antibacterial analyses. The results obtained here are consistent with the acquired data by HPLC. For instance, linezolid antibacterial activity was significantly higher over time compared to the control, as shown in Figure 7. In this context, it is concluded that a sustained release at a relatively constant dose from PGAH-Li maintains antibiotic integrity, comprising better activity over time, as shown in Figure 7B,C. On the contrary, in the control sample, linezolid displayed higher activity in the first hour; however, it loses effectiveness over time, as depicted in Figure 7A,C. The control inhibition zone in the first hour was close to ~30 mm, but over time was decreasing, reaching ~8 mm at 48 h. In contrast, PGAH-Li started with an inhibition zone of ~11 mm and progressively rose to complete an inhibition zone of 23 mm at 48 h. These results are in concordance with the quantitative analysis of antibacterial activity against the *E. faecium* that is exhibited in Figure 7D. The data revealed that, in the control, the bacterial colony forming unit (CFU) increases over time, demonstrating that the antibiotic loses its activity until 72 h. Conversely, the assay with the PGAH-Li release medium significantly inhibits bacterial proliferation, suggesting that the linezolid acted as a bacteriostatic agent against *Enterococcus faecium* [37]. An additional experiment with PGAH without linezolid was performed. However, the antibacterial activity was not observed (data not shown). These data suggest that the hydrogel could improve the bioavailability of linezolid.

3.9. Cytotoxicity Studies

As potential biomaterials, it is pivotal that the designed formulations be innocuous. Therefore, the cytotoxicity of each hydrogel was evaluated on fibroblast cells. The biocompatibility of the sterilized PSAH, PGAH, and PAAH was investigated by a cell viability assay using L929 fibroblast cells after 24 h. Figure 8 displayed cell viability after exposure to three different concentrations of the respective formulation (a concentration range of 500–2500 µg·mL^{-1}). As specified in Figure 8, at 500 µg·mL^{-1}, the fibroblast cell viability is nearly 100% for three hydrogels. When drastically increasing the hydrogel concentration from three to five-fold, the fibroblast cell viability only declines vaguely. That is to say, for all cases, the cell viability was not less than 87%. The results revealed that the prepared hydrogels have minimum toxicity to the fibroblast cell. These data could guarantee that these hydrogels can be potential candidates for medical applications.

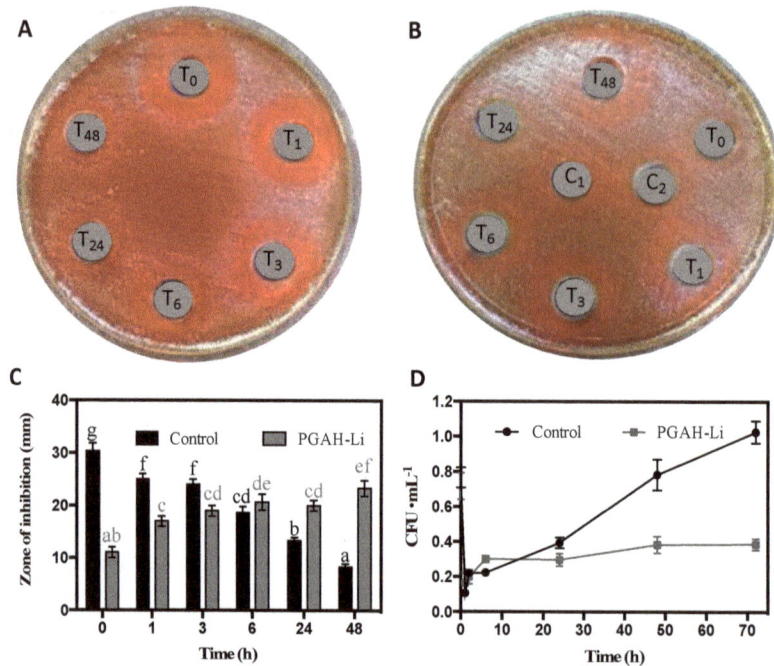

Figure 7. Screening of the antibacterial effect of PGAH-Li. Control (**A**); PGAH-Li (**B**); T_0: 0 h, T_1: 1 h, T_3: 3 h, T_4: 6 h, T_{24}: 24 h, T_{48}: 48 h; the antibacterial effect was expressed as the inhibition area against *E. faecium* (**C**); quantitative test of antibacterial activity against *E. faecium* (**D**). (Equal letters above the bars indicate that there are no statistically significant differences using Tukey's HSD procedure, at 95% confidence level). C_1 and C_2 in Figure 7B are positive controls of 15 and 10 µg·mL^{-1} linezolid, respectively.

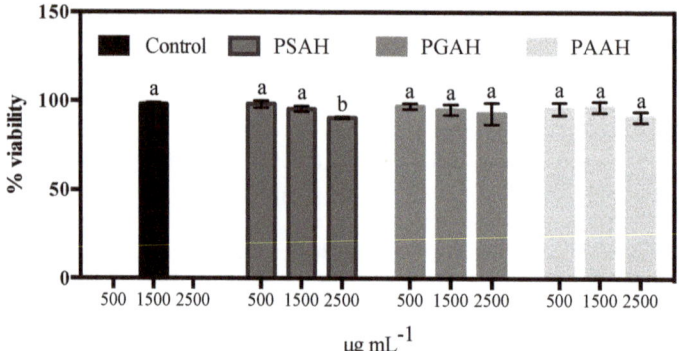

Figure 8. Percentage of cell viability obtained from the MTT assay of the L929 fibroblast cells compared to that of a negative control (without hydrogel). Each bar indicates mean ± relative standard deviations (RSD) of three replications. Bars not labeled by the same letter represent statistically significant differences with the negative control at $p \leq 0.05$ using ANOVA followed by Tukey's HSD test.

4. Conclusions

A series of hydrogels based on PVA and ADAs of variable chain lengths with sustained release of linezolid properties were successfully synthesized. The hydrogels were prepared by crosslinking of PVA and different ADAs of varying chain lengths, such as SA, GA, and AA, respectively. The swelling response, FT-IR, TGA, mechanical properties, and SEM analysis validate the formation of the three hydrogels. The swelling index data evidenced that all the proposed hydrogels are responsive to pH. Moreover, the swelling index depends on the type of ADA and crosslinking degree. The series of hydrogels showed a sustained release rate of linezolid according to the results shown in the chromatographic analysis. The three hydrogels displayed significant differences regarding the release rate of linezolid. This difference seems to be ruled by the intermolecular interactions between linezolid and hydrogel matrix morphology, crosslinking degree, and mechanical properties. These mentioned features have a direct relation with ADA type used as crosslinker. ADAs can confer unique physicochemical and mechanical properties based on their specific structure. Therefore, the ADAs could play a key role in the release profile of the drug. The linezolid release kinetic of PSAH-Li and PGAH-Li were found to follow the Korsmeyer–Peppas release model, and the release mechanism in both cases was Fickian diffusion. On the contrary, the Higushi model was the best fit for PAAH-Li, and their mechanism for linezolid release was pseudo-Fickian. The antibacterial assays confirmed that the sustained release of linezolid from PGAH-Li has a better antibacterial activity compared with the conventional release. This suggests that the hydrogel has the capability to improve the bioavailability of linezolid. The set of proposed hydrogels showed good biocompatibility with L929 mouse connective tissue fibroblasts. The results exhibited viability over 87%. In conclusion, drug delivery platforms based on hydrogels of PVA and specific crosslinker agents such as ADAs could be potentially utilized as an antibiotic delivery system in potential infectious processes. Furthermore, this approach could become a strategy to help stop bacterial resistance.

Author Contributions: G.C.-B., A.M., S.V., O.V., G.C.-B., J.C., and E.F.D.-L. contributed to the conceptualization, methodology, validation, formal analysis, and investigation. E.F.D.-L., S.V., and G.C. contributed to the writing—original draft preparation. E.F.D.-L. contributed to supervision, writing—review, and editing, project administration, resources, and funding acquisition. All authors have read and agreed to the published version of the manuscript.

Funding: This research work was financially supported by ANID FONDECYT project No. 11170155 (E.F.D.-L.), project No. 11170008 (O.V.), project No. 11180059 (A.M.), and ANID CONICYT PIA/APOYO CCTE AFB170007 (G.C.-B.).

Conflicts of Interest: The authors declare no conflict of interest.

References

1. Aslam, B.; Wang, W.; Arshad, M.I.; Khurshid, M.; Muzammil, S.; Rasool, M.H.; Nisar, M.A.; Alvi, R.F.; Aslam, M.A.; Qamar, M.U.; et al. Antibiotic resistance: A rundown of a global crisis. *Infect. Drug Resist.* **2018**, *11*, 1645–1658. [CrossRef] [PubMed]
2. Mwangi, J.; Yin, Y.; Wang, G.; Yang, M.; Li, Y.; Zhang, Z.; Lai, R. The antimicrobial peptide ZY4 combats multidrug-resistant Pseudomonas aeruginosa and Acinetobacter baumannii infection. *Proc. Natl. Acad. Sci. USA* **2019**, *116*, 26516–26522. [CrossRef] [PubMed]
3. Taghabue, A.; Rappuoli, R. Changing Priorities in Vaccinology: Antibiotic Resistance Moving to the Top. *Front. Immunol.* **2018**, *9*, 1068. [CrossRef]
4. Adesida, S.A.; Ezenta, C.C.; Adagbada, A.O.; Aladesokan, A.A.; Coker, A.O. Carriage of Multidrug Resistant Enterococcus Faecium and Enterococcus Faecalis among Apparently Healthy Humans. *Afr. J. Infect. Dis.* **2017**, *11*, 83–89. [CrossRef] [PubMed]
5. Barbachyn, M.R.; Ford, C.W. Oxazolidinone Structure—Activity Relationships Leading to Linezolid. *Chemin* **2003**, *34*, 2010–2023. [CrossRef]
6. Hashemian, S.M.; Farhadi, T.; Ganjparvar, M. Linezolid: A review of its properties, function, and use in critical care. *Drug Des. Dev. Ther.* **2018**, *12*, 1759–1767. [CrossRef] [PubMed]
7. Stebbins, N.D.; Ouimet, M.A.; Uhrich, K.E. Antibiotic-containing polymers for localized, sustained drug delivery. *Adv. Drug Deliv. Rev.* **2014**, *78*, 77–87. [CrossRef] [PubMed]

8. Forero-Doria, O.; Polo, E.; Marican, A.; Guzmán, L.; Venegas, B.; Vijayakumar, S.; Wehinger, S.; Guerrero, M.; Gallego, J.; Durán-Lara, E.F. Supramolecular hydrogels based on cellulose for sustained release of therapeutic substances with antimicrobial and wound healing properties. *Carbohydr. Polym.* **2020**, *242*, 116383. [CrossRef]
9. Hoque, J.; Bhattacharjee, B.; Prakash, R.G.; Paramanandham, K.; Haldar, J. Dual Function Injectable Hydrogel for Controlled Release of Antibiotic and Local Antibacterial Therapy. *Biomacromolecules* **2017**, *19*, 267–278. [CrossRef]
10. Li, S.; Dong, S.; Xu, W.; Tu, S.; Yan, L.; Zhao, C.; Ding, J.; Chen, X. Antibacterial Hydrogels. *Adv. Sci.* **2018**, *5*, 1700527. [CrossRef]
11. Catoira, M.C.; Fusaro, L.; Di Francesco, D.; Ramella, M.; Boccafoschi, F. Overview of natural hydrogels for regenerative medicine applications. *J. Mater. Sci. Mater. Med.* **2019**, *30*, 115. [CrossRef]
12. Avila-Salas, F.; Nuñez, Y.A.R.; Marican, A.; Castro, R.; Villaseñor, J.; Santos, L.; Wehinger, S.; Durán-Lara, E.F. Rational Development of a Novel Hydrogel as a pH-Sensitive Controlled Release System for Nifedipine. *Polymers* **2018**, *10*, 806. [CrossRef]
13. Martin-Serrano, Á.; Gómez, R.; Ortega, P.; de la Mata, F.J. Nanosystems as Vehicles for the Delivery of Antimicrobial Peptides (AMPs). *Pharmaceutics* **2019**, *11*, 448. [CrossRef]
14. Avila-Salas, F.; Marican, A.; Pinochet, S.; Carreño, G.; Rigos, A.E.; Venegas, B.; Donoso, W.; Cabrera, G.; Vijayakumar, S.; Durán-Lara, E.F. Film Dressings Based on Hydrogels: Simultaneous and Sustained-Release of Bioactive Compounds with Wound Healing Properties. *Pharmaceutics* **2019**, *11*, 447. [CrossRef] [PubMed]
15. Rizwan, M.; Yahya, R.; Hassan, A.; Yar, M.; Azzahari, A.D.; Selvanathan, V.; Sonsudin, F.; Abouloula, C.N. pH Sensitive Hydrogels in Drug Delivery: Brief History, Properties, Swelling, and Release Mechanism, Material Selection and Applications. *Polymrews* **2017**, *9*, 137. [CrossRef] [PubMed]
16. Nuñez, Y.A.R.; Castro, R.; Arenas, F.; López-Cabaña, Z.E.; Carreño, G.; Carrasco-Sánchez, V.; Marican, A.; Villaseñor, J.; Vargas, E.; Santos, L.S.; et al. Preparation of Hydrogel/Silver Nanohybrids Mediated by Tunable-Size Silver Nanoparticles for Potential Antibacterial Applications. *Polymers* **2019**, *11*, 716. [CrossRef] [PubMed]
17. Sunitha, K.; Sadhana, R.; Mathew, D.; Nair, C.P.R. Novel superabsorbent copolymers of partially neutralized methacrylic acid and acrylonitrile: Synthesis, characterization and swelling characteristics. *Des. Monomers Polym.* **2015**, *18*, 512–523. [CrossRef]
18. Singh, A.; Vaishagya, K.; Verma, R.K.; Shukla, R. Temperature/pH-Triggered PNIPAM-Based Smart Nanogel System Loaded With Anastrozole Delivery for Application in Cancer Chemotherapy. *AAPS PharmSciTech* **2019**, *20*, 213. [CrossRef]
19. Blacklow, S.O.; Li, J.; Freedman, B.R.; Zeidi, M.; Chen, C.; Mooney, D.J. Bioinspired mechanically active adhesive dressings to accelerate wound closure. *Sci. Adv.* **2019**, *5*, eaaw3963. [CrossRef] [PubMed]
20. Dwivedi, R.; Singh, A.; Dhillon, A. pH-responsive drug release from dependal-M loaded polyacrylamide hydrogels. *J. Sci. Adv. Mater. Devices* **2017**, *2*, 45–50. [CrossRef]
21. Owonubi, S.J.; Aderibigbe, B.A.; Mukwevho, E.; Sadiku, E.R.; Ray, S.S. Characterization and in vitro release kinetics of antimalarials from whey protein-based hydrogel biocomposites. *Int. J. Ind. Chem.* **2018**, *9*, 39–52. [CrossRef]
22. Mosmann, T. Rapid colorimetric assay for cellular growth and survival: Application to proliferation and cytotoxicity assays. *J. Immunol. Methods* **1983**, *65*, 55–63. [CrossRef]
23. Valdés, O.; Ávila-Salas, F.; Marican, A.; Fuentealba, N.; Villaseñor, J.; Arenas-Salinas, M.; Argandoña, Y.; Durán-Lara, E.F. Methamidophos removal from aqueous solutions using a super adsorbent based on crosslinked poly(vinyl alcohol) hydrogel. *J. Appl. Polym. Sci.* **2017**, *135*, 45964. [CrossRef]
24. Engberg, K.; Frank, C.W. Protein diffusion in photopolymerized poly(ethylene glycol) hydrogel networks. *Biomed. Mater.* **2011**, *6*, 55006. [CrossRef]
25. Reguieg, F.; Ricci, L.; Bouyacoub, N.; Belbachir, M.; Bertoldo, M. Thermal characterization by DSC and TGA analyses of PVA hydrogels with organic and sodium MMT. *Polym. Bull.* **2019**, *77*, 929–948. [CrossRef]
26. Wang, J.; Zhang, W.; Li, W.; Xing, W. Preparation and characterization of chitosan-poly (vinyl alcohol)/polyvinylidene fluoride hollow fiber composite membranes for pervaporation dehydration of isopropanol. *Korean J. Chem. Eng.* **2015**, *32*, 1369–1376. [CrossRef]
27. Sonker, A.K.; Tiwari, N.; Nagarale, R.K.; Verma, V. Synergistic effect of cellulose nanowhiskers reinforcement and dicarboxylic acids crosslinking towards polyvinyl alcohol properties. *J. Polym. Sci. Part. A Polym. Chem.* **2016**, *54*, 2515–2525. [CrossRef]

28. Sonker, A.K.; Rathore, K.; Nagarale, R.K.; Verma, V. Crosslinking of Polyvinyl Alcohol (PVA) and Effect of Crosslinker Shape (Aliphatic and Aromatic) Thereof. *J. Polym. Environ.* **2017**, *26*, 1782–1794. [CrossRef]
29. Miranda, C.; Castaño, J.; Valdebenito-Rolack, E.; Sanhueza, F.; Toro, R.; Bello-Toledo, H.; Uarac, P.; Saez, L. Copper-Polyurethane Composite Materials: Particle Size Effect on the Physical-Chemical and Antibacterial Properties. *Polymers* **2020**, *12*, 1934. [CrossRef] [PubMed]
30. Wu, X.; Li, W.; Chen, K.; Zhang, D.; Xu, L.; Yang, X. A tough PVA/HA/COL composite hydrogel with simple process and excellent mechanical properties. *Mater. Today Commun.* **2019**, *21*, 100702. [CrossRef]
31. Abebe, M.W.; Appiah-Ntiamoah, R.; Kim, H. Gallic acid modified alginate self-adhesive hydrogel for strain responsive transdermal delivery. *Int. J. Biol. Macromol.* **2020**, *163*, 147–155. [CrossRef]
32. Oyen, M.L. Mechanical characterization of hydrogel materials. *Inter. Mater. Rev.* **2014**, *59*, 44–59. [CrossRef]
33. Kumar, A.; Behl, T.; Chadha, S. Synthesis of physically crosslinked PVA/Chitosan loaded silver nanoparticles hydrogels with tunable mechanical properties and antibacterial effects. *Int. J. Biol. Macromol.* **2020**, *149*, 1262–1274. [CrossRef] [PubMed]
34. Kord, B.; Malekian, B.; Yousefi, H.A.; Najafi, A. Preparation and characterization of nanofibrillated Cellulose/Poly (Vinyl Alcohol) composite films. *Maderas. Ciencia Tecnología* **2016**, *18*, 743–752. [CrossRef]
35. Singh, B.; Pal, L. Sterculia crosslinked PVA and PVA-poly(AAm) hydrogel wound dressings for slow drug delivery: Mechanical, mucoadhesive, biocompatible and permeability properties. *J. Mech. Behav. Biomed. Mater.* **2012**, *9*, 9–21. [CrossRef] [PubMed]
36. Canaparo, R.; Foglietta, F.; Giuntini, F.; Della Pepa, C.; Dosio, F.; Serpe, L. Recent Developments in Antibacterial Therapy: Focus on Stimuli-Responsive Drug-Delivery Systems and Therapeutic Nanoparticles. *Molecules* **2019**, *24*, 1991. [CrossRef] [PubMed]
37. Gould, K. Clinical update on linezolid in the treatment of Gram-positive bacterial infections. *Infect. Drug Resist.* **2012**, *5*, 87–102. [CrossRef]

Publisher's Note: MDPI stays neutral with regard to jurisdictional claims in published maps and institutional affiliations.

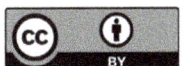

© 2020 by the authors. Licensee MDPI, Basel, Switzerland. This article is an open access article distributed under the terms and conditions of the Creative Commons Attribution (CC BY) license (http://creativecommons.org/licenses/by/4.0/).

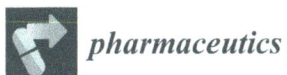

Review

Polymeric Nanomaterials for Efficient Delivery of Antimicrobial Agents

Yin Wang [1] and Hui Sun [2,*]

[1] School of Public Health and Management, Ningxia Medical University, Yinchuan 750004, China; wy9522@126.com
[2] State Key Laboratory of High-Efficiency Coal Utilization and Green Chemical Engineering, Ningxia University, Yinchuan 750021, China
* Correspondence: sunhui@nxu.edu.cn; Tel.: +86-15216719170

Citation: Wang, Y.; Sun, H. Polymeric Nanomaterials for Efficient Delivery of Antimicrobial Agents. *Pharmaceutics* **2021**, *13*, 2108. https://doi.org/10.3390/pharmaceutics13122108

Academic Editor: Umile Gianfranco Spizzirri and Patrick J. Sinko

Received: 5 November 2021
Accepted: 3 December 2021
Published: 7 December 2021

Publisher's Note: MDPI stays neutral with regard to jurisdictional claims in published maps and institutional affiliations.

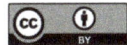

Copyright: © 2021 by the authors. Licensee MDPI, Basel, Switzerland. This article is an open access article distributed under the terms and conditions of the Creative Commons Attribution (CC BY) license (https://creativecommons.org/licenses/by/4.0/).

Abstract: Bacterial infections have threatened the lives of human beings for thousands of years either as major diseases or complications. The elimination of bacterial infections has always occupied a pivotal position in our history. For a long period of time, people were devoted to finding natural antimicrobial agents such as antimicrobial peptides (AMPs), antibiotics and silver ions or synthetic active antimicrobial substances including antimicrobial peptoids, metal oxides and polymers to combat bacterial infections. However, with the emergence of multidrug resistance (MDR), bacterial infection has become one of the most urgent problems worldwide. The efficient delivery of antimicrobial agents to the site of infection precisely is a promising strategy for reducing bacterial resistance. Polymeric nanomaterials have been widely studied as carriers for constructing antimicrobial agent delivery systems and have shown advantages including high biocompatibility, sustained release, targeting and improved bioavailability. In this review, we will highlight recent advances in highly efficient delivery of antimicrobial agents by polymeric nanomaterials such as micelles, vesicles, dendrimers, nanogels, nanofibers and so forth. The biomedical applications of polymeric nanomaterial-based delivery systems in combating MDR bacteria, anti-biofilms, wound healing, tissue engineering and anticancer are demonstrated. Moreover, conclusions and future perspectives are also proposed.

Keywords: antimicrobial agent; polymeric nanomaterial; self-assembly; antimicrobial peptide; silver nanoparticle; anti-biofilm; wound healing; multidrug resistance

1. Introduction

Infectious diseases induced by bacteria, virus and fungi have been considered as one of the biggest enemies that threatened the lives of human beings for a long time [1]. Since the discovery of penicillin in 1928, antibiotics have played an unprecedented role in saving lives of human beings and caused revolutionary changes in medicine. However, with overuse and improper use of antibiotics, the emergence of bacterial drug resistance is becoming a severe problem. In particular, combating MDR bacteria such as methicillin-resistant *Staphylococcus aureus* (*S. aureus*) (MRSA) has drawn wide attention and efforts [2,3]. Non-antibiotic antimicrobial agents such as AMPs [4–6], silver nanoparticles (AgNPs) [7–9], metal oxides [10–12], antimicrobial peptoids [13,14] and polymers [15–18] are alternatives for treating infectious diseases that kill bacteria in a physical manner and avoid the generation of drug resistance. For instance, cationic compounds including AMPs, antimicrobial peptoids and polymers, as well as their corresponding nanostructures, strongly interacted with the negatively charged cell membrane of bacteria, resulting in the disruption of the cell membrane and outflow of the content of bacteria [19,20]. Metal (oxide) nanoparticles such as widely studied AgNPs kill bacteria via heavy metal ions induced by the denaturation of proteins or genetic materials, while ZnO and TiO$_2$ nanoparticles eliminate bacteria by reacting with reactive oxygen species (ROS) generated from photocatalytic process [12,21].

Moreover, emerging antimicrobial agents including gases, photothermal sensitizers and carbon materials were also developed to combat bacterial infections [17,22–24].

The efficient delivery of antimicrobial agents to the target preventing the defense system of bacteria including efflux pump, degrading enzymes and resistance genes is critical for reducing the emergence of drug resistance [25–27]. Polymeric nanomaterials are promising vehicles for the efficient delivery of antimicrobial agents due to their tailorable chemical compositions, microstructures and biological properties for a wide range of biomedical applications [28–30]. For instance, low dimensional nanostructures including dendrimers [31,32], polymeric nanoparticles [33,34], micelles [35,36], vesicles [37,38] and nanogels [39,40] have shown superiorities in the delivery of antimicrobial agents to the areas of infections and on-demand release. Polymeric nanofibers and hydrogels are beneficial for the long-term release of antimicrobial agents and wound coverage [41,42]. Very recently, metal organic frameworks (MOFs) have attracted attention as emerging carriers for the efficient delivery of metal ions, metal nanoparticles, antibiotics and enzymes due to their highly porous structures [43–46]. There are several advantages of using polymeric nanomaterials as carriers to accomplish the on-demand delivery of antimicrobial agents: (i) reduced dosage and drug resistance; (ii) increased in vivo circulation stability; (iii) enhanced penetration ability; (iv) prolonged antimicrobial performance; and (v) improved bioavailability. Therefore, apart from the wide attentional broad spectrum antimicrobial properties, biomedical applications including combating MDR bacteria, anti-biofilm, anticancer, wound healing and tissue engineering based on the polymeric antimicrobial agent delivery systems have been rapidly developed [47–50].

In this review, we aim to present the state of the art of polymeric nanomaterials as carriers for the efficient delivery of antimicrobial agents from the following aspects: (1) classification of polymeric nanoparticles based on their nanostructures; (2) the structural features and corresponding advantages in delivery of antimicrobial agents; and (3) biomedical applications benefiting from the constructed delivery systems, as illustrated in Figure 1.

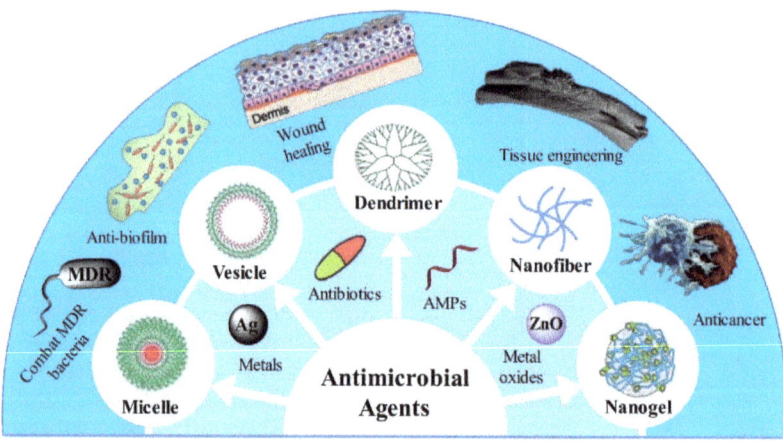

Figure 1. Schematic illustration of polymeric nanomaterials for efficient delivery of antimicrobial agents and their biomedical applications.

2. Efficient Delivery of Antimicrobial Agents by Diverse Polymeric Nanostructures
2.1. Self-Assembled Polymeric Nanoparticles

Polymer self-assembly has been recognized as one of the most versatile strategies for preparing soft nanomaterials with various morphologies and functionalities from small building blocks [51–56]. Typically, polymer micelles and vesicles are the most easily obtained and widely studied nano-objects due to their well-organized structures [57–60]. Polymer micelles are formed by the regular arrangement of building blocks with hydrophobic components forming the cores and hydrophilic polymer chains covering the surface. Moreover, the hydrophobic cores facilitated the efficient encapsulation of hydrophobic drugs [61,62], while polymer vesicles are hollow bilayer nanostructures with hydrophobic membranes, hydrophilic coronas and interior cavities, endowing them with superiorities in loading and delivering hydrophobic, hydrophilic and large-sized cargoes [63–66]. The design of polymer vesicles for meeting the requirements of various applications mainly focuses on the chemical composition and structure of coronas and membranes, such as permeability and homogeneity of the membrane, symmetricity of the corona and so forth [67–69]. Despite the wide applications of polymer micelles and vesicles in cancer therapy, gene delivery and cell imaging, they also exhibit considerable potentials in the efficient delivery of antimicrobial agents [36,70,71].

Polymer micelles, core-shell nanostructures that usually self-assembled from amphiphilic block copolymers, are regarded as one of the most extensively studied nanostructures for antimicrobial agent delivery [35,72]. Typically, hydrophobic antibiotics, AMPs and AgNPs can be loaded in the hydrophobic core, and amphiphilic antimicrobial molecules are usually decorated on the surface of polymer micelles by covalent bonding or electrostatic interaction [73–76]. For instance, a poor water-soluble anti-fungi agent, amphotericin B, could be encapsulated in the core of micelles and showed ultra-long sustained release for 150 h, resulting in reduced hemotoxicity and comparable anti-fungi activity compared with free amphotericin B [77]. Xiong and coworkers [78] functionalized terpyridine on the surface of polymer micelles; after chelating with Fe(II), the micelles displayed excellent biofilm inhibition activity up to 99.9% at a concentration of 128 µM. Recently, Lee et al. [79] prepared AMP-covered micelles by the co-assembly of chimeric antimicrobial lipopeptide and a biodegradable amphiphilic polymer (poly-(lactic-*co*-glycolic acid)-*b*-poly(ethylene glycol), (PLGA-*b*-PEG)). The chimeric peptide HnMc and PEG formed the shell of the micelles in which PEG protected HnMc from proteolytic degradation. Moreover, HnMc on the surface could help micelles in preferentially binding and killing bacteria. Due to the synergy between HnMc and PEG, the micelles targeted a wide range of bacteria preferentially including *Escherichia coli* (*E. coli*), *Listeria monocytogenes*, *Pseudomonas aeruginosa* (*P. aeruginosa*) and *S. aureus* instead of mammalian cells. Moreover, in vivo experiments also demonstrated superior anti-inflammatory effects of the micelles in a mouse model of drug-resistant *P. aeruginosa* lung infection with highly targeted abilities, as shown in Figure 2.

Very recently, Wooley and coworkers [80] fabricated spherical micelles, cylinders and nanoplates derived from the crystallization-driven self-assembly (CDSA) of an amphiphilic block copolymer composed of zwitterionic poly(D-glucose carbonate) and semicrystalline poly(L-lactide) segments (PDGC-*b*-PLLA). As illustrated in Figure 3, fluorescent molecule and cysteine were modified on the polymer in order to afford tracing ability and to chelate with silver ions, respectively. The morphology of the nanostructures could be well controlled by the hydrophilic-to-hydrophobic ratios, which exhibited negligible cytotoxicity, immunotoxicity and cytokine adsorption. However, the nanostructures offered substantial silver ion loading capacity, extended release and in vitro antimicrobial activity. Compared with spherical micelles, the cylinders and nanoplates exhibited enhanced association with uroepithelial cells due to their high aspect ratio, resulting in improved inhibition of the growth of *E. coli* in recurrent urinary tract infections.

Compared with polymer micelles, polymer vesicles are closed hollow spheres with more complicated structures usually acting as simple mimics of biological cells [81]. There are three compartmentalized regions that should be considered for realizing different functions, namely the inner hydrophilic cavity, hydrophobic membrane and hydrophilic corona in contact with external environments [82]. Therefore, both hydrophilic and hydrophobic compounds and even nanoparticles could be encapsulated in the interior cavity or membrane of vesicles, respectively. Moreover, hydrophilic molecules could also be linked onto the coronas of polymer vesicles by covalent bonding. Considering the structural feasibility of polymer vesicles, a large variety of antimicrobial agents could be loaded and delivered to combat bacteria with high loading efficiency, controlled release manner, targeting capability and improved bioavailability [83,84]. For example, Du and coworkers [35] deposited ultrafine AgNPs with a diameter of 1.9 ± 0.4 nm on the membrane of polymer vesicles by in situ reduction of silver ions to inhibit the growth of Gram-negative and Gram-positive bacteria. Battaglia et al. [71] reported the intracellular delivery of metronidazole or doxycycline to *P. gingivalis*-infected oral epithelial cells by polymer vesicles, which were disassembled in early endosomes due to the acidic condition, resulting in the release of loaded cargoes.

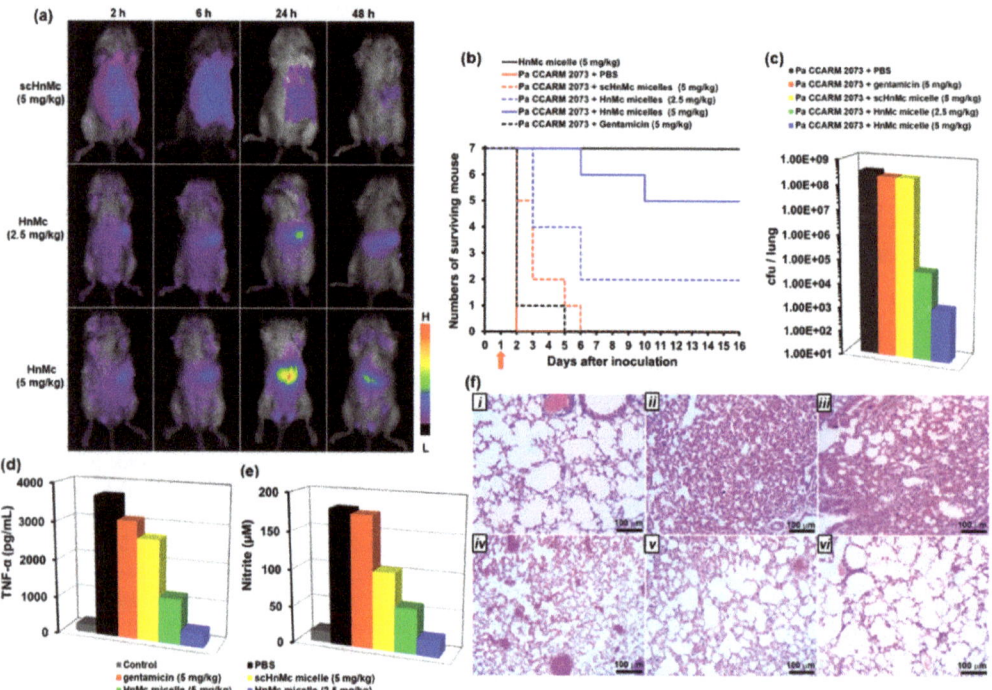

Figure 2. Targeted antibacterial activity of HnMc micelles in the mouse model of drug resistant *P. aeruginosa* lung infection. (**a**) Fluorescent imaging of infected mice after intravenous injection of fluorescent IR820-loaded HnMc micelles. (**b**) Survival rate of infected mice after administration of HnMc micelles. (**c**) Number of remaining cells in the infected lungs after administration of HnMc micelles. Inhibitory effects of HnMc micelles on the expression of TNF-α (**d**) and nitric oxide (**e**) in the blood of infected mice. (**f**) H&E-stained lung tissues. (**i**): control; (**ii**): *P. aeruginosa* + PBS; (**iii**): *P. aeruginosa* + gentamicin (5 mg kg^{-1}); (**iv**): *P. aeruginosa* + scrambled HnMc micelle (5 mg kg^{-1}); (**v**): *P. aeruginosa* + HnMc micelle (2.5 mg kg^{-1}); and (**vi**): *P. aeruginosa* + HnMc micelle (5 mg kg^{-1}) (reproduced with permission from Park et al. [79], ACS Applied Materials & Interfaces; published by American Chemical Society, 2020).

Recently, Liu and coworkers [85] designed enzyme-responsive polymer vesicles for bacterial strain-selective delivery of antimicrobials, as shown in Figure 4. Both hydrophilic and hydrophobic antimicrobials including vancomycin, gentamicin, quinupristin and dalfopristin could be encapsulated either in the interior cavity or membrane of the polymer vesicles with high efficiency. The PEG chains covered on the surface of the vesicle could reduce cytotoxicity and improve biocompatibility, while the self-immolative side chains could be degraded by penicillin Gamidase (PGA) and β-lactamase (Bla), which are overexpressed by drug resistant bacterial strains. Without the trigger by PGA and Bla, the encapsulated antimicrobials were well protected by vesicles. Upon being exposed to drug-resistant bacteria, the membrane of the vesicle was degraded, resulting in the sustained release of antimicrobials, as well as the elimination of bacteria. Considering that Bla is the main cause of bacterial resistance to β-lactam antibiotic drugs that are secreted by MRSA, selective antimicrobial activity of the antimicrobials-loaded vesicles was achieved.

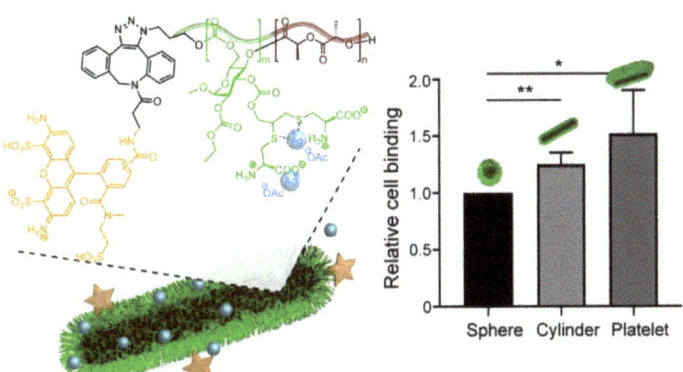

Figure 3. Polymer micelles, cylinders and nanoplates derived from the CDSA of PDGC-*b*-PLLA and their antimicrobial activity (* $p < 0.05$ and ** $p < 0.01$ by *t* test) (reproduced with permission from Song et al. [80], Nano Letters; published by American Chemical Society, 2021).

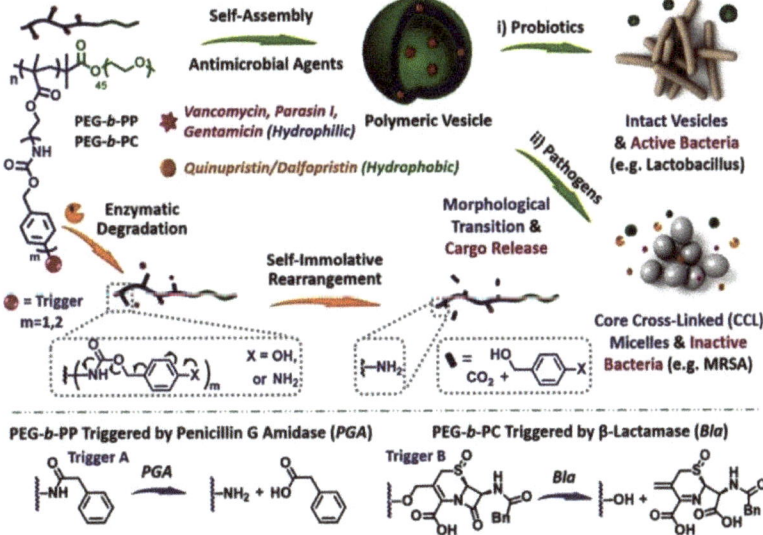

Figure 4. Enzyme-responsive polymer vesicles for bacterial strain-selective delivery of antimicrobials (reproduced with permission from Li et al. [85], Angewandte Chemie International Edition; published by Wiley, 2015).

Loading bioactive enzymes by polymer vesicles to generate antimicrobial active species triggered by external stimuli is another effective method for combating bacteria. For example, Blackman et al. [86] prepared glucose oxidase-loaded semipermeable polymer vesicles by polymerization-induced self-assembly inspired by honey. Hydrogen peroxide, an effective antimicrobial agent, could be generated in response to glucose to switch on antimicrobial activity of the vesicles. In the absence of glucose, the vesicles were completely nontoxic to bacteria, while the vesicles showed seven-log reduction in bacterial growth at high glucose concentrations against a range of Gram-negative and Gram-positive bacterial pathogens including *S. aureus*, *S. epidermidis*, *E. coli* and *Klebsiella pneumoniae* (*K. pneumonia*), even the MRSA clinical isolate. More importantly, the toxicity of the vesicle toward human fibroblasts at different dosage and glucose concentrations was also evaluated, demonstrating that the optimal concentration of the vesicle was 0.69 mg mL^{-1} at physiological blood glucose level to effectively eliminate bacteria while preserving good compatibility to mammalian cells.

2.2. Dendrimers

Dendrimers are highly branched, globular macromolecules with many arms emanating from a central core, which have shown unique structural properties such as high degree of branching, multivalency, globular architecture and well-defined molecular weight, rendering them promising scaffolds for drug delivery [87,88]. Many commercial drugs with anticancer and antimicrobial activity have been successfully loaded within dendrimers including poly(amidoamine) (PAMAM), poly(propylene imine) (PPI) and poly(etherhydroxylamine) (PEHAM), either via physical interactions or by chemical bonding to improve their water solubility [89]. Dendrimers themselves could be used as effective antimicrobial agents [90]. For instance, those with positively charged surfaces usually have strong interaction with negatively charged bacterial cell membranes, while those with metal cores can release active antimicrobial agents such as metal ions and ROS, resulting in the death of bacteria [91].

Moreover, antimicrobial agents including antibiotics, AMPs, AgNPs and metal oxide nanoparticles could be also effectively loaded by dendrimers [89,92]. For example, Tang et al. [93] prepared silver-dendrimer nanocomposites by loading AgNPs in low generation poly(amido amine) dendrimers. The AgNPs were formed by an in situ reduction of silver ions enriched by the amine groups of dendrimers. The factors that influenced the size of AgNPs were discussed, and the average diameter of the AgNPs could be controlled from 7.6 to 16.2 nm. The synthesized silver-dendrimer nanocomposite was used as antimicrobial agent in the fabrication of cotton fabrics, which exhibited excellent antimicrobial activity against both of *E. coli* and *S. aureus*. Recently, Huang and coworkers [94] reported PLGA nanoparticles and PAMAM dendrimers in order to effectively encapsulate and deliver platensimycin, a potent inhibitor for the synthesis of bacterial fatty acid, respectively, to combat MDR bacteria. Benefiting from the improved pharmacokinetics, both the platensimycin-loaded PLGA nanoparticles and PAMAM dendrimers showed enhanced antimicrobial activity and reduced cytotoxicity compared with free platensimycin, resulting in an efficient inhibition of *S. aureus* biofilm formation and the full survival of MRSA-infected mice.

Dendrimers are ideal platforms for compacting and delivering deoxyribonucleic acids (DNAs) and ribonucleic acids (RNAs) for gene therapy due to their hyperbranched structure and strong positive charges, especially PAMAM [95,96]. Recently, antisense therapy strategy has been developed to treat bacterial infections facilitated by the dendrimers-based antisense delivery system [97]. For example, the G3 PAMAM dendrimer has good antimicrobial activity, as shown in Figure 5. However, the cytotoxicity of the G3 PAMAM dendrimer toward mammalian cells is also high. Luo et al. [98] conjugated LED209, a specific inhibitor of quorum sensor QseC of Gram-negative bacteria, onto the surface of G3 PAMAM to generate PAMAM-LED209 in order to reduce cytotoxicity to mammalian cells while retaining the excellent antibacterial activity of the G3 PAMAM dendrimer. In addition, PAMAM-LED209 also inhibited the virulence gene expression of Gram-negative bacteria and prevented the generation of drug resistance. As shown in Figure 5, compared with the control group (Figure 5A), *entero-hemorrhagic E. coli* (*EHEC*) were severely damaged after being treated with G3 PAMAM and G3 PAMAM-LED209 for 300 min (Figure 5B,C), demonstrating that G3 PAMAM-LED209 retained strong antibacterial activity toward resistant Gram-negative bacteria after functionalization of LED209. The induction of the resistance of G3 PAMAM-LED209 was also evaluated after 15 reproductions of bacteria, as illustrated in Figure 5D. The minimal inhibition concentration (MIC) of G3 PAMAM-LED209 barely changed, while the MIC values of classical antimicrobials, including ceftazidime, ampicillin and levofloxacin, increased by 8-fold to 64-fold. The cytotoxicity and antibacterial activity of terminally modified PAMAM are related to the conjugated ligand and degree of modification, as shown in Figure 5E. With an increase in modification ratio, the cytotoxicity of G3 PAMAM-PEG and G3 PAMAM-LED209 decreased dramatically to being almost nontoxic and then increased, while the antimicrobial activity of the G3 PAMAM-PEG and G3 PAMAM-LED209 decreased with an increase in modification ratio due to the shielding of positive charges. Therefore, there is an optimal modification ratio range for balancing cytotoxicity and antimicrobial activity, as pointed out by the arrow in Figure 5E. Moreover, the antibacterial potency of G3 PAMAM-LED209 is also higher than that of G3 PAMAM-PEG, which is indicated by area A and B in Figure 5E, demonstrating better biocompatibility and higher antibacterial potency than compared to G3 PAMAM-PEG.

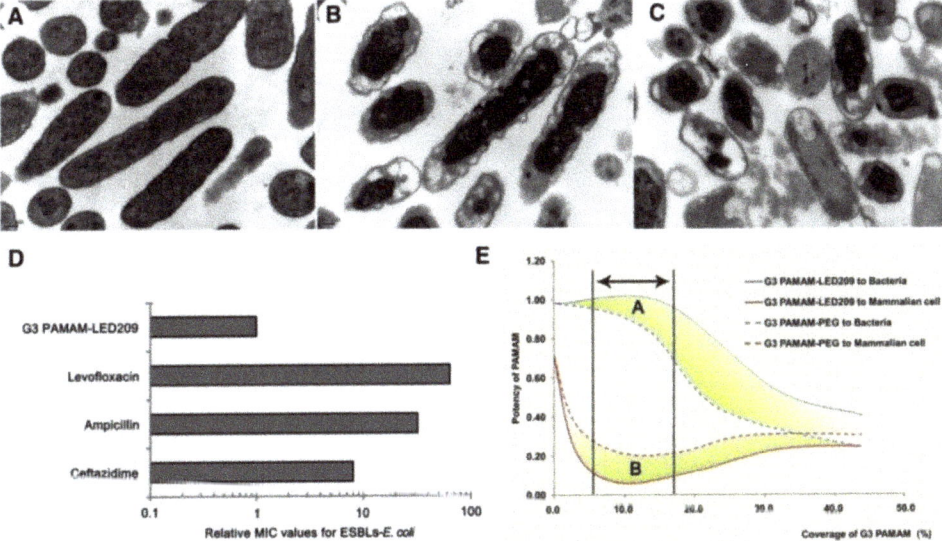

Figure 5. The morphology of EHEC was investigated by transmission electron microscopy (TEM) after different treatments for 300 min. (**A**) Control; (**B**) 75 μg mL^{-1} of G3 PAMAM; and (**C**) 150 μg mL^{-1} of G3 PAMAM-LED209. (**D**) Induction of resistance to G3 PAMAM-LED209. (**E**) The influence of the conjugated ligand and degree of modification on cytotoxicity and antibacterial activity of terminally modified G3 PAMAM dendrimer. Area A and B showed increased antibacterial activity and reduced cytotoxicity with respect to G3 PAMAM-LED209 and G3 PAMAM-PEG, respectively (reproduced with permission from Xue et al. [98], Nanomedicine: Nanotechnology, Biology and Medicine; published by Elsevier, 2015).

2.3. Polymer Nanofibers

Polymer nanofibers are one dimensional nanostructures with large aspect ratio and high surface area and have shown significant potential for delivering antimicrobial agents locally into an infected area, especially in wound healing [42,99]. Typically, there are several methods for preparing nanofibers including self-assembly [100], template synthesis [101], phase separation [102] and electrospinning [103], among which electrospinning is a superior technique for preparing nanofibers with desired chemical compositions and diameters due to its simplicity and versatility [104–106]. Antimicrobial agents including antibiotics, AMPs, AgNPs and metal oxide nanoparticles could be incorporated into nanofibers by mixing with polymer precursors followed by electrospinning or attaching onto the surface of the nanofibers by noncovalent interactions or chemical bonds [107]. For instance, Schiffman et al. [108] immobilized zeolites nanoparticles with high silver ion change capability onto the surface of chitosan nanofibers. After ion exchange, silver ions were loaded in the zeolites to function as molecular delivery vehicles, and their ion release profiles and ability to inhibit *E. coli* were evaluated as a function of time. Interestingly, the zeolites immobilized on the nanofibers showed significantly enhanced antibacterial activity 11-times greater than that of the pure zeolites due to high porosity and hydrophilicity of the nanofibers.

Recently, Tu and coworkers [109] reported the in situ deposition of AgNPs on gold/polydopamine core-shell nanoparticles encapsulated by poly(lactic acid) (PLA) nanofibers (PLA-Au@PDA@Ag), which could be applied to biological coatings for bacteriostatic functionality. The schematic illustration of the preparation and antimicrobial capability of the PLA-Au@PDA@Ag is presented in Figure 6. Chloroauric acid was reduced by ascorbic acid to afford gold nanoparticles. Following the polymerization of dopamine on the surface, Au@PDA core-shell nanoparticles formed, which were then mixed with PLA solution to produce PLA-Au@PDA hybrid nanofibers by electrospinning. Later, PLA-Au@PDA hybrid nanofibers were immersed in silver nitrate solution for in situ reduction of adsorbed silver ions into AgNPs to yield PLA-Au@PDA@Ag nanofibers. The hydrophilicity of the PLA-Au@PDA@Ag nanofibers significantly improved compared to that of PLA nanofibers, resulting in the promoted release of silver ions. Benefiting from the synergy between AuNPs, PDA and AgNPs, including AuNPs providing effective contact with microorganisms, PDA as binder was used to immobilize AgNPs and facilitated the release of silver ions; the PLA-Au@PDA@Ag nanofibers showed significant antibacterial ability against both of E. coli and S. aureus.

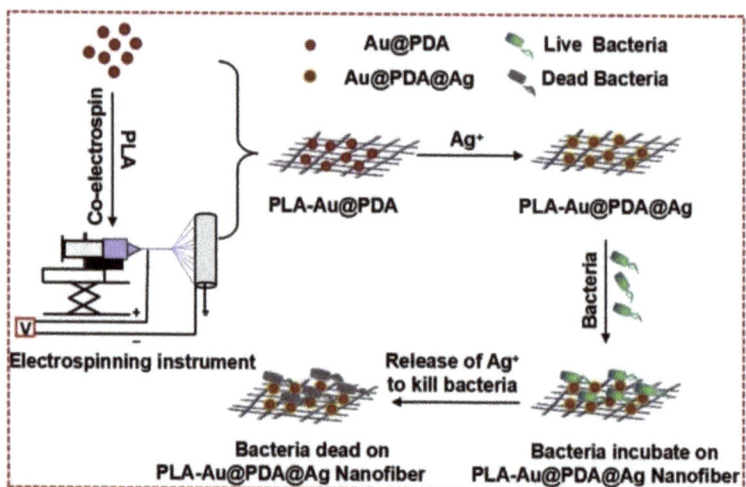

Figure 6. Schematic diagram illustrating the preparation of PLA-Au@PDA@Ag nanofibers and their antibacterial capacity (reproduced with permission from Zhang et al. [109], Colloids and Surfaces B: Biointerfaces; published by Elsevier, 2019).

Due to their large exposed surface area and nanoporosity, polymer nanofiber meshes have shown distinct advantages in wound healing compared with hydrogels, films and foams [110]. The extracellular matrix (ECM) mimicking the structure of nanofibers facilitated the interaction with cells in the wound bed. Moreover, small molecules such as water, oxygen, nutrients and metabolic wastes could be efficiently exchanged due to the highly porous structure of nanofibers [111]. In order to promote the healing rate and elimination of bacteria, functional agents including enzymes, drugs and antimicrobial agents have been incorporated in polymer nanofibers. Rath et al. [112] loaded ZnO nanoparticles and cefazolin in the gelatin nanofibers to accelerate wound healing and prevented infection concurrently. Cefazolin was used to inhibit bacterial reproduction, while zinc cations could be released from ZnO nanoparticles to raise re-epithelialization, reduce inflammation and inhibit bacterial growth. Moreover, ROS was also produced by ZnO nanoparticles, thereby optimizing cell adhesion, proliferation and migration via growth factor mediated pathways, promoting the regeneration of the ECM.

2.4. Polymer Nanogels

Polymer nanogels are a class of nanoparticles composed of nanosized physically or chemically cross-linked hydrophilic or amphiphilic polymer networks [113]. They are of wide interest in various fields including drug delivery due to their flexible nanosize, good stability and high loading capacity, etc. [114]. As their analogues, polymer hydrogels have been widely used in antimicrobial applications due to their high water content, three-dimensional structure and stimuli-responsive sol-gel transition behavior [115]. There are several reviews summarizing the recent advances of antimicrobial polymer hydrogels [116–118]. Therefore, we will not discuss this part and focus on the nanogels as carriers for antimicrobial agent delivery in this section.

The stimuli-responsive swelling and collapsing of nanogels triggered by external stimuli including pH, temperature, enzymes or ionic strength render them ideal candidates in on-demand delivery and release of antimicrobial agents [119]. For instance, AMPs could be encapsulated in nanogels with high loading content via strong electrostatic interaction with negatively charged polymer chains, and they can be released when triggered by salt ions in physiological conditions [120,121]. El-Feky et al. [122] loaded silver sulfadiazine in alginate coated chitosan nanogels to heal burn wounds, and the nanogels showed a release profile of an initial burst followed by a slow and continuous release, resulting in excellent in vivo therapeutic efficacy.

In addition, loading and delivery of antimicrobials including berberine, cyclodextrin, tetracycline hydrochloride and lincomycin hydrochloride by nanogels to combat bacteria and MDR bacteria were widely studied by Paunov, Schaefer and so forth [123–126]. Wang and coworkers [127] designed a lipase-sensitive polymeric triple-layered nanogel (TLN) formed by a cross-linked polyphosphoester core, poly(ε-caprolactone) (PCL) fence and PEG shell to encapsulate and deliver vancomycin, as illustrated in Figure 7. In aqueous solutions, hydrophobic PCL segments collapsed and covered the core to form a densely packed molecular fence to prevent the leakage of vancomycin. Once TLN was exposed to lipase secreting bacteria, the PCL chains were degraded to trigger the release of vancomycin, resulting in the inhibition of bacterial growth. They found that all encapsulated vancomycins were released within 24 h in the presence of *S. aureus*. Moreover, lipase secreting bacteria inside the cells could also be inhibited by TLN, demonstrating the versatility of the strategy of lipase-induced on-demand delivery and release of antimicrobials.

Recently, Knowles et al. [128] synthesized hybrid organic/inorganic AgNPs loaded nanofibrillar silk microgels to effectively eradicate bacteria by a two-step mechanism including bacterial adherence and consequent eradication. Compared with conventional AgNPs and silver ions, the hemolysis and cytotoxicity of hybrid microgels toward mammalian cell lines were significantly reduced due to the protection of the silk matrix. van Rijn and coworkers [129] prepared injectable nanogels loaded with hydrophobic triclosan in hydrophobic domains inside the nanogel networks through intraparticle self-assembly of aliphatic chains, which enhanced antimicrobial efficiency of triclosan up to 1000 times. As shown in Figure 8, a three-stage antimicrobial mechanism of the nanogels was proposed. Firstly, the nanogels attached onto the surfaces of the bacteria via electrostatic interaction to disturb the balance of charge density of the cell membranes. Secondly, bacterial cell membranes were destroyed by the insertion of hydrophobic aliphatic chains. Thirdly, loaded triclosan was released from the hydrophobic domains inside the nanogels and injected into the bacterial cell membranes, resulting in the death of bacteria. This approach dramatically increases the effective concentration of triclosan inside the bacteria. Moreover, both the MIC and minimal bactericidal concentration (MBC) against Gram-positive *S. aureus* and *S. epidermidis* decreased by three orders of magnitude compared with free triclosan, resulting in a decrease in the dosage of triclosan and reduction in drug resistance.

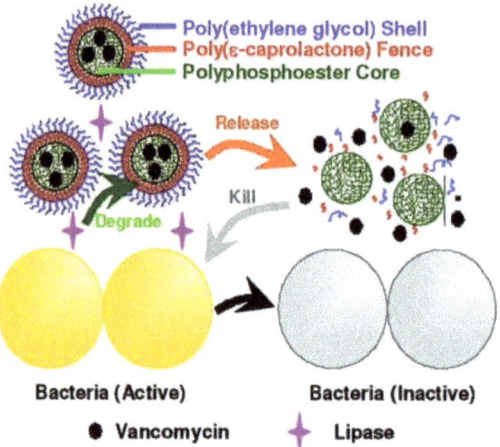

Figure 7. Schematic illustration of the on-demand delivery of vancomycin triggered by bacterial lipase to treat the bacterial infections using TLNs, which contains a bacterial lipase-sensitive PCL interlayer between the cross-linked polyphosphoester core and the shell of the PEG (reproduced with permission from Xiong et al. [127], Journal of the American Chemical Society; published by American Chemical Society, 2012).

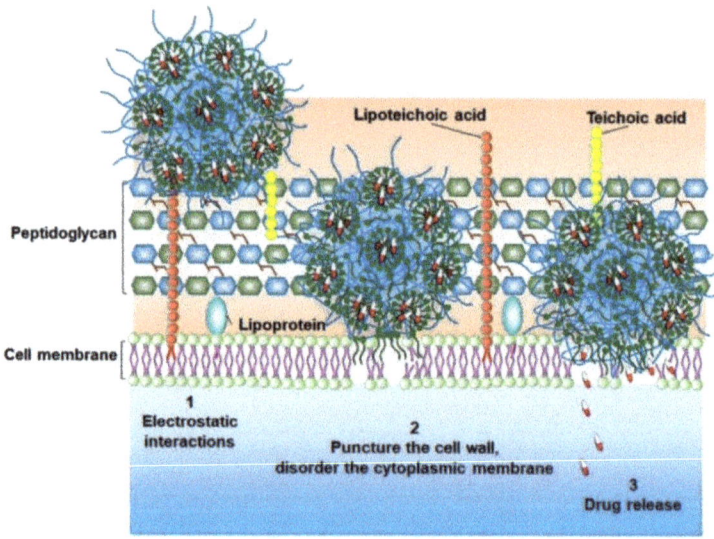

Figure 8. Schematic illustration of the bactericidal mechanism of Triclosan-loaded nanogels (adapted from Zu et al. [129], ACS Applied Polymer Materials; published by American Chemical Society, 2020).

2.5. Hybrid Delivery Systems

Incorporating polymer nanoparticles including dendrimers, micelles and vesicles with high dimensional polymeric nanomaterials such as nanofibers, hydrogels and coatings as hybrid delivery systems could combine the advantages of both and achieve the hierarchical release of antimicrobial agents [130–133]. For example, Zhang and coworkers [130] developed a bioadhesive nanoparticle-hydrogel hybrid in order to enhance localized antimicrobial drug delivery. The antimicrobials ciprofloxacin was loaded in polymer nanoparticles that were embedded in hydrogels adhering to biological surfaces. Hydrogel network properties could be tailored independently for adhesion, which maintained controlled and prolonged ciprofloxacin release profiles from nanoparticles. Imae et al. [131] immobilized AgNPs-loaded amine-terminated fourth generation poly(amido amine) dendrimers onto the viscose rayon cellulose fibers, which exhibited excellent biocidal activity against *E. coli* with low weight percentage of silver of 0.2%. Du and coworkers [132] embedded penicillin encapsulated polypeptide polymersomes in the hydrogels to achieve quick and long-term antibacterial capability in which penicillin could be released from the hydrogel networks for quick bacteria elimination while the intrinsic antibacterial property of the polymersomes ensured long-term antibacterial activity. However, despite the advantages of hybrid delivery systems, the development of incorporation of different polymeric nanostructures as hybrid delivery platforms is still in its infancy, which may bring new opportunities in efficient loading and delivery of antimicrobial agents.

3. Biomedical Applications of Polymeric Nanomaterials Based Antimicrobial Agent Delivery Systems

3.1. Combating MDR Bacteria

The generation of drug resistance of pathogens is typically caused by the accumulation of drug resistant genes through mutation with the long-term use, especially overuse and improper use of antibiotics [25]. Therefore, the exploration of highly efficient delivery system to reduce dosage and improve bioavailability of antibiotics, as well as the delivery of non-antibiotic antimicrobial agents including AMPs, AgNPs, metal oxides, gases and so forth, is a promising strategy for reducing drug resistance [134,135]. Polymeric nanomaterial-based antimicrobial agent delivery systems have widely been used in combating MDR bacteria [136,137]. For instance, Liu et al. [138] conjugated quercetin and acetylcholine on the surface of selenium nanoparticles to combat MDR bacteria, which could effectively eliminate MRSA by destroying the membrane due to the synergy between quercetin, acetylcholine and selenium nanoparticles. Cationic polymeric star-shaped nanoparticles or dendrimers have also shown excellent antimicrobial activity against MDR bacteria even without loading antimicrobial agents [139–141], demonstrating the great potentials of polymeric nanomaterials in combating MDR bacteria.

Hu et al. [142] prepared polyprodrug antimicrobials to combat MRSA by membrane damage and concurrent drug release, as shown in Figure 9. Triclosan was covalently linked with acrylic acid to produce a triclosan prodrug monomer (TMA). Then, TMA was copolymerized with quaternized N,N-dimethylaminoethyl methacrylate (QDMA), affording PQDMA-b-PTMA, which could self-assemble into prodrug micelles with positively charged surfaces. The hydrophilic–hydrophobic balance of the prodrug micelles was optimized to enhance interaction with bacterial cell membranes, resulting in improved antimicrobial activity. They proposed that the antimicrobial mechanism was as follows: (1) the prodrug micelles attached onto the surface of MRSA due to strong electrostatic interaction; (2) the prodrug micelles fused with and inserted into the cell membrane of MRSA; (3) the cell membrane of MRSA was damaged due to charge disorder, and prodrug micelles were encapsulated into the cell; (4) prodrug micelles were disassembled, and the linkage between triclosan and acrylic acid was broken due to the reductive milieu environment, resulting in the in situ release of triclosan and death of MRSA. It was noteworthy that no detectable resistance was observed due to the synergistic antibacterial mechanism, and prodrug micelles exhibited remarkable bacterial inhibition and low hemolysis toward red blood cells compared with commercial triclosan and vancomycin.

The combination of different classes of antimicrobial agents such as antimicrobials and AgNPs could afford synergistic effects, resulting in the efficient inhibition of MDR bacteria that is far better than its individual components [143,144]. Webster and coworkers [145] prepared polymer vesicles to co-deliver ampicillin and AgNPs simultaneously in the hydrophilic cavity and hydrophobic membrane, respectively. The AgNPs-embedded polymersomes exhibited potent antibacterial activity against *E. coli* transformed with a gene for ampicillin resistance in a dose-dependent fashion, while the free ampicillin, AgNPs decorated polymersomes without ampicillin and ampicillin loaded polymersomes without AgNPs had no effect on bacterial growth. TEM images in Figure 10 revealed that the interactions between vesicles, AgNPs and bacterial cells might result in the deformation and disruption of bacterial envelopes and consequently result in the death of bacteria. Later, the same group [146] functionalized proline-rich AMP PR-39 on the corona of polymer vesicles with AgNPs embedded in the membrane to combat MRSA with a AMP/AgNPs ratio-dependent behavior. A ratio of AgNPs-to-AMP of 1:5.8 corresponding to 11.6 µg mL^{-1} of AgNPs and 14.3×10^{-6} M of AMP exhibited the best MRSA inhibition activity, demonstrating the potentials of binary or ternary antimicrobial agent co-delivery systems in combating MDR bacteria.

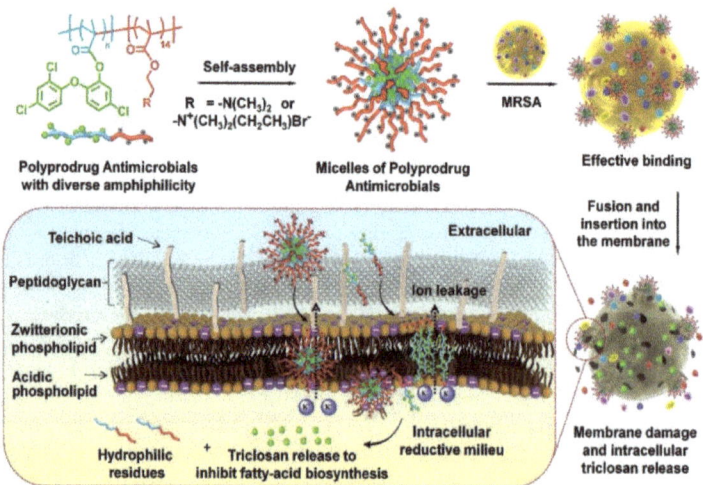

Figure 9. The polyprodrug antimicrobials with optimized hydrophilic–hydrophobic balance for efficiently eradicating MRSA with remarkable membrane damage and concurrent drug release profiles (reproduced with permission from Cao et al. [142], Small; published by Wiley, 2018).

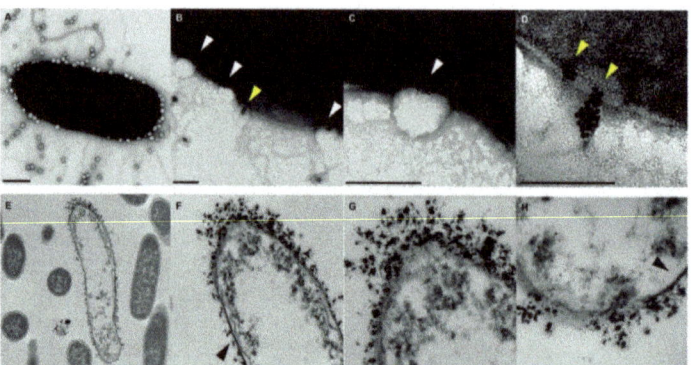

Figure 10. TEM images of bacteria-polymer vesicles interactions. Scale bars are 100 nm for (**A–D,F–H**) and 500 nm for (**E**), respectively. White arrows pointed out the indentation of bacterial cell membrane in regions of AgNPs loaded polymer vesicles; yellow arrows implied the polarization indicative of hydrophobic interactions of AgNPs inside the vesicles; black arrows revealed that the regions of the outer membrane with little AgNPs loaded polymer vesicles contact appeared morphologically normal (reproduced with permission from Geilich et al. [145], Nanoscale; published by Royal Society of Chemistry, 2015).

3.2. Anti-Biofilm

Biofilms are matrix-enclosed communities of bacteria that show increased drug resistance and capability to evade the immune system [47]. It has been widely recognized that bacteria exist in the form of biofilms in many instances, which is hard to eliminate due to the protection of extracellular polymeric substances (EPS), a complex matrix composed of proteins, nucleic acids, phospholipids, polysaccharides, blood components and humic substances produced by bacteria [147]. Therefore, it is difficult for antimicrobials to penetrate the EPS to kill bacteria, resulting in the occurrence of drug resistance. The efficient delivery of antimicrobial agents by polymeric nanomaterials is considered a promising strategy for penetrating the biofilm and delivering antimicrobial agents to the deep end of the matrix to kill pathogens [148–150]. For example, Deoxyribonuclease I functionalized ciprofloxacin-loaded PLGA nanoparticles were prepared to target and disassemble the *P. aeruginosa* biofilm by degrading extracellular DNA that stabilizes the biofilm matrix and released ciprofloxacin inside the biofilm to effectively eliminate *P. aeruginosa*, as reported by Torrents and coworkers [151].

Webster et al. [152] prepared bifunctional polymersomes with methicillin encapsulated in the hydrophilic cavity and superparamagnetic iron oxide nanoparticles (SPIONs) embedded in the membrane, as illustrated in Figure 11. The iron oxide-encapsulated polymersomes (IOPs) penetrated into the *S. epidermidis* biofilm with high efficiency, promoted by external magnetic field. Comparing with individual SPIONs, methicillin and SPION co-encapsulated polymersomes showed enhanced penetration capability up to 20 μm due to the improved relaxivity and magneticity (Figure 11c). Thus, methicillin could be released into the deep end of the biofilm, resulting in the effective eradication of pathogens. The confocal microscopy images and the 3D reconstructions of z-stacks of the bacterial biofilm revealed the capability of IOPs to eradicate biofilms with and without methicillin, as shown in Figure 11d. When there was no methicillin, only bacteria in the bottom layer of the biofilm were killed. On the contrary, all bacteria throughout the biofilm were eliminated by the methicillin loaded IOPs. These organic/inorganic hybrid nanocarriers showed great promise as new weapons for eradicating persistent biofilm or drug-resistant bacteria.

Recently, Du and coworkers [153] reported the treatment of periodontitis by efficiently disrupting biofilms using a dual corona antimicrobials-loaded polymer vesicle with stealthy poly(ethylene oxide) (PEO) corona to penetrate the biofilm and antibacterial polypeptide corona to provide intrinsic antimicrobial activity, as shown in Figure 12. The dual corona polymer vesicles were prepared by the co-assembly of two polymers PCL-*b*-poly(lysine-*stat*-phenylalanine) [PCL-*b*-P(Lys-*stat*-Phe)] and PEO-*b*-PCL with the same hydrophobic biodegradable PCL segment and different hydrophilic chains. Ciprofloxacin could be efficiently encapsulated in the cavity of the vesicles. Due to the protein-repelling ability of PEO, dual corona polymer vesicles penetrated the EPS of the biofilms with high efficiency, while the positive charged P(Lys-*stat*-Phe) allowed the vesicle to target and kill bacteria via electrostatic interaction. In addition, the encapsulated ciprofloxacin could be released as the polymer vesicle reached the deep end of the biofilm, resulting in a reduced dosage of the antimicrobials up to 50% to eradicate *E. coli* or *S. aureus* biofilms. In vivo experiment results demonstrated excellent performance of the dual corona vesicles in reducing dental plaque and alleviating inflammation using a rat periodontitis model.

Despite the strategy of delivering antibiotics to the deep end of biofilms by polymeric nanocarriers in order to reduce dosage and enhance antimicrobial activity, the efficient delivery of non-antibiotic antimicrobial agents including AMPs, AgNPs, photosensitizers and so forth for eliminating biofilms was also widely studied [154–156]. For instance, Haldar et al. [157] fabricated biodegradable polymer-coated AgNPs nanocomposite to eradicate biofilms, which reduced MRSA burden both on the catheter (>99.99% reduction) and in tissues surrounding the catheter (>99.999% reduction) in a mice model. Ji and coworkers [158] developed targeted photodynamic therapy strategies by using a supramolecular delivery system for the treatment of biofilms. The photosensitizer Chlorin e6 was grafted onto α-cyclodextrin, and the targeting group AMP Magainin I was covalently bound with PEG. Taking advantage of supramolecular recognition between α-cyclodextrin and PEG, targeting supramolecular micelles loaded with Chlorin e6 were formed, which exhibited excellent bacterial targeting effects and enhanced biofilm eradication ability against *P. aeruginosa* biofilm and MRSA biofilm. These results proved the versatility and great potential of polymeric nanomaterial-based antimicrobial agent delivery systems for eradicating biofilms.

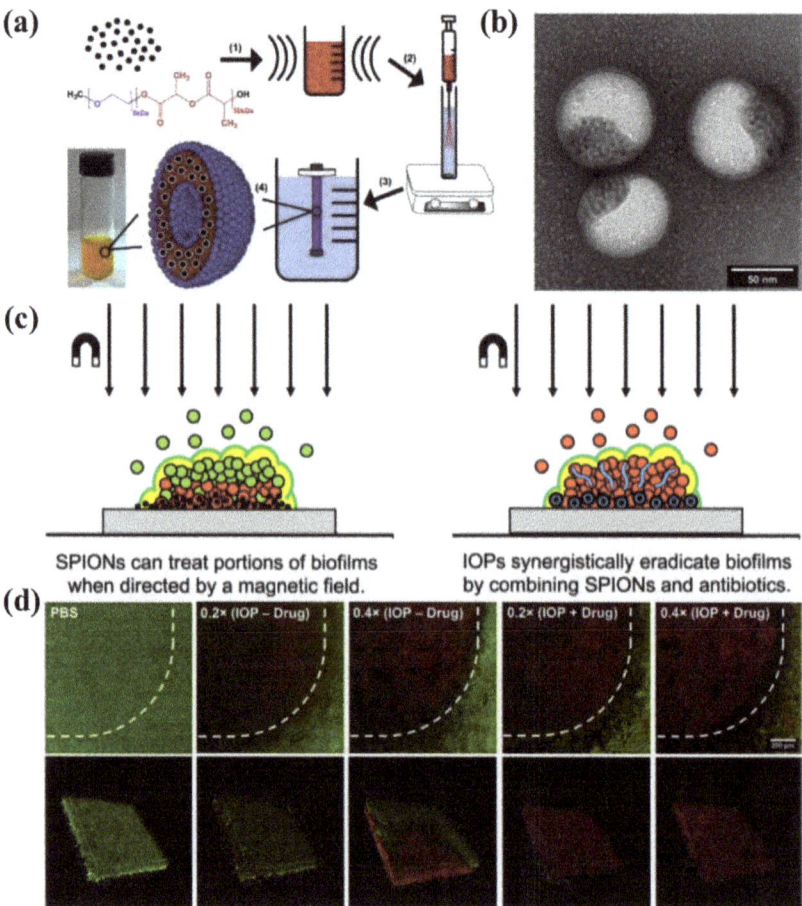

Figure 11. (a) Synthesis of IOPs loaded with SPION and methicillin. (1) 5 nm monodisperse hydrophobic SPIONs are combined with mPEG-PDLLA co-polymer in organic solvent and ultrasonicated to create a uniform suspension. (2) This organic phase is injected through an atomizer into an actively stirring aqueous phase containing PBS and methicillin. (3) The mixture is dialyzed against pure PBS to remove the organic solvent and unencapsulated drug to yield (4) highly stable polymersome solution. (b) TEM image of SPIONs loaded polymersomes. (c) Magnetic field induced treatment of biofilm using SPIONs and/or antimicrobials. (d) Confocal microscopy images of LIVE/DEAD staining of *S. epidermidis* biofilms treated with IOPs with an external magnetic field (reproduced with permission from Geilich et al. [152], Biomaterials; published by Elsevier, 2017).

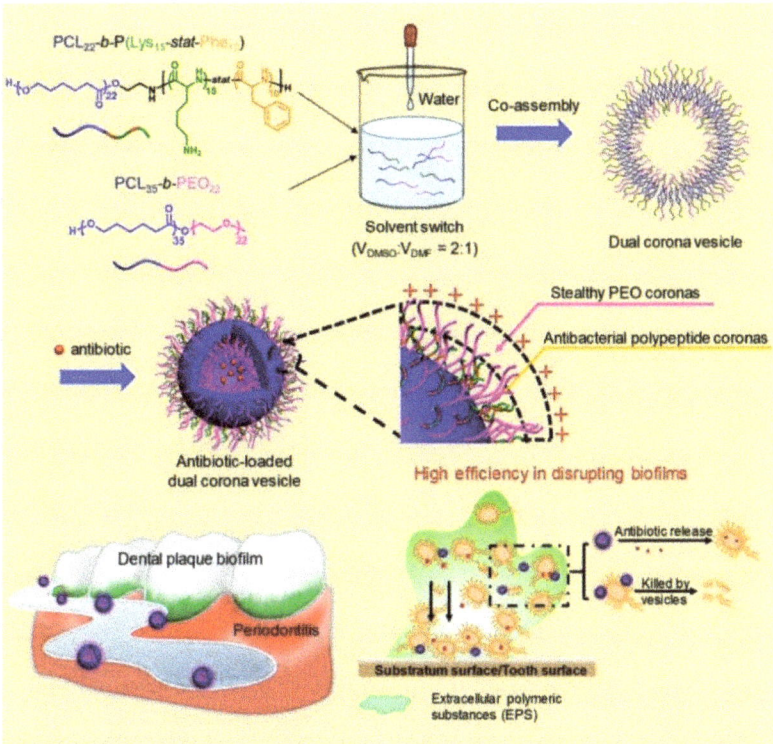

Figure 12. Schematic model showing the treatment of periodontitis by efficiently disrupting biofilms via antimicrobials-loaded multifunctional dual corona vesicles (reproduced with permission from Xi et al. [153], ACS Nano; published by American Chemical Society, 2019).

3.3. Wound Healing

Wound infections induced by pathogens have become one of the main problems in wound care management systems, which impede the healing process and may result in life threatening complications. One of the approaches for treating wound infection is the use of wound dressings with antibacterial agents possessing broad-spectrum antimicrobial activity [159]. Typically, the moisture environment provided by the dressing has been shown to promote ulcer healing and to reduce pain experienced by patients [160]. Moreover, there are other requirements for wound dressings such as separating the wound with external environments and providing good breathability to promote wound healing. Polymeric nanomaterial-based delivery systems have shown considerable potentials in wound healing, especially polymer nanofibers and hydrogels [99,161]. For example, Lakshminarayanan et al. [162] prepared polydopamine crosslinked polyhydroxy antimicrobials loaded gelatin nanofiber mats for advanced wound dressings with long-term antimicrobial activity up to 20 days. The morphology of the nanofiber mats was retained for 1 month in an aqueous environment and showed comparable wound closure compared to commercially available silver-based dressings. Cai and coworkers [163] prepared composite hydrogels embedded with copper nanoparticles that could effectively convert NIR laser irradiation energy into localized heat for photothermal therapy. The synergistic effect of photothermal performance and rapid release of copper ions upon laser irradiation were responsible for excellent antimicrobial activity, reduced inflammatory response and promoted angiogenesis ability.

Antimicrobial agents including AMPs [49], antibiotics [164], AgNPs [165], metal oxide such as ZnO [166], photothermal sensitizers including porphyrin [167] and heavy metal ions [163] are usually used to improve the antimicrobial activity of polymeric wound dressings by covalent linkage, physical interaction or encapsulation. For example, Liu et al. [168] decorated chloramine on the surface of chitosan films by electrostatic interaction to heal MRSA infected wounds. Zhou and coworkers [167] prepared porphyrin containing alternating copolymer vesicles for the disinfection of drug-resistant bacteria infected wounds via photothermal effect. Fahimirad et al. [169] loaded recombinant LL37 AMP into chitosan nanoparticles for the elimination of MRSA infection during wound healing process with ultrahigh encapsulation efficiency of 78.52% and improved the activity and stability of LL37 AMP under thermal, salts and acidic pH treatments. Guo et al. [170] prepared injectable antimicrobial conductive quaternized chitosan hydrogels by loading graphene oxide via covalent bond for drug resistant bacterial disinfection and infectious wound healing, and the hybrid hydrogels showed excellent performance in the treatment of MRSA infected full-thickness defect mouse model.

Very recently, polymer vesicles loaded with antimicrobials have been explored as dressings in promoting wound healing by spraying onto wounds [167,171–173]. Du and coworkers [173] reported bifunctional polymer vesicles loaded with antimicrobials and antioxidant for healing infected diabetic wounds, as presented in Figure 13. As one of the chronically infected wounds, the diabetic wounds are difficult to heal due to high ROS concentration and recurrent infections, resulting in the occurrence of diabetic ulcers and chronic diabetic complications with very high mortality rate. Therefore, scavenging ROS is very important in the treatment of diabetic wounds. In this study, well-dispersed ceria nanoparticles were deposited on the membrane of ciprofloxacin-loaded polymer vesicles (CIP-Ceria-PVs). The CIP-Ceria-PVs could inhibit peroxide free radicals up to 50% at extremely low cerium concentrations of 1.25 µg mL^{-1}, protecting normal L02 cells from the damage of peroxide free radicals. Moreover, CIP-Ceria-PVs exhibited enhanced antimicrobial activity compared with free ciprofloxacin due to scavenging ROS. In vivo studies in Figure 13b demonstrated the excellent wound healing capability of CIP-Ceria-PVs, and the diabetic wound was completely healed within 14 days. At the same time, they developed a H$_2$S delivery polymer vesicle, which was capable of long-term H$_2$S generation to promote the proliferation, migration of epidermal and endothelial cells and angiogenesis, accelerating the complete healing of diabetic wounds [172].

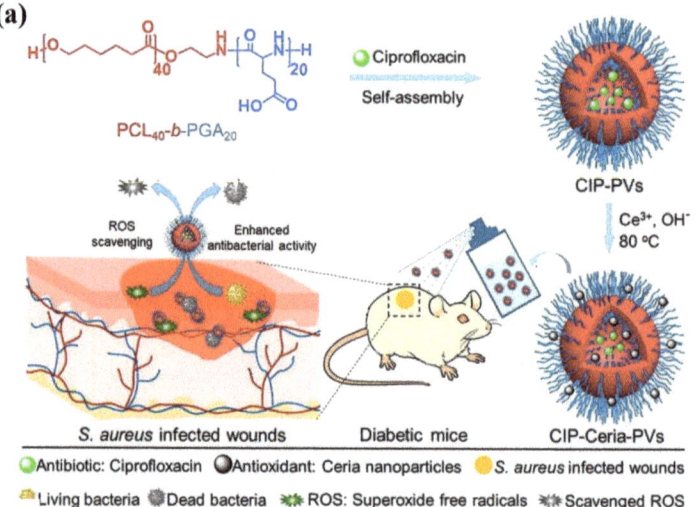

Figure 13. Cont.

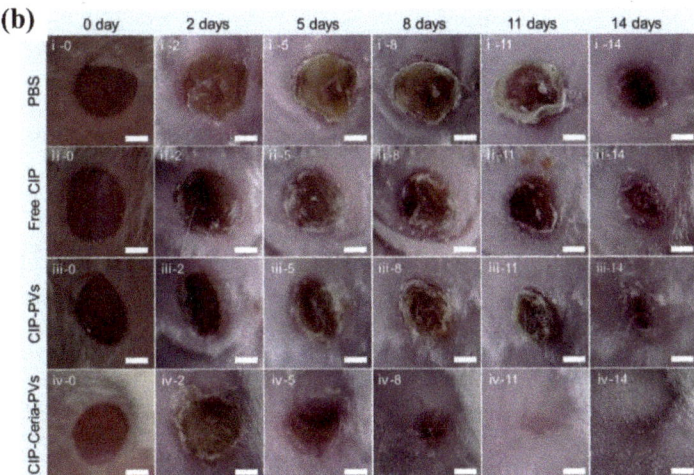

Figure 13. (a) Illustration of the preparation of CIP-Ceria-PVs and the combined antioxidant-antimicrobials treatment of infected diabetic wounds. (b) Digital images of infected diabetic wounds at different time intervals under treatment. Scale bar: 2 cm (reproduced with permission from Wang et al. [173], ACS Nano; published by American Chemical Society, 2021).

3.4. Tissue Engineering

The regeneration of adult tissue following an injury or degeneration is quite a limited process. Usually, the injury site is vulnerable to bacterial infections, which causes complications and delay of the regeneration of tissues [174]. Therefore, the prerequisite of tissue regeneration is to eliminate localized bacterial infections, followed by the delivery of bioactive molecules such as growth factor to the defected tissues. Antimicrobial polymer coatings on the surface of implants can provide appropriate biointerfaces to promote the regeneration of tissues. For instance, ZnO nanoparticles embedded PLA was dip coated on magnesium alloy, which helped to control the degradation and increase antibacterial activity [175]. Suteewong et al. [176] deposited polymethylmethacrylate (PMMA)/chitosan-silver hybrid nanoparticles on rubber substrate, which exhibited enhanced antibacterial activity toward *E. coli* and *S. aureus* and reduced cytotoxicity to L-929 fibroblast cells, demonstrating the potential of this hybrid nanoparticle coating at soft substrates. In addition, antimicrobial agents loaded with polymer nanomaterials can be used as bioadhesives to repair damaged soft tissues. Gu and coworkers [177] developed fast and high strength bioadhesives based on polysaccharides and peptide dendrimers with inherent hemostatic ability and antibacterial properties. Moreover, the bioadhesive showed a remarkable 5-fold increase in adhesion strength comparing with commercial bioadhesive Coseal.

Biocompatible polymeric nanoparticles have been investigated as delivery vehicles for various tissue engineering applications [178]. For example, Du and coworkers [179] prepared antibacterial peptide-mimetic alternating copolymers (PMACs) vesicles loaded with growth factor for bone regeneration. They designed a series of PMACs with different repeating units, and the PMAC with a repeating unit of 14 exhibited the best antibacterial activity against both *E. coli* and *S. aureus* with ultralow MICs of 8.0 μg mL^{-1}. After self-assembling into vesicles in pure water, the antimicrobial activity of the vesicles was well-preserved. Growth factor could be encapsulated in antimicrobial vesicles and released during the long-term antibacterial process to promote the regeneration of bone with a 20 mm defect model in rabbits. Micro-CT, bone mineral content and BMD were used to evaluate the repair of bone defects with scaffolds at 4 weeks and 6 weeks after implantation. After 6 weeks, the defect in the rabbit bone was completely repaired, demonstrating the excellent bone repair capability of antimicrobial growth factor-loaded vesicles.

3.5. Anticancer

The anticancer application of antimicrobial agents is an attracting field since cancers are often accompanied by inflammation, and the drug resistance of cancer cells is becoming increasingly concerning [180]. Theoretically, antimicrobial agents that kill bacteria via non-selective behaviors such as damage of the cell membrane [181], elevating temperature [182] and induced degeneration of proteins and genetic materials [183] can also kill cancer cells. For instance, Shim et al. [183] prepared AgNPs loaded chitosan-alginate composite, exhibiting broad-spectrum antimicrobial activity and high toxicity toward breast cancer cell line MDA-MB-231; Jothivenkatachalam and coworkers [184] fabricated chitosan-copper nanocomposite for the inhibition of various microorganisms and A549 cancer cells by photocatalytic effect. In addition, AMPs with specific sequences and proper positive charge densities have shown anticancer and antiviral activities, such as cecropin A and B, magainins, melittin, defensins, lactoferricin and so forth, as summarized by Hoskin's and Franco's group, respectively [181,185]. However, the AMPs are vulnerable to enzymes and can easily cause immune responses; thus, the delivery system is critical for in vivo applications of AMPs. Hazekawa et al. [186] conjugated antimicrobial human peptide, LL-37 peptide fragment analog, with a PLGA copolymer. The formed micellar system significantly improved the permeability of the peptide to cancer cells, and the proliferation, migration and invasion in various cancer cell lines were effectively exhibited. The intracellular delivery of peptides by polymer carriers in oncology applications has been summarized by Pun et al. very recently [187].

Another strategy for eliminating cancer cells using antimicrobial delivery systems is the co-delivery of antimicrobial and anticancer agents simultaneously or loading anticancer drugs with antimicrobial carriers [188,189]. For instance, Du and coworkers [190] proposed the concept of "armed" carrier to co-deliver anticancer and antiepileptic drugs with antibacterial polypeptide-grafted chitosan-based nanocapsules. Mahkam et al. [191] designed pH-responsive antibacterial clay/polymer nanocomposite as a carrier to deliver anticancer drug methotrexate and antibacterial agent ciprofloxacin with an ultrahigh efficiency of >90%, which showed enhanced antimicrobial and anticancer activity compared with free methotrexate and ciprofloxacin, demonstrating the potential of antibacterial nanocarriers in cancer therapy. Lei and coworkers [192] developed a class of multifunctional polymeric hybrid micelles (PHM) with high antibacterial activity for the efficient delivery of siRNA to cancer cells, as illustrated in Figure 14. The PHM was prepared by the co-assembly of EHP-FA and EHE, for which their structures were presented in Figure 14A. Due to the existence of positively charged poly(ethylene imine) (PEI) and poly-ε-L-lysine (EPL), the PHM showed high antibacterial activity against *S. aureus* in vitro and in vivo. On the contrary, PHM exhibited good hemocompatibility and lower cytotoxicity toward A549, HeLa, HepG2 and C2C12 cells benefiting from the shield effect of PEG. siRNA could be complexed onto PHM by electrostatic interaction, and PHM with folic acid decorated on the surface could effectively target FA receptor overexpressed HeLa cells and other low-expressed cancer cells, resulting in the targeted delivery of siRNA. In vitro experiments revealed that the PHM showed a high p65 gene silencing efficiency above 90% in various cancer cells, which is significantly higher than EHP-FA and EHE, demonstrating the potential of PHM as a safe and effective siRNA vector with high antibacterial activity for multifunctional gene therapy.

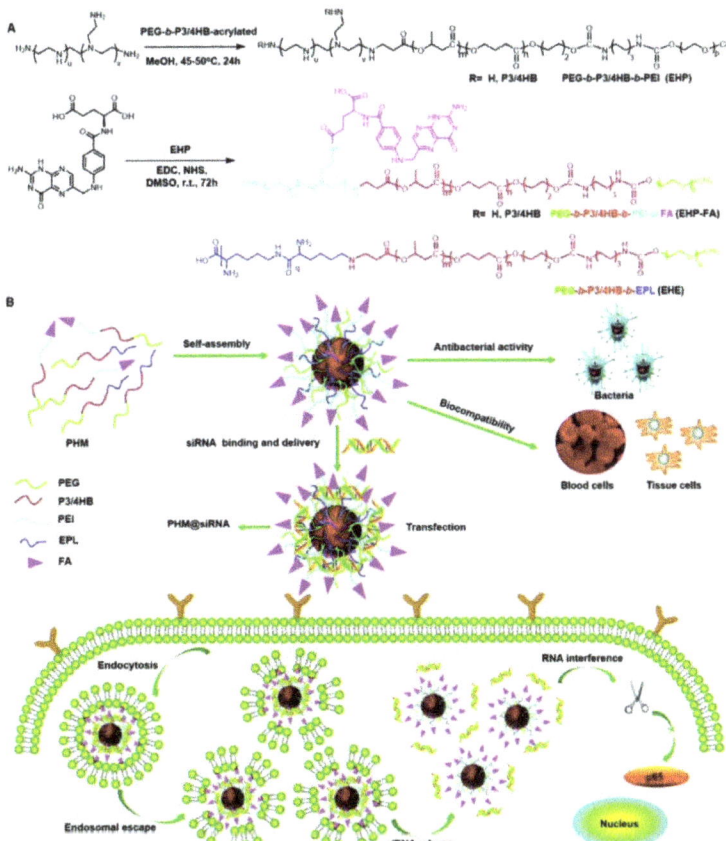

Figure 14. Scheme showing the synthesis and potential application of the PHM copolymer in siRNA delivery. (**A**) EHP and EHP-FA were synthesized by Michael addition and esterification reaction, respectively; PHM micelles were prepared by mixing EHP-FA and EHE copolymer; (**B**) schematic illustration of the application of PHM in siRNA delivery (reproduced with permission from Zhou et al. [192], Nanoscale; published by Royal Society of Chemistry, 2018).

4. Conclusions and Future Perspectives

In summary, the recent progress of efficient loading, delivery and controlled release of antimicrobial agents in vivo or in vitro by polymeric nanomaterial-based delivery systems have been concluded. A large diversity of antimicrobial agents including antibiotics, AMPs, AgNPs, metal nanoparticles, metal oxides, gases, photosensitizers and so forth could be loaded and delivered by polymeric nanomaterials either by physical interactions or covalent bonding while maintaining the intrinsic antimicrobial activity of these antimicrobial agents. In order to fit the physiochemical properties of different kinds of antimicrobial agents to construct highly efficient delivery systems with superiorities such as high loading content and efficiency, good stability and on demand release, polymeric nanomaterials with different chemical compositions and nanostructures including micelles, vesicles, dendrimers, nanofibers and nanogels etc. are developed. Benefiting from the versatility of polymeric nanomaterials, the antimicrobial agent delivery systems have shown significant potentials in a wide variety of biomedical applications, such as combating MDR bacteria, anti-biofilm, wound healing, tissue engineering and anticancer. Despite the rapid development of this field, the in vivo and intracellular delivery of antimicrobial agents is still in its early stage, and there are numerous challenges that should be considered in the future, which may bring new opportunities in the biomedical applications of antimicrobial agent-based delivery systems.

Non-covalent interactions such as hydrogen bonding, π-π stacking and coordination should be introduced to enhance the interactions between antimicrobial agents and the polymeric nanocarriers to increase loading content and efficiency. The strong interactions could also prevent the leakage of cargoes before reaching the target and enhance the stability of the delivery system. Modulation of the properties of different kinds of antimicrobial agents and the structural features of carriers may maximize the efficiency of the loaded antimicrobial agents. Targeting the infected area and high selectivity toward bacteria rather than mammalian cells should always be considered, which is very important for the reduction in side effects and drug resistance. Moreover, external stimuli, especially non-invasive stimuli-triggered release of loaded antimicrobial agents (in other words, the switchable antimicrobial activity of the delivery system), are also helpful for the reduction in side effects and drug resistance. However, the spatial and temporal sensitivity of the stimuli-triggered response still needs to be improved to meet practical applications. Furthermore, the generations of antimicrobial active species such as ROS or change of the micro-circumstance including elevating temperature triggered by stimuli or chemicals secreted by bacteria are also effective methods for eliminating bacteria without the generation of drug resistance. Regardless of the generation of drug resistance, taking advantage of the synergistic effect of multiple antibacterial agents is an effective strategy for eradicating MDR bacteria. In addition, the combination of antibacteria and anticancer simultaneously will be of great significance in cancer therapy.

The biosafety of polymeric nanomaterial-based delivery systems has always been selectively ignored in previous studies. Although many biodegradable polymers have been used, the cytotoxicity and hemolytic activity of the polymeric carriers, especially those with positively charged surfaces, should be evaluated systematically. In addition, the word "biocompatibility" is a comprehensive evaluation of in vivo delivery systems. If we claim that the carrier is biocompatible, numerous parameters should be evaluated more than cytotoxicity and hemolytic activity. The in vivo delivery of antimicrobial agents has been reported in many studies. However, very few investigated the stability of the delivery system in physiological conditions and the interactions between the carriers and proteins, salts, glucose, fatty acids, antigens and so forth. Moreover, the immune response of the delivery systems is also hardly investigated. Considering the complexity of the physiological condition, it is necessary to reveal the stability and true circulation behavior of the delivery systems in vivo and not only borrowing the results of in vitro experiments. Furthermore, the full life-cycle assessment of polymeric carriers should be conducted to explore blood circulation behavior, biodistribution, metabolism and organic accumulations, etc., which will be very valuable for the instructive design of polymer carriers to promote the clinical applications of polymeric nanomaterials-based antimicrobial delivery systems.

Author Contributions: Conceptualization, supervision and writing—review and editing, H.S.; resources and visualization, Y.W.; writing—original draft preparation, H.S. and Y.W. All authors have read and agreed to the published version of the manuscript.

Funding: This research was funded by Natural Science Foundation of Ningxia, grant number 2020AAC03003 and 2021AAC03026.

Institutional Review Board Statement: Not applicable.

Informed Consent Statement: Not applicable.

Acknowledgments: This work was supported by the Natural Science Foundation of Ningxia (2020AAC03003 and 2021AAC03026). H.S. thanks the Ningxia Youth Talent Support Project of Science and Technology and Young Scholars of Western China of CAS.

Conflicts of Interest: The authors declare no conflict of interest.

References

1. Fournier, P.-E.; Drancourt, M.; Colson, P.; Rolain, J.-M.; La Scola, B.; Raoult, D. Modern clinical microbiology: New challenges and solutions. *Nat. Rev. Microbiol.* **2013**, *11*, 574–585. [CrossRef]
2. Ghosh, C.; Sarkar, P.; Issa, R.; Haldar, J. Alternatives to Conventional Antibiotics in the Era of Antimicrobial Resistance. *Trends Microbiol.* **2019**, *27*, 323–338. [CrossRef]
3. Monserrat-Martinez, A.; Gambin, Y.; Sierecki, E. Thinking Outside the Bug: Molecular Targets and Strategies to Overcome Antibiotic Resistance. *Int. J. Mol. Sci.* **2019**, *20*, 1255. [CrossRef]
4. Faya, M.; Kalhapure, R.S.; Kumalo, H.M.; Waddad, A.Y.; Omolo, C.; Govender, T. Conjugates and nano-delivery of antimicrobial peptides for enhancing therapeutic activity. *J. Drug Deliv. Sci. Technol.* **2018**, *44*, 153–171. [CrossRef]
5. Martin-Serrano, A.; Gomez, R.; Ortega, P.; Javier de la Mata, F. Nanosystems as Vehicles for the Delivery of Antimicrobial Peptides (AMPs). *Pharmaceutics* **2019**, *11*, 448. [CrossRef]
6. Cui, Z.; Luo, Q.; Bannon, M.S.; Gray, V.P.; Bloom, T.G.; Clore, M.F.; Hughes, M.A.; Crawford, M.A.; Letteri, R.A. Molecular engineering of antimicrobial peptide (AMP)-polymer conjugates. *Biomater. Sci.* **2021**, *9*, 5069–5091. [CrossRef]
7. Chung, I.-M.; Park, I.; Seung-Hyun, K.; Thiruvengadam, M.; Rajakumar, G. Plant-Mediated Synthesis of Silver Nanoparticles: Their Characteristic Properties and Therapeutic Applications. *Nanoscale Res. Lett.* **2016**, *11*, 40. [CrossRef]
8. Tang, S.; Zheng, J. Antibacterial Activity of Silver Nanoparticles: Structural Effects. *Adv. Healthc. Mater.* **2018**, *7*, 1701503. [CrossRef] [PubMed]
9. Yin, I.X.; Zhang, J.; Zhao, I.S.; Mei, M.L.; Li, Q.; Chu, C.H. The Antibacterial Mechanism of Silver Nanoparticles and Its Application in Dentistry. *Int. J. Nanomed.* **2020**, *15*, 2555–2562. [CrossRef]
10. Chen, H.; Wang, R.; Zhang, J.; Hua, H.; Zhu, M. Synthesis of core-shell structured ZnO@m-SiO$_2$ with excellent reinforcing effect and antimicrobial activity for dental resin composites. *Dent. Mater.* **2018**, *34*, 1846–1855. [CrossRef]
11. Rodrigues, G.R.; Lopez-Abarrategui, C.; de la Serna Gomez, I.; Dias, S.C.; Otero-Gonzalez, A.J.; Franco, O.L. Antimicrobial magnetic nanoparticles based-therapies for controlling infectious diseases. *Int. J. Pharm.* **2019**, *555*, 356–367. [CrossRef] [PubMed]
12. Ziental, D.; Czarczynska-Goslinska, B.; Mlynarczyk, D.T.; Glowacka-Sobotta, A.; Stanisz, B.; Goslinski, T.; Sobotta, L. Titanium Dioxide Nanoparticles: Prospects and Applications in Medicine. *Nanomaterials* **2020**, *10*, 387. [CrossRef] [PubMed]
13. Zhen, J.-B.; Kang, P.-W.; Zhao, M.-H.; Yang, K.-W. Silver Nanoparticle Conjugated Star PCL-b-AMPs Copolymer as Nanocomposite Exhibits Efficient Antibacterial Properties. *Bioconjugate Chem.* **2020**, *31*, 51–63. [CrossRef] [PubMed]
14. Chen, H.; Battalapalli, D.; Draz, M.S.; Zhang, P.; Ruan, Z. The application of cell-penetrating-peptides in antibacterial agents. *Curr. Med. Chem.* **2021**, *28*, 5896–5925. [CrossRef]
15. Sun, H.; Hong, Y.; Xi, Y.; Zou, Y.; Gao, J.; Du, J. Synthesis, Self-Assembly, and Biomedical Applications of Antimicrobial Peptide-Polymer Conjugates. *Biomacromolecules* **2018**, *19*, 1701–1720. [CrossRef]
16. Sun, H.; Wang, Y.; Song, J. Polymer Vesicles for Antimicrobial Applications. *Polymers* **2021**, *13*, 2903. [CrossRef] [PubMed]
17. Duncan, M.J.; Wheatley, P.S.; Coghill, E.M.; Vornholt, S.M.; Warrender, S.J.; Megson, I.L.; Morris, R.E. Antibacterial efficacy from NO-releasing MOF-polymer films. *Mater. Adv.* **2020**, *1*, 2509–2519. [CrossRef]
18. Jin, G.; Gao, Z.; Liu, Y.; Zhao, J.; Ou, H.; Xu, F.; Ding, D. Polymeric Nitric Oxide Delivery Nanoplatforms for Treating Cancer, Cardiovascular Diseases, and Infection. *Adv. Healthc. Mater.* **2021**, *10*, 2001550. [CrossRef] [PubMed]
19. Simonson, A.W.; Aronson, M.R.; Medina, S.H. Supramolecular Peptide Assemblies as Antimicrobial Scaffolds. *Molecules* **2020**, *25*, 2751. [CrossRef] [PubMed]
20. Mahata, D.; Mandal, S.M. Molecular self-assembly of copolymer from renewable phenols: New class of antimicrobial ointment base. *J. Biomater. Sci. Polym. Ed.* **2018**, *29*, 2187–2200. [CrossRef] [PubMed]
21. Krol, A.; Pomastowski, P.; Rafinska, K.; Railean-Plugaru, V.; Buszewski, B. Zinc oxide nanoparticles: Synthesis, antiseptic activity and toxicity mechanism. *Adv. Colloid Interface Sci.* **2017**, *249*, 37–52. [CrossRef]
22. Shi, L.; Chen, J.; Teng, L.; Wang, L.; Zhu, G.; Liu, S.; Luo, Z.; Shi, X.; Wang, Y.; Ren, L. The Antibacterial Applications of Graphene and Its Derivatives. *Small* **2016**, *12*, 4165–4184. [CrossRef]
23. Han, W.; Wu, Z.; Li, Y.; Wang, Y. Graphene family nanomaterials (GFNs)—Promising materials for antimicrobial coating and film: A review. *Chem. Eng. J.* **2019**, *358*, 1022–1037. [CrossRef]
24. Jiang, L.; Gan, C.R.R.; Gao, J.; Loh, X.J. A Perspective on the Trends and Challenges Facing Porphyrin-Based Anti-Microbial Materials. *Small* **2016**, *12*, 3609–3644. [CrossRef] [PubMed]
25. Engler, A.C.; Wiradharma, N.; Ong, Z.Y.; Coady, D.J.; Hedrick, J.L.; Yang, Y.-Y. Emerging trends in macromolecular antimicrobials to fight multi-drug-resistant infections. *Nano Today* **2012**, *7*, 201–222. [CrossRef]
26. Richter, A.P.; Brown, J.S.; Bharti, B.; Wang, A.; Gangwal, S.; Houck, K.; Hubal, E.A.C.; Paunov, V.N.; Stoyanov, S.D.; Velev, O.D. An environmentally benign antimicrobial nanoparticle based on a silver-infused lignin core. *Nat. Nanotechnol.* **2015**, *10*, 817–823. [CrossRef]
27. Boge, L.; Hallstensson, K.; Ringstad, L.; Johansson, J.; Andersson, T.; Davoudi, M.; Larsson, P.T.; Mahlapuu, M.; Hakansson, J.; Andersson, M. Cubosomes for topical delivery of the antimicrobial peptide LL-37. *Eur. J. Pharm. Biopharm.* **2019**, *134*, 60–67. [CrossRef] [PubMed]
28. Zhang, L.; Pornpattananangkul, D.; Hu, C.M.J.; Huang, C.M. Development of Nanoparticles for Antimicrobial Drug Delivery. *Curr. Med. Chem.* **2010**, *17*, 585–594. [CrossRef]
29. Halbus, A.F.; Horozov, T.S.; Paunov, V.N. Colloid particle formulations for antimicrobial applications. *Adv. Colloid Interface Sci.* **2017**, *249*, 134–148. [CrossRef]

30. Gao, W.; Chen, Y.; Zhang, Y.; Zhang, Q.; Zhang, L. Nanoparticle-based local antimicrobial drug delivery. *Adv. Drug Deliv. Rev.* **2018**, *127*, 46–57. [CrossRef]
31. Kalhapure, R.S.; Suleman, N.; Mocktar, C.; Seedat, N.; Govender, T. Nanoengineered Drug Delivery Systems for Enhancing Antibiotic Therapy. *J. Pharm. Sci.* **2015**, *104*, 872–905. [CrossRef] [PubMed]
32. Yan, Y.; Zhang, J.; Ren, L.; Tang, C. Metal-containing and related polymers for biomedical applications. *Chem. Soc. Rev.* **2016**, *45*, 5232–5263. [CrossRef] [PubMed]
33. Chan, C.-F.; Huang, K.-S.; Lee, M.-Y.; Yang, C.-H.; Wang, C.-Y.; Lin, Y.-S. Applications of Nanoparticles for Antimicrobial Activity and Drug Delivery. *Curr. Org. Chem.* **2014**, *18*, 204–215. [CrossRef]
34. Zazo, H.; Colino, C.I.; Lanao, J.M. Current applications of nanoparticles in infectious diseases. *J. Control. Release* **2016**, *224*, 86–102. [CrossRef]
35. Lu, H.; Fan, L.; Liu, Q.; Wei, J.; Ren, T.; Du, J. Preparation of water-dispersible silver-decorated polymer vesicles and micelles with excellent antibacterial efficacy. *Polym. Chem.* **2012**, *3*, 2217–2227. [CrossRef]
36. Basnet, P.; Skalko-Basnet, N. Nanodelivery Systems for Improved Topical Antimicrobial Therapy. *Curr. Pharm. Des.* **2013**, *19*, 7237–7243. [CrossRef]
37. Sun, H.; Fan, L.; Zou, K.; Zhu, H.; Du, J. Decoration of homopolymer vesicles by antibacterial ultrafine silver nanoparticles. *RSC Adv.* **2014**, *4*, 41331–41335. [CrossRef]
38. Walvekar, P.; Gannimani, R.; Salih, M.; Makhathini, S.; Mocktar, C.; Govender, T. Self-assembled oleylamine grafted hyaluronic acid polymersomes for delivery of vancomycin against methicillin resistant Staphylococcus aureus (MRSA). *Colloids Surf. B* **2019**, *182*, 110388. [CrossRef] [PubMed]
39. Lim, Y.H.; Tiemann, K.M.; Heo, G.S.; Wagers, P.O.; Rezenom, Y.H.; Zhang, S.; Zhang, F.; Youngs, W.J.; Hunstad, D.A.; Wooley, K.L. Preparation and In Vitro Antimicrobial Activity of Silver-Bearing Degradable Polymeric Nanoparticles of Polyphosphoester-block-Poly(L-lactide). *ACS Nano* **2015**, *9*, 1995–2008. [CrossRef] [PubMed]
40. Zare, E.N.; Makvandi, P.; Ashtari, B.; Rossi, F.; Motahari, A.; Perale, G. Progress in Conductive Polyaniline-Based Nanocomposites for Biomedical Applications: A Review. *J. Med. Chem.* **2020**, *63*, 1–22. [CrossRef] [PubMed]
41. Mikhalevich, V.; Craciun, I.; Kyropoulou, M.; Palivan, C.G.; Meier, W. Amphiphilic Peptide Self-Assembly: Expansion to Hybrid Materials. *Biomacromolecules* **2017**, *18*, 3471–3480. [CrossRef]
42. Kong, H.; Jang, J. Antibacterial properties of novel poly(methyl methacrylate) nanofiber containing silver nanoparticles. *Langmuir* **2008**, *24*, 2051–2056. [CrossRef]
43. Quiros, J.; Boltes, K.; Aguado, S.; Guzman de Villoria, R.; Jose Vilatela, J.; Rosal, R. Antimicrobial metal-organic frameworks incorporated into electrospun fibers. *Chem. Eng. J.* **2015**, *262*, 189–197. [CrossRef]
44. Gallis, D.F.S.; Butler, K.S.; Agola, J.O.; Pearce, C.J.; McBride, A.A. Antibacterial Countermeasures via Metal-Organic Framework Supported Sustained Therapeutic Release. *ACS Appl. Mater. Interfaces* **2019**, *11*, 7782–7791. [CrossRef] [PubMed]
45. Kaur, N.; Tiwari, P.; Kapoor, K.S.; Saini, A.K.; Sharma, V.; Mobin, S.M. Metal-organic framework based antibiotic release and antimicrobial response: An overview. *Crystengcomm* **2020**, *22*, 7513–7527. [CrossRef]
46. Yang, J.; Yang, Y.-W. Metal-Organic Frameworks for Biomedical Applications. *Small* **2020**, *16*, 1906846. [CrossRef] [PubMed]
47. Kasimanickam, R.K.; Ranjan, A.; Asokan, G.V.; Kasimanickam, V.R.; Kastelic, J.P. Prevention and treatment of biofilms by hybrid- and nanotechnologies. *Int. J. Nanomed.* **2013**, *8*, 2809–2819. [CrossRef]
48. Bai, M.; Li, C.; Cui, H.; Lin, L. Preparation of self-assembling Litsea cubeba essential oil/ diphenylalanine peptide micro/nanotubes with enhanced antibacterial properties against Staphylococcus aureus biofilm. *LWT—Food Sci. Technol.* **2021**, *146*, 111394. [CrossRef]
49. Patrulea, V.; Borchard, G.; Jordan, O. An Update on Antimicrobial Peptides (AMPs) and Their Delivery Strategies for Wound Infections. *Pharmaceutics* **2020**, *12*, 840. [CrossRef]
50. Drayton, M.; Kizhakkedathu, J.N.; Straus, S.K. Towards Robust Delivery of Antimicrobial Peptides to Combat Bacterial Resistance. *Molecules* **2020**, *25*, 3048. [CrossRef] [PubMed]
51. Du, J.; Sun, H. Polymer/TiO$_2$ hybrid vesicles for excellent UV screening and effective encapsulation of antioxidant agents. *ACS Appl. Mater. Interfaces* **2014**, *6*, 13535–13541. [CrossRef] [PubMed]
52. Xiao, Y.; Sun, H.; Du, J. Sugar-Breathing Glycopolymersomes for Regulating Glucose Level. *J. Am. Chem. Soc.* **2017**, *139*, 7640–7647. [CrossRef] [PubMed]
53. Sun, H.; Jiang, J.; Xiao, Y.; Du, J. Efficient Removal of Polycyclic Aromatic Hydrocarbons, Dyes, and Heavy Metal Ions by a Homopolymer Vesicle. *ACS Appl. Mater. Interfaces* **2018**, *10*, 713–722. [CrossRef] [PubMed]
54. Warren, N.J.; Armes, S.P. Polymerization-Induced Self-Assembly of Block Copolymer Nano-objects via RAFT Aqueous Dispersion Polymerization. *J. Am. Chem. Soc.* **2014**, *136*, 10174–10185. [CrossRef]
55. Qiu, H.; Hudson, Z.M.; Winnik, M.A.; Manners, I. Multidimensional hierarchical self-assembly of amphiphilic cylindrical block comicelles. *Science* **2015**, *347*, 1329–1332. [CrossRef] [PubMed]
56. Sun, H.; Du, J. Intramolecular Cyclization-Induced Crystallization-Driven Self-Assembly of an Amorphous Poly(amic acid). *Macromolecules* **2020**, *53*, 11033–11039. [CrossRef]
57. Shah, A.; Shahzad, S.; Munir, A.; Nadagouda, M.N.; Khan, G.S.; Shams, D.F.; Dionysiou, D.D.; Rana, U.A. Micelles as Soil and Water Decontamination Agents. *Chem. Rev.* **2016**, 6042–6074. [CrossRef]
58. Sun, H.; Du, J. Plasmonic vesicles with tailored collective properties. *Nanoscale* **2018**, *10*, 17354–17361. [CrossRef]

59. Sun, H.; Zhu, Y.; Yang, B.; Wang, Y.; Wu, Y.; Du, J. Template-free fabrication of nitrogen-doped hollow carbon spheres for high-performance supercapacitors based on a scalable homopolymer vesicle. *J. Mater. Chem. A* **2016**, *4*, 12088–12097. [CrossRef]
60. Wang, F.; Xiao, J.; Chen, S.; Sun, H.; Yang, B.; Jiang, J.; Zhou, X.; Du, J. Polymer Vesicles: Modular Platforms for Cancer Theranostics. *Adv. Mater.* **2018**, *30*, e1705674. [CrossRef] [PubMed]
61. Owen, S.C.; Chan, D.P.Y.; Shoichet, M.S. Polymeric micelle stability. *Nano Today* **2012**, *7*, 53–65. [CrossRef]
62. Cabral, H.; Miyata, K.; Osada, K.; Kataoka, K. Block Copolymer Micelles in Nanomedicine Applications. *Chem. Rev.* **2018**, *118*, 6844–6892. [CrossRef] [PubMed]
63. Zhu, Y.; Yang, B.; Chen, S.; Du, J. Polymer vesicles: Mechanism, preparation, application, and responsive behavior. *Prog. Polym. Sci.* **2017**, *64*, 1–22. [CrossRef]
64. Otrin, L.; Witkowska, A.; Marusic, N.; Zhao, Z.; Lira, R.B.; Kyrilis, F.L.; Hamdi, F.; Ivanov, I.; Lipowsky, R.; Kastritis, P.L.; et al. En route to dynamic life processes by SNARE-mediated fusion of polymer and hybrid membranes. *Nat. Commun.* **2021**, *12*, 4972. [CrossRef] [PubMed]
65. Zhou, X.; Cornel, E.J.; Fan, Z.; He, S.; Du, J. Bone-Targeting Polymer Vesicles for Effective Therapy of Osteoporosis. *Nano Lett.* **2021**, *21*, 7998–8007. [CrossRef] [PubMed]
66. Xi, D.; Xiao, M.; Cao, J.; Zhao, L.; Xu, N.; Long, S.; Fan, J.; Shao, K.; Sun, W.; Yan, X.; et al. NIR Light-Driving Barrier-Free Group Rotation in Nanoparticles with an 88.3% Photothermal Conversion Efficiency for Photothermal Therapy. *Adv. Mater.* **2020**, *32*, 1907855. [CrossRef]
67. Sun, H.; Wang, F.; Du, J. Preparation, application and perspective in polymer vesicles with an inhomogeneous membrane. *Sci. Sin. Chim.* **2019**, *49*, 877–890. [CrossRef]
68. Liu, D.; Sun, H.; Xiao, Y.; Chen, S.; Cornel, E.J.; Zhu, Y.; Du, J. Design principles, synthesis and biomedical applications of polymer vesicles with inhomogeneous membranes. *J. Control. Release* **2020**, *326*, 365–386. [CrossRef]
69. Wei, P.; Cornel, E.J.; Du, J. Breaking the Corona Symmetry of Vesicles. *Macromolecules* **2021**, *54*, 7603–7611. [CrossRef]
70. Chen, J.; Wang, F.; Liu, Q.; Du, J. Antibacterial polymeric nanostructures for biomedical applications. *Chem. Commun.* **2014**, *50*, 14482–14493. [CrossRef] [PubMed]
71. Wayakanon, K.; Thornhill, M.H.; Douglas, C.W.I.; Lewis, A.L.; Warren, N.J.; Pinnock, A.; Armes, S.P.; Battaglia, G.; Murdoch, C. Polymersome-mediated intracellular delivery of antibiotics to treat Porphyromonas gingivalis-infected oral epithelial cells. *FASEB J.* **2013**, *27*, 4455–4465. [CrossRef] [PubMed]
72. Glisoni, R.J.; Sosnik, A. Encapsulation of the Antimicrobial and Immunomodulator Agent Nitazoxanide within Polymeric Micelles. *J. Nanosci. Nanotechnol.* **2014**, *14*, 4670–4682. [CrossRef] [PubMed]
73. Lin, W.; Huang, K.; Li, Y.; Qin, Y.; Xiong, D.; Ling, J.; Yi, G.; Tang, Z.; Lin, J.; Huang, Y.; et al. Facile In Situ Preparation and In Vitro Antibacterial Activity of PDMAEMA-Based Silver-Bearing Copolymer Micelles. *Nanoscale Res. Lett.* **2019**, *14*, 256. [CrossRef] [PubMed]
74. Morteza, M.; Roya, S.; Hamed, H.; Amir, Z.; Abolfazl, A. Synthesis and evaluation of polymeric micelle containing piperacillin/tazobactam for enhanced antibacterial activity. *Drug Deliv.* **2019**, *26*, 1292–1299. [CrossRef]
75. Chen, M.; Wei, J.; Xie, S.; Tao, X.; Zhang, Z.; Ran, P.; Li, X. Bacterial biofilm destruction by size/surface charge-adaptive micelles. *Nanoscale* **2019**, *11*, 1410–1422. [CrossRef] [PubMed]
76. Rigo, S.; Huerlimann, D.; Marot, L.; Malmsten, M.; Meier, W.; Palivan, C.G. Decorating Nanostructured Surfaces with Antimicrobial Peptides to Efficiently Fight Bacteria. *ACS Appl. Bio Mater.* **2020**, *3*, 1533–1543. [CrossRef]
77. Diaz, I.L.; Parra, C.; Linarez, M.; Perez, L.D. Design of Micelle Nanocontainers Based on PDMAEMA-b-PCL-b-PDMAEMA Triblock Copolymers for the Encapsulation of Amphotericin B. *AAPS PharmSciTech* **2015**, *16*, 1069–1078. [CrossRef] [PubMed]
78. Qao, J.; Purro, M.; Liu, Z.; Xiong, M.P. Terpyridine-Micelles for Inhibiting Bacterial Biofilm Development. *ACS Infect. Dis.* **2018**, *4*, 1346–1354. [CrossRef]
79. Park, S.-C.; Ko, C.; Hyeon, H.; Jang, M.-K.; Lee, D. Imaging and Targeted Antibacterial Therapy Using Chimeric Antimicrobial Peptide Micelles. *ACS Appl. Mater. Interfaces* **2020**, *12*, 54306–54315. [CrossRef]
80. Song, Y.; Elsabahy, M.; Collins, C.A.; Khan, S.; Li, R.; Hreha, T.N.; Shen, Y.; Lin, Y.-N.; Letteri, R.A.; Su, L.; et al. Morphologic Design of Silver-Bearing Sugar-Based Polymer Nanoparticles for Uroepithelial Cell Binding and Antimicrobial Delivery. *Nano Lett.* **2021**, *21*, 4990–4998. [CrossRef]
81. Song, J.; Zhou, J.; Duan, H. Self-Assembled Plasmonic Vesicles of SERS-Encoded Amphiphilic Gold Nanoparticles for Cancer Cell Targeting and Traceable Intracellular Drug Delivery. *J. Am. Chem. Soc.* **2012**, *134*, 13458–13469. [CrossRef] [PubMed]
82. Blanazs, A.; Armes, S.P.; Ryan, A.J. Self-Assembled Block Copolymer Aggregates: From Micelles to Vesicles and their Biological Applications. *Macromol. Rapid Commun.* **2009**, *30*, 267–277. [CrossRef]
83. Deng, Y.; Li, J.; Yu, J.; Zhao, J.; Tang, J. Silver nanoparticles well-dispersed in amine-functionalized, one-pot made vesicles as an effective antibacterial agent. *Mater. Sci. Eng. C* **2016**, *60*, 92–99. [CrossRef] [PubMed]
84. Li, Y.-M.; Liu, S.-Y. Enzyme-triggered Transition from Polymeric Vesicles to Core Cross-linked Micelles for Selective Release of Antimicrobial Agents. *Acta Polym. Sin.* **2017**, *7*, 1178–1190. [CrossRef]
85. Li, Y.; Liu, G.; Wang, X.; Hu, J.; Liu, S. Enzyme-Responsive Polymeric Vesicles for Bacterial-Strain-Selective Delivery of Antimicrobial Agents. *Angew. Chem. Int. Ed.* **2016**, *55*, 1760–1764. [CrossRef] [PubMed]
86. Blackman, L.D.; Oo, Z.Y.; Qu, Y.; Gunatillake, P.A.; Cass, P.; Locock, K.E.S. Antimicrobial Honey-Inspired Glucose-Responsive Nanoreactors by Polymerization-Induced Self-Assembly. *ACS Appl. Mater. Interfaces* **2020**, *12*, 11353–11362. [CrossRef] [PubMed]
87. Cheng, Y.; Zhao, L.; Li, Y.; Xu, T. Design of biocompatible dendrimers for cancer diagnosis and therapy: Current status and future perspectives. *Chem. Soc. Rev.* **2011**, *40*, 2673–2703. [CrossRef] [PubMed]

88. Kesharwani, P.; Jain, K.; Jain, N.K. Dendrimer as nanocarrier for drug delivery. *Prog. Polym. Sci.* **2014**, *39*, 268–307. [CrossRef]
89. Svenson, S. Dendrimers as versatile platform in drug delivery applications. *Eur. J. Pharm. Biopharm.* **2009**, *71*, 445–462. [CrossRef]
90. Alfei, S.; Schito, A.M. From Nanobiotechnology, Positively Charged Biomimetic Dendrimers as Novel Antibacterial Agents: A Review. *Nanomaterials* **2020**, *10*, 2022. [CrossRef]
91. Abd-El-Aziz, A.S.; Agatemor, C. Emerging Opportunities in the Biomedical Applications of Dendrimers. *J. Inorg. Organomet. Polym. Mater.* **2018**, *28*, 369–382. [CrossRef]
92. Chen, S.; Huang, S.; Li, Y.; Zhou, C. Recent Advances in Epsilon-Poly-L-Lysine and L-Lysine-Based Dendrimer Synthesis, Modification, and Biomedical Applications. *Front. Chem.* **2021**, *9*, 659304. [CrossRef]
93. Tang, J.; Chen, W.; Su, W.; Li, W.; Deng, J. Dendrimer-Encapsulated Silver Nanoparticles and Antibacterial Activity on Cotton Fabric. *J. Nanosci. Nanotechnol.* **2013**, *13*, 2128–2135. [CrossRef]
94. Liu, X.; Wang, Z.; Feng, X.; Bai, E.; Xiong, Y.; Zhu, X.; Shen, B.; Duan, Y.; Huang, Y. Platensimycin-Encapsulated Poly(lactic-co-glycolic acid) and Poly(amidoamine) Dendrimers Nanoparticles with Enhanced Anti-Staphylococcal Activity In Vivo. *Bioconjugate Chem.* **2020**, *31*, 1425–1437. [CrossRef] [PubMed]
95. Li, J.; Liang, H.; Liu, J.; Wang, Z. Poly (amidoamine) (PAMAM) dendrimer mediated delivery of drug and pDNA/siRNA for cancer therapy. *Int. J. Pharm.* **2018**, *546*, 215–225. [CrossRef] [PubMed]
96. Lim, D.G.; Rajasekaran, N.; Lee, D.; Kim, N.A.; Jung, H.S.; Hong, S.; Shin, Y.K.; Kang, E.; Jeong, S.H. Polyamidoamine-Decorated Nanodiamonds as a Hybrid Gene Delivery Vector and siRNA Structural Characterization at the Charged Interfaces. *ACS Appl. Mater. Interfaces* **2017**, *9*, 31543–31556. [CrossRef] [PubMed]
97. Pashaei-Asl, R.; Khodadadi, K.; Pashaei-Asl, F.; Haqshenas, G.; Ahmadian, N.; Pashaiasl, M.; Baghdadabadi, R.H. Legionella Pneumophila and Dendrimers-Mediated Antisense Therapy. *Adv. Pharm. Bull.* **2017**, *7*, 179–187. [CrossRef]
98. Xue, X.Y.; Mao, X.G.; Li, Z.; Chen, Z.; Zhou, Y.; Hou, Z.; Li, M.K.; Meng, J.R.; Luo, X.X. A potent and selective antimicrobial poly(amidoamine) dendrimer conjugate with LED209 targeting QseC receptor to inhibit the virulence genes of gram negative bacteria. *Nanomedicine* **2015**, *11*, 329–339. [CrossRef]
99. Homaeigohar, S.; Boccaccini, A.R. Antibacterial biohybrid nanofibers for wound dressings. *Acta Biomater.* **2020**, *107*, 25–49. [CrossRef] [PubMed]
100. Schnaider, L.; Brahmachari, S.; Schmidt, N.W.; Mensa, B.; Shaham-Niv, S.; Bychenko, D.; Adler-Abramovich, L.; Shimon, L.J.W.; Kolusheva, S.; DeGrado, W.F.; et al. Self-assembling dipeptide antibacterial nanostructures with membrane disrupting activity. *Nat. Commun.* **2017**, *8*, 1365. [CrossRef]
101. Feng, L.; Li, S.; Li, H.; Zhai, J.; Song, Y.; Jiang, L.; Zhu, D. Super-Hydrophobic Surface of Aligned Polyacrylonitrile Nanofibers. *Angew. Chem. Int. Ed.* **2002**, *41*, 1221–1223. [CrossRef]
102. Ma, P.X.; Zhang, R.Y. Synthetic nano-scale fibrous extracellular matrix. *J. Biomed. Mater. Res.* **1999**, *46*, 60–72. [CrossRef]
103. Elbahri, M.; Homaeigohar, S.; Abdelaziz, R.; Dai, T.; Khalil, R.; Zillohu, A.U. Smart Metal–Polymer Bionanocomposites as Omnidirectional Plasmonic Black Absorber Formed by Nanofluid Filtration. *Adv. Funct. Mater.* **2012**, *22*, 4771–4777. [CrossRef]
104. Pant, B.; Park, M.; Park, S.-J. Drug Delivery Applications of Core-Sheath Nanofibers Prepared by Coaxial Electrospinning: A Review. *Pharmaceutics* **2019**, *11*, 305. [CrossRef] [PubMed]
105. Xue, J.; Wu, T.; Dai, Y.; Xia, Y. Electrospinning and Electrospun Nanofibers: Methods, Materials, and Applications. *Chem. Rev.* **2019**, *119*, 5298–5415. [CrossRef] [PubMed]
106. Wang, M.; Wang, K.; Yang, Y.; Liu, Y.; Yu, D.-G. Electrospun Environment Remediation Nanofibers Using Unspinnable Liquids as the Sheath Fluids: A Review. *Polymers* **2020**, *12*, 103. [CrossRef]
107. Agarwal, S.; Greiner, A.; Wendorff, J.H. Functional materials by electrospinning of polymers. *Prog. Polym. Sci.* **2013**, *38*, 963–991. [CrossRef]
108. Rieger, K.A.; Cho, H.J.; Yeung, H.F.; Fan, W.; Schiffman, J.D. Antimicrobial Activity of Silver Ions Released from Zeolites Immobilized on Cellulose Nanofiber Mats. *ACS Appl. Mater. Interfaces* **2016**, *8*, 3032–3040. [CrossRef] [PubMed]
109. Zhang, Q.; Wang, Y.; Zhang, W.; Hickey, M.E.; Lin, Z.; Tu, Q.; Wang, J. In situ assembly of well-dispersed Ag nanoparticles on the surface of polylactic acid-Au@polydopamine nanofibers for antimicrobial applications. *Colloids Surf. B* **2019**, *184*, 110506. [CrossRef]
110. Abrigo, M.; McArthur, S.L.; Kingshott, P. Electrospun Nanofibers as Dressings for Chronic Wound Care: Advances, Challenges, and Future Prospects. *Macromol. Biosci.* **2014**, *14*, 772–792. [CrossRef] [PubMed]
111. Czaja, W.K.; Young, D.J.; Kawecki, M.; Brown, R.M. The Future Prospects of Microbial Cellulose in Biomedical Applications. *Biomacromolecules* **2007**, *8*, 1–12. [CrossRef] [PubMed]
112. Rath, G.; Hussain, T.; Chauhan, G.; Garg, T.; Goyal, A.K. Development and characterization of cefazolin loaded zinc oxide nanoparticles composite gelatin nanofiber mats for postoperative surgical wounds. *Mater. Sci. Eng. C* **2016**, *58*, 242–253. [CrossRef]
113. Oh, J.K.; Drumright, R.; Siegwart, D.J.; Matyjaszewski, K. The development of microgels/nanogels for drug delivery applications. *Prog. Polym. Sci.* **2008**, *33*, 448–477. [CrossRef]
114. Karimi, M.; Ghasemi, A.; Zangabad, P.S.; Rahighi, R.; Basri, S.M.M.; Mirshekari, H.; Amiri, M.; Pishabad, Z.S.; Aslani, A.; Bozorgomid, M.; et al. Smart micro/nanoparticles in stimulus-responsive drug/gene delivery systems. *Chem. Soc. Rev.* **2016**, *45*, 1457–1501. [CrossRef]
115. Veiga, A.S.; Schneider, J.P. Antimicrobial Hydrogels for the Treatment of Infection. *Biopolymers* **2013**, *100*, 637–644. [CrossRef]
116. Ng, V.W.L.; Chan, J.M.W.; Sardon, H.; Ono, R.J.; Garcia, J.M.; Yang, Y.Y.; Hedrick, J.L. Antimicrobial hydrogels: A new weapon in the arsenal against multidrug-resistant infections. *Adv. Drug Deliv. Rev.* **2014**, *78*, 46–62. [CrossRef] [PubMed]

117. Yang, K.; Han, Q.; Chen, B.; Zheng, Y.; Zhang, K.; Li, Q.; Wang, J. Antimicrobial hydrogels: Promising materials for medical application. *Int. J. Nanomed.* **2018**, *13*, 2217–2263. [CrossRef] [PubMed]
118. Kundu, R.; Payal, P. Antimicrobial Hydrogels: Promising Soft Biomaterials. *Chemistryselect* **2020**, *5*, 14800–14810. [CrossRef]
119. Sivaram, A.J.; Rajitha, P.; Maya, S.; Jayakumar, R.; Sabitha, M. Nanogels for delivery, imaging and therapy. *Wiley Interdiscip. Rev. Nanomed. Nanobiotechnol.* **2015**, *7*, 509–533. [CrossRef]
120. Nordstrom, R.; Nystrom, L.; Andren, O.C.J.; Malkoch, M.; Umerska, A.; Davoudi, M.; Schmidtchen, A.; Malmsten, M. Membrane interactions of microgels as carriers of antimicrobial peptides. *J. Colloid Interface Sci.* **2018**, *513*, 141–150. [CrossRef]
121. Nordstrom, R.; Andren, O.C.J.; Singh, S.; Malkoch, M.; Davoudi, M.; Schmidtchen, A.; Malmsten, M. Degradable dendritic nanogels as carriers for antimicrobial peptides. *J. Colloid Interface Sci.* **2019**, *554*, 592–602. [CrossRef]
122. El-Feky, G.S.; El-Banna, S.T.; El-Bahy, G.S.; Abdelrazek, E.M.; Kamal, M. Alginate coated chitosan nanogel for the controlled topical delivery of Silver sulfadiazine. *Carbohydr. Polym.* **2017**, *177*, 194–202. [CrossRef] [PubMed]
123. Al-Awady, M.J.; Fauchet, A.; Greenway, G.M.; Paunov, V.N. Enhanced antimicrobial effect of berberine in nanogel carriers with cationic surface functionality. *J. Mater. Chem. B* **2017**, *5*, 7885–7897. [CrossRef]
124. Kettel, M.J.; Heine, E.; Schaefer, K.; Moeller, M. Chlorhexidine Loaded Cyclodextrin Containing PMMA Nanogels as Antimicrobial Coating and Delivery Systems. *Macromol. Biosci.* **2017**, *17*, 1600230. [CrossRef]
125. Al-Awady, M.J.; Weldrick, P.J.; Hardman, M.J.; Greenway, G.M.; Paunov, V.N. Amplified antimicrobial action of chlorhexidine encapsulated in PDAC-functionalized acrylate copolymer nanogel carriers. *Mater. Chem. Front.* **2018**, *2*, 2032–2044. [CrossRef]
126. Weldrick, P.J.; Iveson, S.; Hardman, M.J.; Paunov, V.N. Breathing new life into old antibiotics: Overcoming antibacterial resistance by antibiotic-loaded nanogel carriers with cationic surface functionality. *Nanoscale* **2019**, *11*, 10472–10485. [CrossRef]
127. Xiong, M.-H.; Bao, Y.; Yang, X.-Z.; Wang, Y.-C.; Sun, B.; Wang, J. Lipase-Sensitive Polymeric Triple-Layered Nanogel for "On-Demand" Drug Delivery. *J. Am. Chem. Soc.* **2012**, *134*, 4355–4362. [CrossRef] [PubMed]
128. Schnaider, L.; Toprakcioglu, Z.; Ezra, A.; Liu, X.; Bychenko, D.; Levin, A.; Gazit, E.; Knowles, T.P.J. Biocompatible Hybrid Organic/Inorganic Microhydrogels Promote Bacterial Adherence and Eradication In Vitro and In Vivo. *Nano Lett.* **2020**, *20*, 1590–1597. [CrossRef] [PubMed]
129. Zu, G.; Steinmueller, M.; Keskin, D.; van der Mei, H.C.; Mergel, O.; van Rijn, P. Antimicrobial Nanogels with Nanoinjection Capabilities for Delivery of the Hydrophobic Antibacterial Agent Triclosan. *ACS Appl. Polym. Mater.* **2020**, *2*, 5779–5789. [CrossRef]
130. Zhang, Y.; Zhang, J.; Chen, M.; Gong, H.; Tharnphiwatana, S.; Eckmann, L.; Gao, W.; Zhang, L. A Bioadhesive Nanoparticle-Hydrogel Hybrid System for Localized Antimicrobial Drug Delivery. *ACS Appl. Mater. Interfaces* **2016**, *8*, 18367–18374. [CrossRef] [PubMed]
131. Kebede, M.A.; Imae, T.; Wu, C.-M.; Cheng, K.-B. Cellulose fibers functionalized by metal nanoparticles stabilized in dendrimer for formaldehyde decomposition and antimicrobial activity. *Chem. Eng. J.* **2017**, *311*, 340–347. [CrossRef]
132. Hong, Y.; Xi, Y.; Zhang, J.; Wang, D.; Zhang, H.; Yan, N.; He, S.; Du, J. Polymersome-hydrogel composites with combined quick and long-term antibacterial activities. *J. Mater. Chem. B* **2018**, *6*, 6311–6321. [CrossRef] [PubMed]
133. Zhou, W.; Jia, Z.; Xiong, P.; Yan, J.; Li, M.; Cheng, Y.; Zheng, Y. Novel pH-responsive tobramycin-embedded micelles in nanostructured multilayer-coatings of chitosan/heparin with efficient and sustained antibacterial properties. *Mater. Sci. Eng. C* **2018**, *90*, 693–705. [CrossRef] [PubMed]
134. Brooks, B.D.; Brooks, A.E. Therapeutic strategies to combat antibiotic resistance. *Adv. Drug Deliv. Rev.* **2014**, *78*, 14–27. [CrossRef] [PubMed]
135. Liu, S.Q.; Venkataraman, S.; Ong, Z.Y.; Chan, J.M.W.; Yang, C.; Hedrick, J.L.; Yang, Y.Y. Overcoming Multidrug Resistance in Microbials Using Nanostructures Self-Assembled from Cationic Bent-Core Oligomers. *Small* **2014**, *10*, 4130–4135. [CrossRef]
136. Lakshminarayanan, R.; Ye, E.; Young, D.J.; Li, Z.; Loh, X.J. Recent Advances in the Development of Antimicrobial Nanoparticles for Combating Resistant Pathogens. *Adv. Healthc. Mater.* **2018**, *7*, 1701400. [CrossRef] [PubMed]
137. Gupta, A.; Mumtaz, S.; Li, C.-H.; Hussain, I.; Rotello, V.M. Combatting antibiotic-resistant bacteria using nanomaterials. *Chem. Soc. Rev.* **2019**, *48*, 415–427. [CrossRef] [PubMed]
138. Huang, X.; Chen, X.; Chen, Q.; Yu, Q.; Sun, D.; Liu, J. Investigation of functional selenium nanoparticles as potent antimicrobial agents against superbugs. *Acta Biomater.* **2016**, *30*, 397–407. [CrossRef]
139. Lam, S.J.; O'Brien-Simpson, N.M.; Pantarat, N.; Sulistio, A.; Wong, E.H.; Chen, Y.Y.; Lenzo, J.C.; Holden, J.A.; Blencowe, A.; Reynolds, E.C.; et al. Combating multidrug-resistant Gram-negative bacteria with structurally nanoengineered antimicrobial peptide polymers. *Nat. Microbiol.* **2016**, *1*, 16162. [CrossRef] [PubMed]
140. Lam, S.J.; Wong, E.H.; O'Brien-Simpson, N.M.; Pantarat, N.; Blencowe, A.; Reynolds, E.C.; Qiao, G.G. Bionano Interaction Study on Antimicrobial Star-Shaped Peptide Polymer Nanoparticles. *ACS Appl. Mater. Interfaces* **2016**, *8*, 33446–33456. [CrossRef]
141. Siriwardena, T.N.; Stach, M.; He, R.; Gan, B.-H.; Javor, S.; Heitz, M.; Ma, L.; Cai, X.; Chen, P.; Wei, D.; et al. Lipidated Peptide Dendrimers Killing Multidrug-Resistant Bacteria. *J. Am. Chem. Soc.* **2017**, *140*, 423–432. [CrossRef]
142. Cao, B.; Xiao, F.; Xing, D.; Hu, X. Polyprodrug Antimicrobials: Remarkable Membrane Damage and Concurrent Drug Release to Combat Antibiotic Resistance of Methicillin-Resistant Staphylococcus aureus. *Small* **2018**, *14*, 1802008. [CrossRef] [PubMed]
143. Lee, N.-Y.; Ko, W.-C.; Hsueh, P.-R. Nanoparticles in the Treatment of Infections Caused by Multidrug-Resistant Organisms. *Front. Pharmacol.* **2019**, *10*, 1153. [CrossRef] [PubMed]
144. Fatima, F.; Siddiqui, S.; Khan, W.A. Nanoparticles as Novel Emerging Therapeutic Antibacterial Agents in the Antibiotics Resistant Era. *Biol. Trace Elem. Res.* **2021**, *199*, 2552–2564. [CrossRef]
145. Geilich, B.M.; van de Ven, A.L.; Singleton, G.L.; Sepúlveda, L.J.; Sridhar, S.; Webster, T.J. Silver nanoparticle-embedded polymersome nanocarriers for the treatment of antibiotic-resistant infections. *Nanoscale* **2015**, *7*, 3511–3519. [CrossRef] [PubMed]

146. Bassous, N.J.; Webster, T.J. The Binary Effect on Methicillin-Resistant Staphylococcus aureus of Polymeric Nanovesicles Appended by Proline-Rich Amino Acid Sequences and Inorganic Nanoparticles. *Small* **2019**, *15*, 1804247. [CrossRef]
147. Forier, K.; Raemdonck, K.; De Smedt, S.C.; Demeester, J.; Coenye, T.; Braeckmans, K. Lipid and polymer nanoparticles for drug delivery to bacterial biofilms. *J. Control. Release* **2014**, *190*, 607–623. [CrossRef] [PubMed]
148. Martin, C.; Low, W.L.; Gupta, A.; Amin, M.C.I.M.; Radecka, I.; Britland, S.T.; Raj, P.; Kenward, K. Strategies for Antimicrobial Drug Delivery to Biofilm. *Curr. Pharm. Des.* **2015**, *21*, 43–66. [CrossRef] [PubMed]
149. Mu, H.; Tang, J.; Liu, Q.; Sun, C.; Wang, T.; Duan, J. Potent Antibacterial Nanoparticles against Biofilm and Intracellular Bacteria. *Sci. Rep.* **2016**, *6*, 18877. [CrossRef]
150. Li, C.; Cornel, E.J.; Du, J. Advances and Prospects of Polymeric Particles for the Treatment of Bacterial Biofilms. *ACS Appl. Polym. Mater.* **2021**, *3*, 2218–2232. [CrossRef]
151. Baelo, A.; Levato, R.; Julian, E.; Crespo, A.; Astola, J.; Gavalda, J.; Engel, E.; Angel Mateos-Timoneda, M.; Torrents, E. Disassembling bacterial extracellular matrix with DNase-coated nanoparticles to enhance antibiotic delivery in biofilm infections. *J. Control. Release* **2015**, *209*, 150–158. [CrossRef]
152. Geilich, B.M.; Gelfat, I.; Sridhar, S.; van de Ven, A.L.; Webster, T.J. Superparamagnetic iron oxide-encapsulating polymersome nanocarriers for biofilm eradication. *Biomaterials* **2017**, *119*, 78–85. [CrossRef] [PubMed]
153. Xi, Y.; Wang, Y.; Gao, J.; Xiao, Y.; Du, J. Dual Corona Vesicles with Intrinsic Antibacterial and Enhanced Antibiotic Delivery Capabilities for Effective Treatment of Biofilm-Induced Periodontitis. *ACS Nano* **2019**, *13*, 13645–13657. [CrossRef]
154. Pircalabioru, G.G.; Chifiriuc, M.-C. Nanoparticulate drug-delivery systems for fighting microbial biofilms: From bench to bedside. *Future Microbiol.* **2020**, *15*, 679–698. [CrossRef]
155. Birk, S.E.; Boisen, A.; Nielsen, L.H. Polymeric nano- and microparticulate drug delivery systems for treatment of biofilms. *Adv. Drug Deliv. Rev.* **2021**, *174*, 30–52. [CrossRef] [PubMed]
156. Porter, G.C.; Schwass, D.R.; Tompkins, J.W.R.; Bobbala, S.K.R.; Medlicott, N.J.; Meledandri, C.J. AgNP/Alginate Nanocomposite hydrogel for antimicrobial and antibiofilm applications. *Carbohydr. Polym.* **2021**, *251*, 117017. [CrossRef] [PubMed]
157. Hoque, J.; Yadav, V.; Prakash, R.G.; Sanyal, K.; Haldar, J. Dual-Function Polymer-Silver Nanocomposites for Rapid Killing of Microbes and Inhibiting Biofilms. *ACS Biomater. Sci. Eng.* **2019**, *5*, 81–91. [CrossRef]
158. Gao, Y.; Wang, J.; Hu, D.; Deng, Y.; Chen, T.; Jin, Q.; Ji, J. Bacteria-Targeted Supramolecular Photosensitizer Delivery Vehicles for Photodynamic Ablation Against Biofilms. *Macromol. Rapid Commun.* **2019**, *40*, 1800763. [CrossRef] [PubMed]
159. Anjum, S.; Gupta, A.; Sharma, D.; Gautam, D.; Bhan, S.; Sharma, A.; Kapil, A.; Gupta, B. Development of novel wound care systems based on nanosilver nanohydrogels of polymethacrylic acid with Aloe vera and curcumin. *Mater. Sci. Eng. C* **2016**, *64*, 157–166. [CrossRef] [PubMed]
160. Wu, J.; Zheng, Y.; Wen, X.; Lin, Q.; Chen, X.; Wu, Z. Silver nanoparticle/bacterial cellulose gel membranes for antibacterial wound dressing: Investigation in vitro and in vivo. *Biomed. Mater.* **2014**, *9*, 035005. [CrossRef]
161. Gupta, A.; Briffa, S.M.; Swingler, S.; Gibson, H.; Kannappan, V.; Adamus, G.; Kowalczuk, M.; Martin, C.; Radecka, I. Synthesis of Silver Nanoparticles Using Curcumin-Cyclodextrins Loaded into Bacterial Cellulose-Based Hydrogels for Wound Dressing Applications. *Biomacromolecules* **2020**, *21*, 1802–1811. [CrossRef]
162. Dhand, C.; Venkatesh, M.; Barathi, V.A.; Harini, S.; Bairagi, S.; Leng, E.G.T.; Muruganandham, N.; Low, K.Z.W.; Fazil, M.H.U.T.; Loh, X.J.; et al. Bio-inspired crosslinking and matrix-drug interactions for advanced wound dressings with long-term antimicrobial activity. *Biomaterials* **2017**, *138*, 153–168. [CrossRef]
163. Tao, B.; Lin, C.; Deng, Y.; Yuan, Z.; Shen, X.; Chen, M.; He, Y.; Peng, Z.; Hu, Y.; Cai, K. Copper-nanoparticle-embedded hydrogel for killing bacteria and promoting wound healing with photothermal therapy. *J. Mater. Chem. B* **2019**, *7*, 2534–2548. [CrossRef]
164. Hu, Y.; Cai, X.; Qu, X.; Yu, B.; Yan, C.; Yang, J.; Li, F.; Zheng, Y.; Shi, X. Preparation of biocompatible wound dressings with long-term antimicrobial activity through covalent bonding of antibiotic agents to natural polymers. *Int. J. Biol. Macromol.* **2019**, *123*, 1320–1330. [CrossRef]
165. Kalantari, K.; Mostafavi, E.; Afifi, A.M.; Izadiyan, Z.; Jahangirian, H.; Rafiee-Moghaddam, R.; Webster, T.J. Wound dressings functionalized with silver nanoparticles: Promises and pitfalls. *Nanoscale* **2020**, *12*, 2268–2291. [CrossRef] [PubMed]
166. Alavi, M.; Nokhodchi, A. An overview on antimicrobial and wound healing properties of ZnO nanobiofilms, hydrogels, and bionanocomposites based on cellulose, chitosan, and alginate polymers. *Carbohydr. Polym.* **2020**, *227*, 115349. [CrossRef]
167. Chen, C.; Chu, G.; Qi, M.; Liu, Y.; Huang, P.; Pan, H.; Wang, Y.; Chen, Y.; Zhou, Y. Porphyrin Alternating Copolymer Vesicles for Photothermal Drug-Resistant Bacterial Ablation and Wound Disinfection. *ACS Appl. Bio Mater.* **2020**, *3*, 9117–9125. [CrossRef]
168. Qu, X.; Liu, H.; Zhang, C.; Lei, Y.; Lei, M.; Xu, M.; Jin, D.; Li, P.; Yin, M.; Payne, G.F.; et al. Electrofabrication of functional materials: Chloramine-based antimicrobial film for infectious wound treatment. *Acta Biomater.* **2018**, *73*, 190–203. [CrossRef]
169. Fahimirad, S.; Ghaznavi-Rad, E.; Abtahi, H.; Sarlak, N. Antimicrobial Activity, Stability and Wound Healing Performances of Chitosan Nanoparticles Loaded Recombinant LL37 Antimicrobial Peptide. *Int. J. Pept. Res. Ther.* **2021**, *27*, 2505–2515. [CrossRef]
170. Liang, Y.; Chen, B.; Li, M.; He, J.; Yin, Z.; Guo, B. Injectable Antimicrobial Conductive Hydrogels for Wound Disinfection and Infectious Wound Healing. *Biomacromolecules* **2020**, *21*, 1841–1852. [CrossRef]
171. Zhou, J.; Yao, D.; Qian, Z.; Hou, S.; Li, L.; Jenkins, A.T.A.; Fan, Y. Bacteria-responsive intelligent wound dressing: Simultaneous In situ detection and inhibition of bacterial infection for accelerated wound healing. *Biomaterials* **2018**, *161*, 11–23. [CrossRef]
172. Liu, D.; Liao, Y.; Cornel, E.J.; Lv, M.; Wu, T.; Zhang, X.; Fan, L.; Sun, M.; Zhu, Y.; Fan, Z.; et al. Polymersome Wound Dressing Spray Capable of Bacterial Inhibition and H_2S Generation for Complete Diabetic Wound Healing. *Chem. Mater.* **2021**, *33*, 7972–7985. [CrossRef]

173. Wang, T.; Li, Y.; Cornel, E.J.; Li, C.; Du, J. Combined Antioxidant-Antibiotic Treatment for Effectively Healing Infected Diabetic Wounds Based on Polymer Vesicles. *ACS Nano* **2021**, *15*, 9027–9038. [CrossRef]
174. Nathanael, A.J.; Oh, T.H. Biopolymer Coatings for Biomedical Applications. *Polymers* **2020**, *12*, 3061. [CrossRef]
175. Mousa, H.M.; Abdal-hay, A.; Bartnikowski, M.; Mohamed, I.M.A.; Yasin, A.S.; Ivanovski, S.; Park, C.H.; Kim, C.S. A Multifunctional Zinc Oxide/Poly(Lactic Acid) Nanocomposite Layer Coated on Magnesium Alloys for Controlled Degradation and Antibacterial Function. *ACS Biomater. Sci. Eng.* **2018**, *4*, 2169–2180. [CrossRef] [PubMed]
176. Suteewong, T.; Wongpreecha, J.; Polpanich, D.; Jangpatarapongsa, K.; Kaewsaneha, C.; Tangboriboonrat, P. PMMA particles coated with chitosan-silver nanoparticles as a dual antibacterial modifier for natural rubber latex films. *Colloids Surf. B* **2019**, *174*, 544–552. [CrossRef]
177. Zhu, H.; Mei, X.; He, Y.; Mao, H.; Tang, W.; Liu, R.; Yang, J.; Luo, K.; Gu, Z.; Zhou, L. Fast and High Strength Soft Tissue Bioadhesives Based on a Peptide Dendrimer with Antimicrobial Properties and Hemostatic Ability. *ACS Appl. Mater. Interfaces* **2020**, *12*, 4241–4253. [CrossRef]
178. Balakrishnan, B. Role of Nanoscale Delivery Systems in Tissue Engineering. *Curr. Pathobiol. Rep.* **2021**. [CrossRef]
179. Zhou, C.; Yuan, Y.; Zhou, P.; Wang, F.; Hong, Y.; Wang, N.; Xu, S.; Du, J. Highly Effective Antibacterial Vesicles Based on Peptide-Mimetic Alternating Copolymers for Bone Repair. *Biomacromolecules* **2017**, *18*, 4154–4162. [CrossRef]
180. Cirillo, S.; Tomeh, M.A.; Wilkinson, R.N.; Hill, C.; Brown, S.; Zhao, X. Designed Antitumor Peptide for Targeted siRNA Delivery into Cancer Spheroids. *ACS Appl. Mater. Interfaces* **2021**, *3*, 49713–49728. [CrossRef] [PubMed]
181. Hoskin, D.W.; Ramamoorthy, A. Studies on anticancer activities of antimicrobial peptides. *Biochim. Biophys. Acta Biomembr.* **2008**, *1778*, 357–375. [CrossRef] [PubMed]
182. Kirar, S.; Chaudhari, D.; Thakur, N.S.; Jain, S.; Bhaumik, J.; Laha, J.K.; Banerjee, U.C. Light-assisted anticancer photodynamic therapy using porphyrin-doped nanoencapsulates. *J. Photochem. Photobiol. B* **2021**, *220*, 112209. [CrossRef] [PubMed]
183. Venkatesan, J.; Lee, J.-Y.; Kang, D.S.; Anil, S.; Kim, S.-K.; Shim, M.S.; Kim, D.G. Antimicrobial and anticancer activities of porous chitosan-alginate biosynthesized silver nanoparticles. *Int. J. Biol. Macromol.* **2017**, *98*, 515–525. [CrossRef] [PubMed]
184. Nithya, A.; Mohan, S.C.; Jeganathan, K.; Jothivenkatachalam, K. A potential photocatalytic, antimicrobial and anticancer activity of chitosan-copper nanocomposite. *Int. J. Biol. Macromol.* **2017**, *104*, 1774–1782. [CrossRef]
185. Felicio, M.R.; Silva, O.N.; Goncalves, S.; Santos, N.C.; Franco, O.L. Peptides with Dual Antimicrobial and Anticancer Activities. *Front. Chem.* **2017**, *5*, 5. [CrossRef]
186. Mori, T.; Hazekawa, M.; Yoshida, M.; Nishinakagawa, T.; Uchida, T.; Ishibashi, D. Enhancing the anticancer efficacy of a LL-37 peptide fragment analog using peptide-linked PLGA conjugate micelles in tumor cells. *Int. J. Pharm.* **2021**, *606*, 120891. [CrossRef]
187. Lv, S.; Sylvestre, M.; Prossnitz, A.N.; Yang, L.F.; Pun, S.H. Design of Polymeric Carriers for Intracellular Peptide Delivery in Oncology Applications. *Chem. Rev.* **2021**, *121*, 11653–11698. [CrossRef] [PubMed]
188. Cortese, B.; D'Amone, S.; Testini, M.; Ratano, P.; Palama, I.E. Hybrid Clustered Nanoparticles for Chemo-Antibacterial Combinatorial Cancer Therapy. *Cancers* **2019**, *11*, 1338. [CrossRef] [PubMed]
189. Zha, J.; Mao, X.; Hu, S.; Shang, K.; Yin, J. Acid- and Thiol-Cleavable Multifunctional Codelivery Hydrogel: Fabrication and Investigation of Antimicrobial and Anticancer Properties. *ACS Appl. Bio Mater.* **2021**, *4*, 1515–1523. [CrossRef]
190. Zhou, C.C.; Wang, M.Z.; Zou, K.D.; Chen, J.; Zhu, Y.Q.; Du, J.Z. Antibacterial Polypeptide-Grafted Chitosan-Based Nanocapsules As an "Armed" Carrier of Anticancer and Antiepileptic Drugs. *ACS Macro Lett.* **2013**, *2*, 1021–1025. [CrossRef]
191. Zeynabad, F.B.; Salehi, R.; Mahkam, M. Design of pH-responsive antimicrobial nanocomposite as dual drug delivery system for tumor therapy. *Appl. Clay Sci.* **2017**, *141*, 23–35. [CrossRef]
192. Zhou, L.; Xi, Y.; Chen, M.; Niu, W.; Wang, M.; Ma, P.X.; Lei, B. A highly antibacterial polymeric hybrid micelle with efficiently targeted anticancer siRNA delivery and anti-infection in vitro/in vivo. *Nanoscale* **2018**, *10*, 17304–17317. [CrossRef]

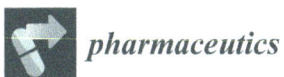

Review

Nanotechnologies: An Innovative Tool to Release Natural Extracts with Antimicrobial Properties

Umile Gianfranco Spizzirri [1,*], Francesca Aiello [1], Gabriele Carullo [2], Anastasia Facente [1] and Donatella Restuccia [1]

[1] Department of Pharmacy, Health and Nutritional Sciences Department of Excellence 2018–2022, University of Calabria, Edificio Polifunzionale, 87036 Rende, Italy; francesca.aiello@unical.it (F.A.); anastasiafacente_93@hotmail.it (A.F.); donatella.restuccia@unical.it (D.R.)

[2] Department of Biotechnology, Chemistry and Pharmacy, Department of Excellence 2018–2022, University of Siena, Via Aldo Moro 2, 53100 Siena, Italy; gabriele.carullo@unisi.it

* Correspondence: g.spizzirri@unical.it; Tel.: +39-0984-493298

Abstract: Site-Specific release of active molecules with antimicrobial activity spurred the interest in the development of innovative polymeric nanocarriers. In the preparation of polymeric devices, nanotechnologies usually overcome the inconvenience frequently related to other synthetic strategies. High performing nanocarriers were synthesized using a wide range of starting polymer structures, with tailored features and great chemical versatility. Over the last decade, many antimicrobial substances originating from plants, herbs, and agro-food waste by-products were deeply investigated, significantly catching the interest of the scientific community. In this review, the most innovative strategies to synthesize nanodevices able to release antimicrobial natural extracts were discussed. In this regard, the properties and structure of the starting polymers, either synthetic or natural, as well as the antimicrobial activity of the biomolecules were deeply investigated, outlining the right combination able to inhibit pathogens in specific biological compartments.

Keywords: nanotechnologies; plant extracts; agro-food-wastes; antimicrobial agents; polymeric nanocarriers

Citation: Spizzirri, U.G.; Aiello, F.; Carullo, G.; Facente, A.; Restuccia, D. Nanotechnologies: An Innovative Tool to Release Natural Extracts with Antimicrobial Properties. *Pharmaceutics* **2021**, *13*, 230. https://doi.org/10.3390/pharmaceutics13020230

Academic Editor: Clive Prestidge
Received: 29 December 2020
Accepted: 3 February 2021
Published: 6 February 2021

Publisher's Note: MDPI stays neutral with regard to jurisdictional claims in published maps and institutional affiliations.

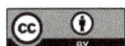

Copyright: © 2021 by the authors. Licensee MDPI, Basel, Switzerland. This article is an open access article distributed under the terms and conditions of the Creative Commons Attribution (CC BY) license (https://creativecommons.org/licenses/by/4.0/).

1. Introduction

Nanotechnology involves different strategies by using natural and synthetic materials in nanoscale dimensions to fabricate devices widely employed in the electronic and food industries, as well as in the pharmaceutical and biomedical fields [1]. Polymeric nanocarriers, due to their high surface area and small dimension (1–100 nm), are able to increase permeability and solubility of the enclosed molecules, making them available for several health applications, including diagnosis, disease treatments, and imaging [2–4]. In addition, effectively modifying the key features of nanocarriers, i.e., size, constituents, shape, and surface properties, it is possible to tune their mechanical, biological, and physicochemical characteristics [5]. In particular, nanotechnologies have gained outstanding consideration in the development of smart and effective pharmaceutical systems able to transport and deliver bioactive components in a specific site, avoiding, at the same time, deterioration due to enzymatic activity and pH values [6]. Among bioactive molecules, natural compounds have always represented the most widely employed substances for their unique therapeutic properties against several diseases [7]. In fact, natural bioactive extracts from plants, herbals, or agro-food by-products represent a rich source of compounds (polyphenols, anthocyanins, flavonoids, and many others) useful in the treatment of various diseases, thus suggesting their addition to pharmaceutical and cosmetic formulations, as well as to nutraceutical supplies [8]. In particular, many nanodevices (i.e., nanofibers and nanoparticles) have been developed to serve as antimicrobial agents to avoid pathogens' proliferation. In literature, a large number of articles can be found, describing the transport of antimicrobial agents, mainly, but not only, to the skin compartment in the wound treatment, in order to prevent infections and/or to accelerate the healing process [9–11].

In this review, highly innovative nanotechnology-based delivery systems loaded with bioactive molecules recovered from natural matrices and showing antimicrobial activity were described. The referenced papers were selected through the articles published from the year 2010 and sorted based on the specific type of nanocarrier.

2. Natural Extracts with Antimicrobial Activity

The search for new therapeutically active compounds has spurred researchers over the years to investigate natural compounds [12–17]. In particular, food and plant wastes represent interesting sources of biologically active molecules [18–24] and have been proposed as indigenous remedies [25,26]. Specifically, secondary metabolites from plants represent valuable bioactive ingredients [27–30] with remarkable antibacterial properties [31,32], useful in the treatment of several diseases. Table 1 summarizes the main natural extracts proposed for their antimicrobial features.

The valuable therapeutic power of *Glycyrrhiza glabra* L. var cordara is well known: its extracts showed a panel of antibacterial features against various bacterial strains (128 < minimal inhibitory concentration (MIC < 512 µg/mL), the activity being mainly related to the pinocembrin, recovered in the extract as free and fatty acids-conjugated form [14]. Similarly, the nutritional properties of the male date palm flower, via defining its antibacterial actions, were also scouted [33]. The chromatographic analysis identified the presence of several phenolic compounds. Among them, quinic acid was recovered as the main component (84.52% w/w) and significantly influenced the nutraceutical and pharmacological properties of the extract.

Thin-layer chromatography (TLC) micro-fractionation of the organic extracts of *Ferula ferulioides* [34], a traditional medicinal plant, served as a guiding tool to isolate two compounds (dalpanitin and vicenin-3), with remarkable antimicrobial activity against drug-resistant *Staphylococcus aureus* [35].

Antimicrobial activity of essential oil (EO) of Cyprus *Citrus aurantium* L. flowers was analyzed, and the recorded minimum inhibitory concentrations (MIC) against Amoxicillin-resistant *Bacillus cereus* was 1.562 mg/mL [36]. Moreover, the extracts of *Psidium* sp., *Mangifera* sp., and *Mentha* sp. and its mixtures displayed antimicrobial effects and strongly reduced *Streptococcus mutans* [37].

The phytochemical study of the aerial part of *Pulicaria undulata* L. led to the isolation of nine compounds. The organic extracts (methanol, ethyl acetate, and dichloromethane) of the aerial parts were assayed by in vitro antimicrobial activity against a panel of sensitive microorganisms [38]. Similarly, the phenolic compounds in the solvent extracts of *Genista saharae* were analyzed. The chloroform extract, containing high amounts of quercetin and naringenin, revealed the antioxidant potential and antibacterial activity against the bacterial strains (MIC 0.02 mg/mL). These results seemed to indicate a high contribution of quercetin and naringenin in the antimicrobial and antioxidant activities recorded [39].

The prevalence of different types of chronic wounds due to the aging population and the increasing incidence of diseases is a worldwide clinical emergency. Various medicinal plants used in folk medicine and showing wound healing and antimicrobial properties have been widely assessed [40].

As known, some mushrooms and numerous other fungi exhibit innovative properties, including antimicrobial features against bacteria, fungi, and protozoans. In particular, in a study, 316 species of 150 genera from 64 fungal families were analyzed, showing antibacterial activity against different bacteria and fungi [41].

The main component of extracts from white guava (*Psidium guajava* L. cv. Pearl) was quercetin-glycosides. In particular, the micro-morphology of both *Escherichia coli* and *S. aureus* was changed with a flavonoids concentration of 5.00 mg/mL and 0.625 mg/mL, extracted from white guava leaves [42].

Table 1. Plant extracts endowed with antimicrobial activity.

Source	Microorganisms	Antibacterial Activity	Ref.
Male date palm flower	Pseudomonas savastanoi, Escherichia coli, Salmonella enterica, Agrobacterium tumefaciens, Bacillus subtilis, Staphylococcus aureus, Micrococcus luteus, Listeria monocytogenes	10.5–12.1 [a]	[33]
Ferula ferulioides	S. aureus	0.00025 > 0.128 [b]	[34]
Derris scandens	S. aureus, Bacillus cereus, E. coli, Pseudomonas aeruginosa	0.06–13 [b]	[35]
C. aurantium flowers	B. cereus	1.562 ≤ 6.250 [b]	[36]
Psidium sp., Mangifera sp. and Mentha sp	Streptococcus sanguinis, Streptococcus mutans	31.63 ± 5.11 [c]	[37]
Pulicaria undulata L	S. aureus, E. coli, Klebsiella pneumoniae, P. aeruginosa	17–18 [d]	[38]
Genista saharae	E. coli, Acinetobacter baumannii, Citrobacter freundii, Proteus mirabilis, Salmonella typhimurium, Enterobacter cloacae, S. aureus, B. cereus, B. subtilis, Enterococcus faecalis, L. monocytogenes	0.01 > 1000 [c]	[39]
Cerbera manghas, Commelina diffusa, Kleinhovia hospita, Mikania micrantha, Omalanthus nutans, Peperomia pellucida, Phymatosorus scolopendria, Piper graeffei, Psychotria insularum, Schizostachyum glaucifolium	S. aureus, E. coli, P. aeruginosa	0.004–0.512 [b]	[40]
Fungi	—	—	[41]
Psidium guajava L. cv. Pearl	E. coli, S. aureus, P. aeruginosa	0.3 – 10.0 [b]	[42]
Polyscias scutellaria Fosberg	A. sp.	225–400 [d]	[43]
Aspidosperma quebracho-blanco, Schinus fasciculatus, S. gracilipes, Amphilophium cynanchoides, Tecoma stans	Pseudomonas corrugate, Pseudomonas syringae pv. tomato, Erwinia carotovora var. carotovora, A. tumefaciens, Xanthomonas campestres pv. vesicatoria	2.2 > 4.0 [b] 2.0–4.8 [a]	[44]
Cardamom (Elettaria cardamomum)	Aggregatibacter actinomycetemcomitans, Fusobacterium nucleatum, Porphyromonas gingivalis, Prevotella intermedia	0.06–1.00 [b]	[45]
Origanum vulgare, Salvia officinalis, Thymus vulgaris	E. coli, Klebsiella oxytoca, K. pneumoniae	2–370 [b]	[46]
Myristica fragrans	S. aureus, methicillin-resistant S. aureus, Streptococcus pyogenes, P. aeruginosa, Candida albicans	0–12 [b] 0–45 [a]	[47]
Euphorbia tirucalli L.	S. aureus, Staphylococcus epidermidis, E. faecalis, E. coli, P. aeruginosa	12.8–16.0 [b]	[48]
Tradescantia zebrina	B. cereus, B. subtilis, M. luteus, S. aureus, S. epidermidis	5 > 10 [b]	[49]

Table 1. Cont.

Source	Microorganisms	Antibacterial Activity	Ref.
Adiantum caudatum	B. subtilis, E. coli, P. aeruginosa	8-22 [a]	[50]
Agastache rugosa Korean Mint	Aeromonas salmonicida, Cronobacter sakazakii, E. coli, Staphylococcus haemolyticus, Aeromonas hydrophila	9.3-28.3 [a]	[51]
Algae and diatoms	E. faecalis, S. aureus, S. epidermidis, Streptococcus agalactiae, Streptococcus pneumoniae, S. pyogenes, Acinetobacter lwoffii, E. coli, K. oxytoca, K. pneumoniae, P. mirabilis, P. aeruginosa, Serratia marcescens	6.0-12.0 [a] 0.062 > 1000 [b]	[52]
Fagus sylvatica L	S. aureus, P. aeruginosa, S. typhimurium, E. coli, Candida	1-3 (MIC) [b]; 3-6 (MBC) [b]	[53]

[a] Inhibition zone; [b] minimal inhibitory concentration (MIC), Minimum bactericidal concentration (MBC) (mg/mL); [c] cell-surface hydrophobicity of bacteria (%); [d] inhibition zone dimension (IZD) (mm).

The traditional use of *Polyscias scutellaria* Fosberg to treat body odor suggested that this plant shows antibacterial properties. Most of the microorganisms hosted by human skin are harmless and even useful against pathogenic bacteria. Furthermore, *Acinetobacter* sp., formerly known as commensal bacteria, evolved into pathogenic bacteria and caused outbreaks in the intensive care unit. In this context, the antibacterial activity of *P. scutellaria* Fosberg extracts against *Acinetobacter* sp. isolated from healthy human armpit was investigated [43].

The ethyl acetate fraction from the leaves of *Schismus fasciculatus* contained kaempferol, quercetin, and agathist flavone, which showed moderate antibacterial activity against different tested strains (IC_{50} 0.9 mg/mL) [44]. In addition, both cardamom (*Elettaria cardamomum*) fruit and seed extracts exerted remarkable antibacterial effect against *Aggregatibacter actinomycetemcomitans*, *Fusobacterium nucleatum*, *Porphyromonas gingivalis*, and *Prevotella intermedia* [45].

The antimicrobial properties of oregano (*Origanum vulgare*), sage (*Salvia officinalis*), and thyme (*Thymus vulgaris*) essential oils (EO) were assayed against *Klebsiella oxytoca* (MIC of 0.9 mg/mL for oregano EO and 8.1 mg/mL for thyme EO) [46].

The water and ethanolic extracts of *Myristica fragrans* (Myristicaceae) wood displayed interesting antimicrobial, anti-inflammatory, and antioxidant activities [47].

The phenolic composition, antimicrobial activities, and antioxidant activity of *Euphorbia tirucalli* L. extracts were evaluated by agar dilution methods, and MIC values were recorded. In all samples, ferulic acid resulted as the main phenolic compound identified and quantified through LC-UV. The extracts demonstrated inhibitory potential against *Staphylococcus epidermidis* and *S. aureus* [48].

The methanol leaf extract of *Tradescantia zebrina* showed the highest antioxidant content and activity, exhibiting antibacterial activity against six species of Gram-positive and two species of Gram-negative bacteria in a range of 5–10 mg/mL [49].

The aqueous extracts of *Adiantum caudatum* leaves, obtained by Soxhlet extraction, resulted as more powerful than the hexanoic one against *Pseudomonas aeruginosa* [50]. The methanol extracts from the flowers of *Agastache rugosa* (Korean mint) showed high antibacterial activities [51]. Finally, the carotenoid fucoxanthin was observed to have a significantly stronger impact on Gram-positive than Gram-negative bacteria [52,53].

3. Agro-Food Wastes as Antimicrobials

The processing of agro-products generates huge amounts of waste materials every year in the form of peels, seeds, and oilseed meals, thus representing serious environmental concerns. Besides, the cost of drying, storage, or transportation poses a severe financial limitation to wastes utilization. To support the transformation and exploitation of these by-products, there is a growing interest in recycling waste biomass of agro-products in particular, considering their therapeutic properties (Table 2).

For example, the major wastes for industrial apple juices are the seeds. After a Soxhlet extraction, oil was recovered, and this apple seed oil was completely active against bacteria, showing MIC values ranged from 0.3–0.6 mg/mL [54].

About a quarter of the total tomato production undergoes processing, leading to derivatives like sauces, canned tomatoes, ketchup, or juices, largely consumed worldwide. At the same time, the tomato industry generates huge quantities of wastes, up to 5–0% of the total production. These by-products are used as livestock feed or discarded in landfills, creating many environmental problems. However, considering that valuable phytochemicals, such as carotenoids, polyphenols, tocopherols, some terpenes, and sterols, resist industrial treatment, tomato by-products represent also a precious resource. An interesting experimental work reported that the most active peel tomato extract against *S. aureus* and *Bacillus subtilis* (MIC: 2.5 mg tomato peels/mL) belonged to the Țărănești roz variety, owing to its high carotenoid amount [55].

Table 2. Agro-food wastes with antimicrobial properties.

Source	Microorganisms	Antimicrobial Activity	Ref.
Apple seeds	Escherichia coli, Salmonella sp., Bacillus subtilis, Staphylococcus aureus, Candida sp., Saccharomyces cerevisiae, Aspergillus flavus, Penicillium citrinum, Mucor sp., Rhizopus sp.	0.3–0.6 [a]	[54]
Tomato peels	S. aureus, B. subtilis, Listeria monocytogenes, E. coli, Pseudomonas aeruginosa, Salmonella typhimurium	2.5–10.0 [a]	[55]
Leaves of fennel and carrot	Salmonella enteritidis, S. aureus, Candida albicans	6.5–50.0 [a]	[56]
Betel leaf stalk	B. subtilis, E.coli, P. aeruginosa, S. aureus	0.025–0.250 [a]	[57]
Olive mill waste	S. aureus, E. coli, Staphylococcus faecalis	11.1–28.8 [b]	[58]
Seed and peel of Citrus sinensis	S. aureus, C. albicans	2.5–40.0 [a] 2.0–14.0 [b]	[59]
Orange peels of Citrus senensis	S. aureus, L. monocytogenes, P. aeruginosa	15–92 [a]	[60]
Grape seeds	E. coli, S. aureus	9–21 [b]	[61]
Grape pomace	S. aureus, E. coli, C. albicans	0.195–100 [a]	[62]
Lavender (Lavandula angustifolia) and melissa (Melissa Officinalis) waste	E. coli, Proteus vulgaris, P. aeruginosa, S. aureus, Enterococcus faecalis, L. monocytogenes, Candida utilis, B. subtilis, Aspergillus niger, Penicillium chrysogenum, S. cerevisiae	8.00–12.00 [a]	[63]
Mango seed kernel	Xanthomonas axonopodis pv. manihotis	3.08–7.10 [b]	[64, 65]
	E. coli, C. albicans	1.10–2.23 [a]	
Vaccinium meridionale Swartz pomace	S. aureus, E. coli	126–520 [c]	[66]
Walnut green husk	Bacillus cereus, B. subtilis, S. aureus, Staphylococcus epidermis, E. coli, P. aeruginosa	20–100 [a]	[67]
Carya illinoinensis	L. monocytogenes, S. aureus, Vibrio parahaemolyticus, B. cereus	0.075–1.870 [a]	[68]
Garlic (Allium sativum L.) husk	P. aeruginosa, Klebsiella pneumoniae	1–10 [a]	[69]
Mangosteen bark, leaf, and fruit pericarp	L. monocytogenes, S. aureus	0.03 > 10 [a]	[70]
Newhall navel orange peel	E. coli, S. aureus, B. subtilis	0.16–30.36 [a]	[71]
Peel of Punica granatum Var. Bhagwa	S. aureus, E. coli, Streptococcus mutans mutans, C. albicans	17–32 [a]	[72]
Brewers' spent grain	S. aureus L. monocytogenes, S. typhimurium, E. coli, P. aeruginosa, C. albicans	0.00097–0.125 [a]	[73]

Table 2. Cont.

Source	Microorganisms	Antimicrobial Activity	Ref.
Agave sisalana Perrine juice (waste)	E. faecalis, C. albicans, P. aeruginosa, Bacillus atrophaeus, Shigella dysenteriae	24–31 [b]	[74]
Orange, yellow lemon, and banana peel	P. aeruginosa, K. pneumoniae, Serratia marcescens, E. coli, P. vulgaris, Salmonella typhi, S. aureus, E. faecalis, Aeromonas hydrophila, Streptococcus pyogenes, L. monocytogenes, Lactobacillus casei	9–35 [b]	[75]
Guava bagasse (Psidium guajava), Cabernet Sauvignon, Pinot Noir (Vitis vinifera), Isabella grape marcs (Vitis labrusca), Petit Verdot grape seeds and red grapes fermentation lees (Vitis vinifera), tomato bagasse (Solanum lycopersicum), kale (Brassica oleracea), beet (Beta vulgaris), broccoli (Brassica oleracea), turnip stems (Brassica rapa), carrot (Daucus carota), radish leaves (Raphanus sativus), pumpkin (Cucurbita sp.), passion fruit hulls (Passiflora edulis), artichoke leaves (Cynara cardunculus), and peanut peels (Arachis hypogaea)	S. aureus, L. monocytogenes, S. Enteritidis, E. coli	10.0–20.0 [d] 0.78–25.00 [a]	[76]
Mango (Mangifera indica L.),	B. subtilis, S. aureus, P. aeruginosa, E. coli	13–18 [b]	[77]
Camu-camu (Myrciaria dubia (Kunth) McVaugh)	E. coli, K. pneumoniae, Morganella morganii, Proteus mirabilis, P. aeruginosa, E. faecalis, L. monocytogenes	0.625 > 20	[78]
Olive mill wastewater	Campylobacter strains	0.25–2.00 [a]	[79]
Coffee pulp and husk	Salmonella choleraesus, S. aureus, P. aeruginosa, L. monocytogenes, E. coli	0.000612–0.001225 [a]	[80]

MIC = minimum inhibitory concentration; MBC = minimum bactericidal concentration; IZ = inhibition zone; GAE = gallic acid equivalent. [a] MIC/MBC (mg/mL); [b] disc diffusion method (mm); [c] µg GAE/mL; [d] IZ (inhibition zone mm).

Fennel and carrot, two species belonging to the Apiaceae family, are, like many others (e.g., tomatoes, potatoes, and onions), the most commonly consumed vegetables worldwide. They are aromatic and have been used as spices and condiments. Their EO, related to the fruits, is well characterized, whereas the chemical composition of the leaves, a by-product, is poor. Wiem Chiboub and co-workers performed a hydrodistillation of fresh leaves of carrot and Daucus carota subsp. sativus orange roots and yellow roots and *F. vulgare* subsp. vulgare var. azoricum and *F. vulgare* subsp. vulgare var. latina. The recorded results showed that the Daucus carota subsp. sativus yellow roots oil was significantly more effective against Gram-negative than Gram-positive bacteria, and the MIC values were in the range 6.25–50 mg/mL [56].

In order to reuse agro-wastes, the betel leaf stalk extract was found to be a potent antimicrobial agent, showing activity against Gram-positive and Gram-negative bacteria. The MIC values were in the range 25–250 µg/mL, measured against ciprofloxacin as a standard [57].

Among agro-food wastes, those derived from the olive oil production represent the most representative, especially in the Mediterranean area. Their composition was found to be rich in hydroxytyrosol and secoiridoids derivatives, important for their healthy properties. Inass et al. investigated the in vitro antimicrobial potential of olive mill wastewater and olive cake extracts. Oleuropein and verbascoside, already pointed out in various studies for their important antimicrobial potential, were also detected in these extracts. Furthermore, the elenolic acid, the main fragment of the oleuropein degradation, was mostly found in the olive cake extract. It can be considered as an important antimicrobial and antiviral agent, justifying the reuse of this kind of wastes [58].

Besides, the fruits belonging to the Citrus sinensis family produce large amounts of wastes, mostly seeds and peels, endowing suitable biological value. Seed oil demonstrated better activities than peel oil, with remarkable inhibitions obtained against *S. aureus* and *Candida albicans* at a concentration as low as 2.5 mg/mL [59]. Furthermore, the orange peel of 12 cultivars of Citrus sinensis from central-eastern was extracted through steam distillation and using hexane. In all the cultivars, the main component was D-limonene (73.9–97%). The antimicrobial activity was investigated against *S. aureus*, *Listeria monocytogenes*, and *P. aeruginosa*. 'Sanguinello' and 'Solarino Moro' essential oils were significantly active against *L. monocytogenes*, while 'Valencia' hexanoic extract against all the tested microorganisms [60].

In this context, the winemaking process is also involved in smart wastes management. Grape seeds are the by-products of the fruit juice and wine industries. Nowadays, more attention is devoted to the valorization of these kinds of wastes due to the valuable phytochemicals content. A study performed on different varieties of grape seeds, extracted with 70% ethanol, showed that all the tested varieties possessed a considerable antibacterial activity. Particularly, the variety Shiraz showed a large zone of inhibition (17 mm) [61]. Different fractions of wine residue (pomace, including seed and skin, seeds, or skin) from two red varieties of *Vitis vinifera* grapes (Pinot noir and Pinot Meunier) grown in New Zealand were extracted using different water-organic solvent mixtures. It was found that all the extracts exhibited antibacterial and antifungal effects, with MIC values ranging between 0.195 and 100 mg/mL [62].

Similarly, lavender and melissa wastes were proved to be rich in polyphenols (especially rosmarinic acid) and exhibited high antimicrobial activity [63]. The processing of jackfruit (*Artocarpus heterophyllus* Lam) yields large amounts of bio-wastes. The ethyl acetate extracts obtained from the peel, fiber, and core of the jackfruit showed antibacterial activity against *Xanthomonas* axonopodis pv. manihotis [64].

Apple and Sabine mango kernel extracts exhibited significantly high inhibition zones of 1.93 and 1.73 compared to Kent and Ngowe with 1.13 and 1.10, respectively, against *E. coli*. For *C. albicans*, the inhibition of Kent mango kernel extract, 1.63, was significantly lower than that of Ngowe, Apple, and Sabine with 2.23, 2.13, and 1.83, respectively [65].

The *Vaccinium meridionale* Swartz pomace is a source of bioactive compounds with remarkable antibacterial activity. Quercetin derivatives represented 100% of the total flavonols in the extracts, and *S. aureus* was the most sensitive strain [66].

The walnut green husk is an agro-forest waste obtained during walnut (*Juglans regia* L.) processing; its aqueous extracts were found to be able to inhibit the growth of Gram-positive bacteria [67]. Another study reported the antioxidant and antimicrobial activities of extracts of pecan nutshell. The MIC and minimum bactericidal concentration (MBC) values against *L. monocytogenes*, *Vibrio parahaemolyticus*, *S. aureus*, and *B. cereus* were significantly lower ($p < 0.05$) for the extract obtained through infusion, followed by atomization in a spray dryer when compared to the other extracts [68]. Water, methanol, ethanol, and 50% (v/v) aqueous solutions of methanol and ethanol extracts of disposed garlic husk displayed antimicrobial activity against Gram-positive bacteria when applied at different concentrations (1–10 mg/mL). These interesting biological properties could be attributed to specific phenolic compounds, such as caffeic, p-coumaric, ferulic, and di-ferulic acids [69].

Extracts prepared from mangosteen bark or fruit pericarp exhibited strong pH-dependent bacteriostatic and bactericidal effects against *L. monocytogenes* and *S. aureus* [70]. Ethyl acetate extract of Newhall orange peel showed the best antimicrobial effect due to the presence of sinensetin, 4′,5,6,7-tetramethoxyflavone, nobiletin, 3,3′,4′,5,6,7-hexamethoxyflavone, and narirutin [71]. *Punica granatum* peels (Bhagwa) furnished extracts, endowing interesting antibacterial properties. LC analysis of the extract recorded the punicalagin (163.52 mg/g of waste) as a major ellagitannin compound. Peel extract exerted high antibacterial activity against both Gram-positive and Gram-negative bacteria [72].

Extracts from brewer's spent grain, the major by-product of the brewing industry, proved to be a rich source of bioactive compounds with antimicrobial activity (especially against *C. albicans*) [73].

The phytochemical screening of the aqueous extract of the Agave sisalana Perrine juice (waste) revealed the presence of saponins, glycosides, phlobatannins, terpenoids, tannins, flavonoids, and cardiac glycosides and had the potential to be used against pathogenic organisms [74].

The antimicrobial activity of three abundantly available fruits peel waste (orange, yellow lemon, and banana) was evaluated on a wide range of microorganisms. Methanol, ethyl acetate, ethanol, and distilled water were used for extraction, and the results showed that, among the used solvents, the extracts exhibiting better performances were in decreasing order: Distilled water > Methanol > Ethanol > Ethyl acetate, reflecting the suitability of solvent for fruit peel extraction. Additionally, the effectiveness of fruit peel extracts was evaluated, showing Yellow lemon > Orange > Banana peel. It was observed that Gram-negative bacteria were more sensitive to the extracts, and, among them, *Klebsiella pneumoniae* showed the highest sensitivity against the extract of yellow lemon peel with the highest zone of inhibition [75]. Beet stalk, peanut peel, Pinot Noir grape marc, Petit Verdot grape seed and marc, red grapes fermentation lees, and guava bagasse wastes showed antimicrobial activity against *S. aureus* and *L. monocytogenes*. Analyses by GC-MS identified relevant concentrations of compounds exhibiting antimicrobial activity, such as caffeic, gallic, ferulic, and r-coumaric acids, and flavonoids quercetin, myricetin, and epicatechin. This study confirmed that agro-industrial wastes from wine and food industries could be used in the research about new antimicrobial compounds to be used as natural preservatives in the food and beverage industry with promising applications also in the pharmaceutical and biomedical fields [76].

With a growing world production, mango represents one of the most important tropical fruits produced worldwide. India is one of the most important producers where any mango-based products are also commonly consumed. Mango is mostly used in food processing industries, such as juice, jam, jelly, and pickle industries. This processed food leads to an enormous generation of mango peel as a waste product. It needs a huge capital to decompose these peels and to make sure that it does not pollute the environment. The

EO of both mango indica cultivars pulp and peel showed a wide range of antibacterial and antifungal activities [77].

The peel of Camu-camu (*Myrciaria dubia* (Kunth) McVaugh) displayed the richest phenolic profile as well as the most significant antibacterial activity (MICs recorded were in the range 0.625–10 mg/mL) [78].

Interesting results showed that the fraction with the highest content of phenolic and secoiridoid compounds from crude olive mill wastewater had a relevant antibacterial activity against a large panel of strains with a strain-dependent character [79].

The natural food colors market is trying to fit the consumer needs by increasingly replacing synthetic additives with natural ones. Besides being a natural product, the biological relevance of the carotenoids is related to their potential antioxidant and antimicrobial features, boosting their wide application in the food and pharmaceutical industry. The production of carotenoids by microorganisms using agricultural waste has been reported, employing coffee pulp and husk using a non-conventional yeast [80]. Despite the high antimicrobial activity exhibited by these extracts, their bioavailability is poor when used as such. In this context, the inclusion of nanocarriers seems to be an innovative tool to overcome this limit.

4. Nanofibers as Carriers of Antimicrobial Natural Products

During the last years, an increasing interest in the biomedical use of polymeric nanofibers was recorded due to their high porosity, outstanding mechanical strength, and simplicity of fabrication [10]. In particular, nanofibers have been proposed as systems for the delivery of bioactive molecules [81] or in regenerative medicine [82] and also as wound dressings devices [83]. Usually, polymeric nanofibers can be fabricated by template synthesis [84], self-assembly [85], phase separation [86], and electrospinning [87]. Among these, the electrospinning technique is the most used strategy for applications in tissue engineering and drug delivery due to its high-throughput, easy handling, and reproducibility (Figure 1).

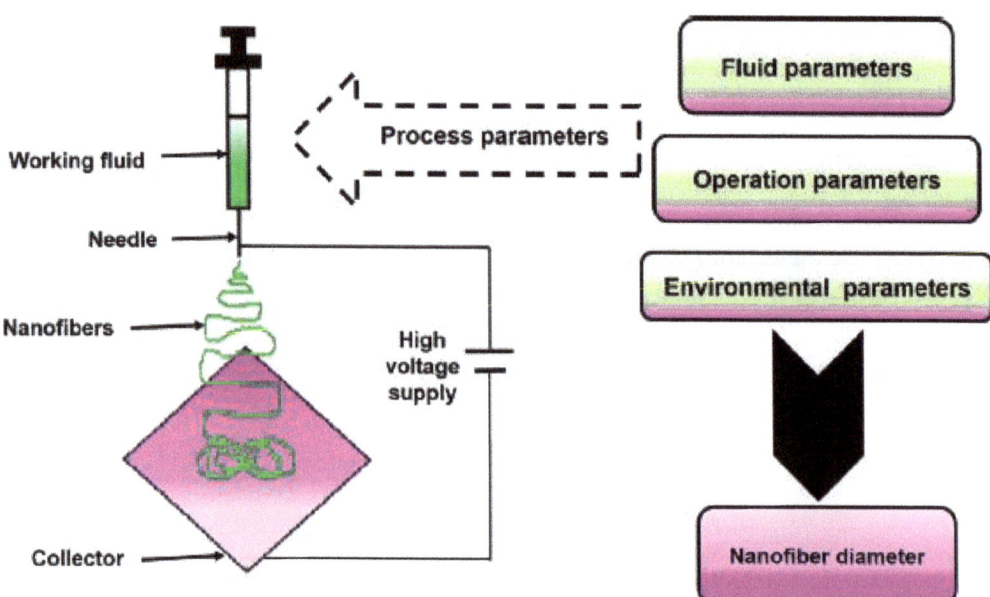

Figure 1. Electrospinning process and the different experimental parameters affecting the diameters of the produced nanofibers. Reproduced with permission from [10], Elsevier, 2020.

Additionally, electrospun meshes significantly increase adhesion and drug loading due to the structural similarity to the extracellular environment of the living tissues [88]. Literature data clearly indicate that electrospun nanofibers have the remarkable potential to amplify effectively the biological properties of medicinal plant extracts, essential oils, or pure single components with antimicrobial features. For this reason, they were largely employed as bioactive molecules to fabricate delivery systems, tissue engineering scaffolds, and regenerative medicine devices (Figure 2) [11].

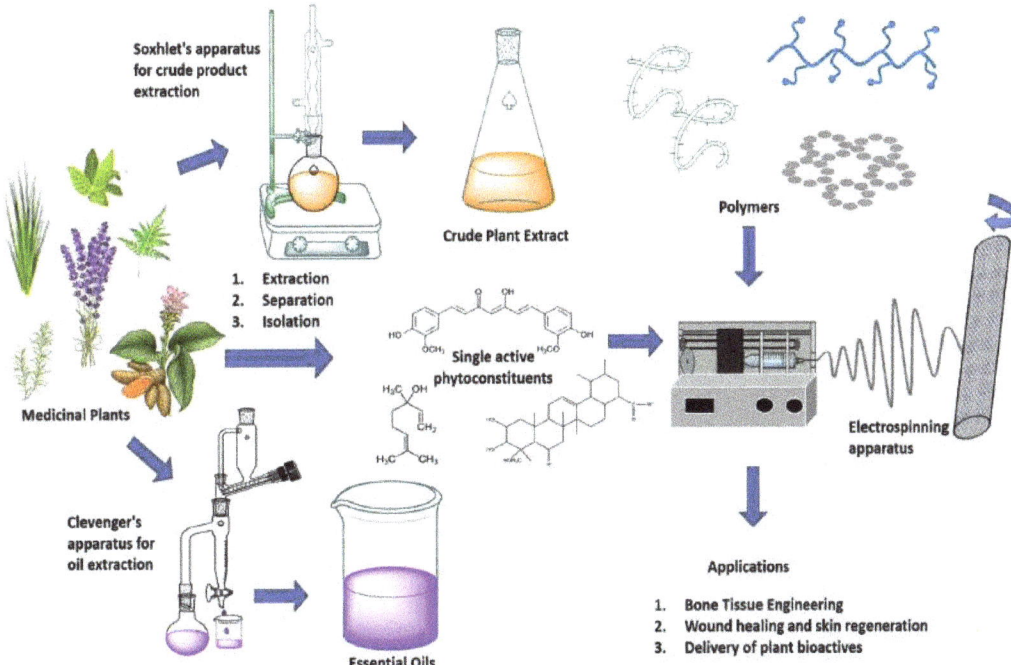

Figure 2. Schematic representation for the use of extracts isolated from medicinal plants and their nanofibers fabrication useful for pharmaceutical and biomedical applications. Reproduced with permission from [11]; Elsevier, 2020.

Specifically, in order to obtain polymeric nanofibers able to protect bioactive molecules and to ensure their controlled and site-specific delivery, both synthetic (polyesters, polyvinyl pyrrolidone (PVP), polyvinyl alcohol (PVA), or polyacrylates) and/or natural (polysaccharides or proteins) macromolecular structures have been proposed [89,90]. Synthetic constituents are usually cheaper and stronger, more easily electrospinnable, and show a precise structure [91]. Among the synthetic polymers used in the preparation of the nanofibers, PVA, PVP, and polyesters, such as polylactic, polylactic-*co*-glycolic acid, polyurethane, and polycaprolactone, were widely used with significant results (Table 3). On the contrary, natural polymers can be obtained by environment-friendly sources, offer good biocompatibility, thus reducing the adverse effects that could be observed when introduced to the human body [65] (Table 4). However, synthetic polymers are often required to strengthen the weak mechanical resistance of natural polymers [66].

Table 3. Synthetic polymers employed in the fabrication of nanofibers for the delivery of antimicrobial natural extracts.

Nanofiber	Incorporated Species	Antimicrobial Activity Against	Applications	Ref.
Polyacrylonitrile	Moringa leaf extracts	Staphylococcus aureus, Escherichia coli	Wound dressing	[92]
Polyacrylonitrile	Syzygium aromaticum oil	S. aureus, Bacillus subtilis, E. coli, Klebsiella pneumoniae	Wound dressing and tissue engineering scaffolds	[93]
Polyacrylonitrile	Lavender essential oil	S. aureus, K. pneumoniae	Antimicrobial activity	[94]
Poly (lactic acid)	Leptospermum scoparium and Melaleuca alternifolia essential oil	Staphylococcus epidermidis	Tissue engineering scaffolds	[95]
Poly (D,L-lactide-co-glycolide)	Methanolic extract of Grewia mollis	S. aureus, E. coli	Wound dressing	[96]
Poly (D,L-lactide-co-glycolide)	Human epidermal growth factor and Aloe vera extract	S. aureus, S. epidermidis	Wound dressing	[97]
Polycaprolactone	Biophytum sensitivum extract	S. aureus, E. coli	Wound dressing	[98]
Polycaprolactone	Gymnema sylvestre	Pseudomonas aeruginosa, E. coli	Wound dressing	[99]
Polycaprolactone	Clerodendrum phlomidis	S. aureus, P. aeruginosa, Salmonella typhi, E. coli	Wound dressing	[100]
Polycaprolactone, gelatin	Althea officinalis	—	Tissue engineering scaffolds	[101]
Polycaprolactone, gelatin	Black pepper oleoresin	S. aureus	Antimicrobial activity	[102]
Polycaprolactone, polyvinyl pyrrolidone	Tecomella undulate extract	P. aeruginosa, S. aureus, E. coli	Wound dressings	[103]
Polycaprolactone, silver nanoparticles	Nepelium lappaceum extract	E. coli, S. aureus, P. aeruginosa	Wound dressings	[104]
Polyurethane	Emu oil	B. subtilis, E. coli	Wound dressings and tissue engineering scaffolds	[105]
Polyurethane	Propolis	E. coli	Wound dressings and tissue engineering scaffolds	[84]
Polyurethane	Agrimonia eupatoria, Satureja hortensis, Hypericum perforatum herbal extract	S. aureus, P. aeruginosa	Wound dressings	[106]
Polyurethane	Szygium aromaticum extract	S. aureus, E. coli	Wound dressings	[107]
Polyurethane/polyethylene terephthalate	Juniperus chinensis extract	S. aureus, K. pneumoniae	Antimicrobial clothing materials, bedding materials	[108]
Polyurethane/carboxymethyl cellulose	Malva sylvestris extract	S. aureus, E. coli	Wound dressings	[109]
Poly (vinyl alcohol)	Lawsonia inermis leaves extract	S. aureus, E. coli	Wound dressings	[110]
Poly (vinyl alcohol)	Tridax procumbens leaves extract	S. aureus, E. coli	Antimicrobial activity	[111]

Table 3. Cont.

Nanofiber	Incorporated Species	Antimicrobial Activity Against	Applications	Ref.
Poly (vinyl alcohol)	*Coptis chinensis* extract	*S. aureus, S. epidermidis*	Medical and cosmetics fields	[112]
Poly (vinyl alcohol)	*Rhodomyrtus tomentosa* extract	*E. coli, P. aeruginosa, B. subtilis, Enterococcu faecalis*	Antimicrobial activity	[113]
Poly (vinyl alcohol)	*Coptidis rhizoma* extract	*S. aureus, S. epidermidis*	Wound dressings	[114]
Poly(vinyl alcohol)/ranocellulose from pineapple	*Stryphodedron barbatimao* extract	—	Antimicrobial activity	[115]
Poly(vinyl alcohol)/guar gum	*Acalypha indica* extract	*E. coli, B. subtilis, S. aureus, Pseudomonas fluorescens*	Wound dressings	[116]
Poly(vinyl alcohol)/sodium alginate	Cinnamon, clove, and lavender oils	*S. aureus*	Wound dressings	[117]
Polyvinylpyrrolidone	*Sophora flavescens* extract	*S. epidermidis*	Antimicrobial air filtration	[118]
Polyvinylpyrrolidone	Cinnamon essential oil	*S. aureus, E. coli, P. aeruginosa, Candida albicans*	Antimicrobial activity	[119]

Table 4. Natural polymers employed in the fabrication of nanofibers for the delivery of antimicrobial natural extracts.

Nanofiber	Incorporated Species	Antimicrobial Activity Against	Applications	Ref.
Cellulose acetate	Lemongrass, cinnamon, and peppermint essential oils	*Escherichia coli, Candida albicans*	Tissue engineering scaffolds	[120]
Cellulose acetate	Rosemary and oregano essential oils	*Staphylococcus aureus, E. coli, C. albicans*	Wound dressings	[121]
Carboxymethyl cellulose/sodium alginate	Olive leaf extract	*S. aureus, E. coli, Enterococcus faecalis, Pseudomonas aeruginosa*	Wound dressings	[122]
Cellulose	*S. persica* extract	*S. aureus, E. coli*	Antimicrobial activity	[123]
Cellulose	*Oryza sativa* and *Tinospora cordifolia* extracts	*E. coli, P. aeruginosa, Bacillus subtilis*	Wound dressing and tissue engineering scaffolds	[124]
Dandelion polysaccharide	*Litsea cubeba* essential oil	*S. aureus*	Antimicrobial activity	[125]

Table 4. Cont.

Nanofiber	Incorporated Species	Antimicrobial Activity Against	Applications	Ref.
Chitosan-ethylenediaminetetra acetic acid/poly(vinyl alcohol)	*Garcinia mangostana* fruit hull extract	*S. aureus*, *E. coli*	Wound dressings	[126]
Chitosan/poly(vinyl alcohol)	*Bidens pilosa* extract	*S. aureus*, *E. coli*	Antimicrobial activity	[127]
Chitosan/poly(vinyl alcohol)/honey	–	*S. aureus*, *E. coli*	Wound dressings	[128,129]
Chitosan/poly(vinyl alcohol)/honey	*Cleome droserifolia* and *Allium sativum* extracts	Multidrug-resistant *P. aeruginosa*, *E. coli*, *S. aureus*, and methicillin-resistant *S. aureus*	Wound dressings	[130]
Chitosan/poly(ethylene oxide)	Cinnamaldehyde essential oil	*P. aeruginosa*	Tissue engineering scaffolds	[131]
Chitosan/poly(ethylene oxide)	Green tea extract	*S. aureus*, *E. coli*	Wound dressings	[132]
Gelatin	*Phaeodactylum tricornuttuma* extract	Multidrug-resistant *P. aeruginosa*, *E. coli*	Wound dressings	[133]
Gelatin	*Centella asiatca*	*S. aureus*, *E. coli*, and *P. aeruginosa*	Wound dressings	[134]
Gelatin	*Curcuma comosa* Roxb. extract	*S. aureus*, *Staphylococcus epidermidis*	Antimicrobial activity	[135]
Gelatin	*Chromolaena odorata* crude extract	*S. aureus*	Antimicrobial activity	[136]
Gelatin/polycaprolactone	*Aloe vera* extract	*S. aureus*, *E. coli*	Tissue engineering scaffolds	[137]
Silk fibroin/poly(ethylene oxide)	Manuka honey	Methicillin-resistant *S. aureus*, *P. aeruginosa*, *E. coli*, *S. aureus*	Wound dressings	[138]
Silk fibroin/polyvinylpyrrolidone	Baicalein	*S. aureus*	Wound dressings	[139]
Silk fibroin/hyaluronic acid	Olive leaf extract	*S. aureus*, *E. coli*	Antimicrobial activity	[140]
Zein/tragacanth gum	Saffron extract	–	Polymeric carrier	[141]
Zein	Propolis extract	*S. aureus*, *S. epidermidis*, *E. coli*, *Salmonella enterica*, *P. aeruginosa*, *C. albicans*	Wound dressings	[142]
Soy protein isolate	Raspberry extract	*S. epidermidis*	Antimicrobial activity	[143]

4.1. Synthetic Polymer-Based Nanofibers

4.1.1. Polyacrylates

Among polyacrylates, polyacrylonitrile (PAN) has been well documented to be a very important material for easy manufacturing of synthetic fibers with unique thermal and mechanical stability, as well as excellent resistance to the solvents [144,145]. In the biomedical field, PAN nanofibers loaded with moringa leaf extracts, rich in phytochemicals, such as zeatin, quercetin, amino acids, and phenolic compounds, have been proposed for wound healing applications [92,146]. The antibacterial properties of the loaded nanofibers were evaluated against *E. coli* and *S. aureus*. Results displayed that the activity of the device strictly depended on the concentration of the extract in the PNA nanofibers, confirming its promising potential as an effective wound dressing. Alternatively, electrospinning PNA nanofibers loaded with *Syzygium aromaticum* oil, containing unexplored natural bioactive molecules (eugenol and caryophyllene), were found to be highly effective against both Gram-positive and Gram-negative bacteria in in vitro delivery studies [93,147]. The release profile of *Syzygium aromaticum* was characterized by an initial burst, followed by controlled diffusion kinetics. Similarly, PNA fibers were loaded with EO of lavender (*Lavendula angustifolia*) [94]. This natural product is largely exploited in aromatherapy as a holistic relaxant and has been exploited for its excellent antimicrobial features. Lavender oil, highly encapsulated in PAN fibers with a loading content equal to 13.6%, displayed a release profile with an initial burst effect, reaching a 35% of active release after 24 h in a buffer medium (pH 7.4). The loaded polymeric device showed also in vitro antibacterial activity after an incubation time of 24 h (MIC equal to 100 mg·mL^{-1}).

4.1.2. Polyesters

Poly (lactic acid) (PLA) is an outstanding polymeric material largely employed in the pharmaceutical and biomedical sectors due to its excellent biodegradability and biocompatibility [148]. PLA represents the most extensively used synthetic polymer in the fabrication of nanofibers [149]. Electrospinning of PLA fibers containing EO derived from *Leptospermum scoparium* and *Melaleuca alternifolia* at different concentrations has been proposed for the treatment of microbial infections induced by *S. epidermidis* [95], a bacterium abundant on human skin and often responsible for infections and formation of biofilms on the medical devices [150]. The antibacterial activity of *Leptospermum scoparium* EO was mainly ascribed to triketone species, such as flavesone and leptospermone [151], while terpinen-4-ol and α-terpinene determined the antimicrobial activity of *Melaleuca alternifolia* EO. Although *Melaleuca alternifolia* oil showed remarkable activity against *S. epidermidis*, its efficacy was largely limited due to the low amount of active molecules available after the electrospinning process. On the contrary, the antimicrobial activity of the PLA-*Leptospermum scoparium* oil system was preserved during the electrospinning process.

In order to improve its water solubility, PLA was successfully modified by hyperbranched polyglycerol, a highly hydrophilic polymer with excellent biocompatibility and water solubility [152]. Nanofibrous dressing with PLA and the hyperbranched polyglycerol blend was fabricated using electrospinning technique and loaded with curcumin, a polyphenolic biologically active ingredient of turmeric isolated from the dry rhizomes of *Curcumin Longa* L. [153]. Curcumin release profiles, recorded at 37°C in PBS and displayed as the increased hydrophilicity of the device, allowed to achieve a complete delivery in 72 h, suggesting its use as potential wound patch dressing for chronic and acute wound diseases.

Alternatively, fibers based on poly(D,L-lactide-*co*-glycolide) (PLGA) have been successfully proposed as delivery systems due to their high biodegradability. In particular, the electrospinning technique was employed to fabricate ultrafine PLGA fiber mats containing a methanolic extract of *Grewia mollis* (7.5% w/w). The antimicrobial effect of the device was tested against pathogenic bacteria, such as *E. coli* and *S. aureus*, suggesting its use in the treatment of dermal bacterial infections or as a wound dressing agent [96]. Garcia-Orue and coworkers developed a PLGA-based nanofibrous membrane in which the antibacterial properties of the natural extract and the ability of the epidermal growth factor to enhance fibroblast proliferation allowed the fabrication of an efficient device against *S. aureus* and *S. epidermidis*, reducing, at the same time, the wound healing time [97].

Polycaprolactone (PCL) represents a biodegradable aliphatic polyester, largely employed to produce nanofibers by electrospinning techniques. The incorporation of suitable natural extracts allowed the fabrication of devices with remarkable antimicrobial properties. Specifically, crude extract of *biophytum sensitivum* was loaded, and experimental release displayed a controlled delivery of the bioactive molecules (59% in 72 h) [98]. The antimicrobial performances of the device were evaluated against some common wound bacteria, such as *S. aureus* (27 mm inhibition) and *E. Coli* (47 mm inhibition). Similarly, electrospun PCL-based nanofiber mats containing natural leaves extracts of *Gymnema sylvestre* [99] or *Clerodendrum phlomidis* [100] were proposed as a wound dressing with remarkable antimicrobial characteristics. The cumulative delivery profiles depicted an intense burst effect, mainly due to bioactive desorption release mechanisms, while a constant delivery of the therapeutic was reached after 24 h.

Althea officinalis extract is also well known as a traditional herbal drug with noteworthy wound healing capacity and antimicrobial properties. In particular, *Althea officinalis* extract was loaded in nanofibers based on PCL and gelatin [101]. The blending of synthetic and natural macromolecules was proposed as an efficient strategy to optimize the mechanical properties of the scaffolds. In addition, the superior viscoelastic properties of PCL with respect to other polyesters made it more compatible with natural macromolecules, allowing the construction of multilayer structures. Cumulative release experiments highlighted a release of bioactive molecules proximately to 100% after 24 h. Similarly, the PCL layer was deposited onto the gelatin films by electrospinning to obtain complex structures able to vehicle black pepper oleoresin bioactive components. Strong antimicrobial properties of the multilayer were recorded over time (10 days) against *S. aureus* [102].

Blended polymer-based electrospun nanofibers have gained great attention because of the mechanical properties of the matrices and easy monitoring of the release profiles, depending on the ratio of the components in the polymer chains. By coupling the strength of PCL with polyvinyl pyrrolidone (PVP), PCL/PVP nanofibers containing crude bark extract of *Tecomella undulata* were fabricated, and their antimicrobial behavior was evaluated against *S. aureus*, *E.coli*, and *P. aeruginosa* [103]. Recently, in order to improve antimicrobial properties of PCL-nanofibers loaded with *Nephelium lappaceum* extract, they were decorated with silver nanoparticles [154], providing a multi-component device with synergistic antibacterial properties [104]. The antimicrobial activity was evaluated against *E. coli*, *S. aureus*, and *P. aeruginosa*, and the results suggested a synergistic effect between silver nanoparticles and extract-loaded nanofibers.

Polyurethane (PU) is a biocompatible hydrophobic polymer, largely used for biomedical and pharmaceutical scopes, owing to its excellent oxygen permeability and good barrier and mechanical properties [155]. Nanofibers based on PU were successfully prepared to load emu oil, a natural mixture derived from the emu (*Dromaius novaehollandiae*), which originated in Australia and positively tested against both Gram-positive (*B. subtilis*) and Gram-negative (*E. coli*) pathogens [105]. Similarly, PU nanofibers were proposed as polymeric carriers of propolis [84], a resinous substance produced by bees from plant exudates, containing different bioactive compounds [156]. In addition, the adhesive properties of propolis afford the point-bonding to the PU nanofibers, improving their mechanical issues. The antimicrobial properties of propolis/PU nanofibers were evaluated against *E. coli*, and the results showed that the bacterial inhibition zone was progressively increased with increasing the propolis amount in the nanocomposite. More recently, herbal extracts of *Agrimonia eupatoria*, *Satureja hortensis*, and *Hypericum perforatum* were loaded on several PU composite nanofibers, and their antimicrobial properties were evaluated against *S. aureus* and *P. aeruginosa* [110]. Finally, antibacterial and elastic nanofibers from thermoplastic PU were produced by coating process with *Syzgium aromaticum* extract, gained by Soxhlet extraction of clove oil [107]. All coated nanofibers (2–10 mg cm^{-2}) showed antibacterial activity against *S. aureus* and *E. coli*.

Nanomaterials to be employed as antimicrobial clothing materials or bedding materials for allergic patients often required a lamination process. In this regard, the nanofibers of PU/*Juniperus chinensis* extracts were prepared by laminating electrospraying PU adhesive resin on polyethylene terephthalate-based fabric and an electrospun PU nanofiber web [108]. The antibacterial experiments performed at 110 and 130°C against *S. aureus* and *K. pneumoniae* confirmed that the combination between laminating and electrospinning represents an interesting way to project useful composites to be employed in the biomedical field. Finally, in order to improve the absorption ability of wound exudates, hydrophilic blend materials based on a different weight ratio between PU and carboxymethyl cellulose (CMC) and containing *Malva sylvestris* extract were prepared. The new materials proved to efficiently deliver the bioactive compounds to diabetic wounds [109]. The release profile of the active compounds resulted in a complete delivery in 85 h, and strong antibacterial activity against *E. coli* and *S. aureus* was recorded.

4.1.3. Poly(Vinyl Alcohol)

Synthetic biodegradable polymers, such as PLA, PLGA, and poly(glycolic acid), are poorly soluble in water. It follows that the production of nanofiber mats often requires the use of organic solvents, incompatible with the preparation of carriers for pharmaceutical and biomedical uses. On the contrary, biocompatible, biodegradable, and no-toxic poly(vinyl alcohol) (PVA) can be easily employed to prepare nanofibers in aqueous environments [157]. Different natural extracts, as sources of antimicrobial molecules, were enclosed in PVA nanofibers. In particular, *Lawsonia inermis* leaves' hydroalcoholic (ethanol/water 90/10 *v/v*) extracts were loaded to achieve antibacterial nanofibers (2.8% *w/w*) with bacteriostatic action towards *E. coli*. and bactericidal efficiency against *S. aureus* [110]. Similarly, the methanolic extracts of *Tridax procumbens* leaves [111] and the aqueous extracts of *Coptis chinensis* [112] were employed to prepare nanofibrous mats with antimicrobial activity. PVA/*Tridax procumbens* nanofibers showed an outstanding zone of inhibitions and improved resistivity power against *S. aureus* and *E. coli*, whereas PVA/*Coptis chinensis* nanofibers, evaluated against different Gram-positive bacteria, displayed the highest antibacterial activity against *S. epidermidis*. The ethyl acetate *Rhodomyrtus tomentosa* extract, rich in myricetin and rhodomyrtosone, was involved in the fabrication of electrospun nanofibers; the antimicrobial experiments against the common human pathogens (*E. coli, P. aeruginosa, B. subtilis*, and *E. faecalis*) displayed a clear inhibition zone (7–12 mm) by loading the extract in the concentration range of 1.5–2.5% (*w/w*) [113]. Finally, nanofibers containing *Coptidis rhizoma* extracts (10, 20, and 30% *w/w*) were fabricated using PVA as a carrier [114]. The release experiments performed at physiological pH of 5.5, set by acetate buffer solution, displayed an initial fast release, followed by a gradual release for 48 h. In addition, high antimicrobial activity was recorded against *S. aureus* (max inhibition zone 17.0 mm) and *S. epidermidis* (max inhibition zone 6.2 mm).

In addition, PVA was employed in combination with a natural polymer to achieve bio-nanocomposites fibrous mats. Specifically, a PVA-based device enclosing nanocellulose from pineapple was loaded with *Stryphodedron barbatimao* extract (water-alcohol solution 96:4 *v/v*) [115], a well-known mixture employed in medicine as an antiseptic, anti-inflammatory, and anti-bacterial remedy [158]. More recently, PVA/guar gum composite nanofibers were proposed as a carrier of alcoholic extract of *Acalypha indica*, a traditionally acclaimed plant for wound healing [116]. The release profiles displayed a constant and slow delivery throughout the experimental time, while a complete release was observed after 38 h. The antimicrobial experiments against *E. coli, B. subtilis, S. aureus, P. fluorescens* highlighted bacteriostatic action against all microbial strains. Finally, several EOs (cinnamon, clove, and lavender at a concentration of 0.5, 1, and 1.5% *w/w*) were involved in the synthesis of PVA/sodium alginate (SA) polymeric nanofibers, allowing the preparation of devices able to efficiently inhibit *S. aureus* [117]. Cinnamon oil (1.5% *w/w*)/PVA/SA nanofibers exhibited the best results (inhibition zone of 2.7 cm).

4.1.4. Polyvinylpyrrolidone

Polyvinylpyrrolidone (PVP) exhibits unique properties because it is biocompatible, water-soluble, and non-toxic, allowing its application in the biomedical area [159].

Sophora flavescens extract was incorporated into PVP nanofibers, and the device was proposed as antimicrobial air filtration [118]. Filtration and antimicrobial performances of the PVP-based nanofiber filter were evaluated, employing *S. epidermidis* bioaerosols as test airborne particles; the results displayed excellent antimicrobial activity and highly effective air filters (99.99% filtration efficiency).

Nutraceutical properties of the cinnamon EO were exploited by enclosing the oil in the PVP-based nanofibers by oil-in-water emulsion electrospinning, and its antimicrobial properties were recorded against *S. aureus, E. coli, P. aeruginosa, C. albicans* [119]. The outstanding antimicrobial activity of the device was proved to be related to the size of the fibers and mainly ascribed to the high eugenol concentration in the cinnamon oil. Experimental tests were highlighted as the antimicrobial activity was recorded with cinnamon EO concentration into PVP in the range 2–4% (*w/w*).

4.2. Natural Polymer-Based Nanofibers

4.2.1. Polysaccharides

Materials based on cellulose acetate (CA) have been largely employed in the biopharmaceutical processing industry as wound dressings, tissue engineering scaffolds, and drug delivery systems [160]. Electrospun CA nanofibers encapsulating lemongrass, cinnamon, and peppermint EOs were employed to fabricate scaffold devices able to inhibit bacteria growth. Results demonstrated the complete inhibition of *E. coli*, while *C. albicans* yeast showed a remarkable resistance, mainly due to its diameter more than four times larger than *E. coli* [120]. More recently, CA-based nanofibers enclosing rosemary and oregano EOs were evaluated against *S. aureus, E. coli*, and *C. albicans* [121]. Nanofibers loaded with the oregano oil (containing a high concentration of carvacrol and thymol) displayed the best anti-biofilm and antimicrobial performances. Electrospun nanofibrous mats based on carboxymethyl cellulose (CMC) and SA were proposed as functional wound dressing materials able to load olive leaf extracts [122]. The antibacterial properties of oleuropein and hydroxytyrosol contained in this aqueous extract allowed to fabricate a device able to inhibit pathogens mostly responsible for infections by skin wounds. The analysis of the release profile from the nanofibers depicted a substantial burst effect (50%) and a complete delivery within 24 h.

Nanofibers have also been proposed as reinforcing agents to improve the mechanical and physical performances of other polymeric devices, such as films, hydrogels, and sponges [161]. Nanocomposites based on CMC and cellulose nanofibers (CNF) were loaded with *Salvadora persica* hydro-alcoholic extract to obtain a device with good antimicrobial properties against both *S. aureus* and *E. coli*. [123]. The incorporation of CNF (5% *w/w*) into the CMC matrix caused a significant improvement of the mechanical properties in comparison with CMC. Similarly, composite biosponges of SA reinforced with CNF were prepared [124], determining a noteworthy enhancement in the mechanical performances and the thermal stability for SA-based composite biosponges. Moreover, the sponges loading with *Oryza sativa* and *Tinospora cordifolia* extracts imparted additional antibacterial functionality to the composite against *E. coli* and *P. aeruginosa*.

The encapsulation into nanofibers of the EOs gained from natural plants often requires a strong electric field and high-voltage. This could lead to adverse reactions, frequently involving the species able to impart pharmacological and nutraceutical properties to the extracts. To overcome this inconvenience, the employment of the β-cyclodextrin represents an endearing strategy [162]. *Litsea cubeba* EO was first encapsulated in the cavity of the β-cyclodextrin, and the inclusion complex was then loaded by electrospinning into nanofibers based on the dandelion polysaccharide [125], a natural polymer used for the preparation of active nanofibers [163]. The release profiles of the EO in PBS solution (pH 7.2) showed a good sustained release (about 70% after 100 h), ensuring also a long-lasting antibacterial effect against *S. aureus*.

Biomedical devices based on chitosan (CT) were exploited for developing nanofibrous wound dressing materials [164]. Additionally, CT is also known for its strong antibacterial activity against different fungi, bacteria, and viruses [165–167]. However, CT viscosity, as well as the high charge of the polysaccharide chains, made difficult the electrospinning process, and the application of highly acidic and toxic solvents was required [168]. These drawbacks can be overcome by co-spinning CT with other spun polymers, such as poly(ethylene oxide) (PEO), PCL, and PVA [169].

CT-ethylenediaminetetraacetic acid and PVA were selected for the preparation of nanofibrous mats to be employed as carriers of extracts gained by maceration (acetone/water 70/30 *v/v*) of *Garcinia mangostana* fruit hull [126], known to exert important antimicrobial properties due to the presence of the α-mangostin (13.20% *w/w*) [170]. α-Mangostin release experiments from the nanofiber mats loaded with the extracts revealed that active molecules were rapidly released, reaching 80% within 1 h. Additionally, the fiber mats loaded with the natural extracts exhibited antibacterial activity against *S. aureus* and *E. coli*. More recently, CT and PVA were successfully used to fabricate electrospun nanofibers containing *Bidens pilosa* extract. Composite nanofibers were effective against *E. coli* (growth inhibition 91% and MIC 10 mg/mL) and *S. aureus* (growth inhibition 86% and MIC 10 mg/mL) bacteria due to the combined effect of CT and natural extract [127]. Polymeric devices with multi-antibacterial activity were prepared by electrospinning of CT and honey, a carbohydrate-rich syrup, showing a relevant wound healing activity and remarkable antibacterial performances [171]. The synthesis of honey-based nanofibers was frequently hard due to the viscosity of the honey that permits its use in the electrospinning process only at small concentrations (<10%) [172]. Electrospinning of CT and honey at high concentration, with PVA and using eco-friendly solvents, was performed, and the antimicrobial activity of the fiber mats was evaluated against *E. coli* and *S. aureus* [128,129]. In addition, two aqueous extracts (*Cleome droserifolia* and *Allium sativum*) were loaded within honey, PVA, and CT nanofibers; in vitro antimicrobial experiments revealed a complete inhibition of *E. coli* and *S. aureus* [130]. However, only the fibers simultaneously loaded with both the extracts exhibited some antimicrobial activity against methicillin-resistant *S. aureus*. In addition, preliminary in vivo study (wound closure rates in mice and histological examination of the wounds) revealed the beneficial effects of the extract-loaded device on the wound healing process in comparison with the untreated control.

Alternatively, CT-based nanofibers can be fabricated employing PEO, which allows the use of solutions at pH 4, thus not requiring an extremely acid environment. CT/PEO solutions were successfully electrospun, by oil-in-water emulsion technique, into fibrous mats and loaded with cinnamaldehyde (0.5 and 5.0% *w/w*), a volatile EO derived from cinnamon bark [131]. The delivery/antimicrobial experiments of cinnamaldehyde EO from the CT/PEO nanofibers displayed a strong inactivation of *P. aeruginosa* (81% after 180 min). Finally, a green tea extract was proposed as an antibacterial enhancer to be enclosed in the electrospinning process involving CT/PEO chains [132]. In vitro tests revealed that this device had an antibacterial effect against *E. coli* and *S. aureus*.

4.2.2. Proteins

Gelatin (GL) is a hydrophilic biopolymer, which has been widely used in the biomedical field [173]. Nanofibrous material based on GL was proposed as a carrier of active ingredients gained from natural sources. Specifically, electrospinning of GL in the presence of a small amount of the *Phaeodactylum tricornutuma* extracts provided a device with remarkable antimicrobial properties against *E. coli* and multidrug-resistant *S. aureus* [133,174]. Similarly, *Centella asiatica*, a traditional herbal medicine able to facilitate the wound-repair process, was involved in the fabrication of GL-based nanofibrous mats [175]. This device exhibited remarkable antimicrobial properties against *S. aureus*, *E. coli*, and *P. aeruginosa* and dermal wound-healing activity in the rat model. More recently, GL fibers loaded with *Curcuma comosa* Roxb. extract displayed antibacterial activities against *S. aureus* (Inhibition zone of 7.77 mm) and *S. epidermidis* (Inhibition zone of 7.73 mm) [135], while the loading of *Chromolaena odorata* crude extract [136] allowed the fabrication of a system with excellent antimicrobial activity against *S. aureus* (100% of inhibition). However, nanofibers only based on natural polymers, such as GL, are often not useful for biomedical applications due to their low mechanical strength and high rate of degradation [103]. Baghersad et al., (2018) fabricated hybrid scaffolds, based on GL, PCL, and aloe vera, as an active extract, displaying good antibacterial activity against *E. coli* (inhibition 85.63%) and *S. aureus* (inhibition > 99%) [137].

Silk fibroin (SF) nanofibers were largely employed in the biomedical field due to their valuable properties, such as biocompatibility, electrospinnability, low inflammatory response, and therapeutic features [176]. SF/PEO nanofibers, incorporating Manuka honey [177], have been successfully fabricated by electrospinning and evaluated as a potential antimicrobial tissue engineering scaffold [138]. Manuka honey/SF nanofibers exhibited antibacterial properties against methicillin-resistant *S. aureus*, *P. aeruginosa*, *E. coli*, and *S. aureus*. Similarly, SF/PVP nanofibers loaded with baicalein, a Chinese herbal extract, were prepared by electrospinning technique and proposed as wound healing devices [139]. Experimental release displayed that almost 65% of baicalein was delivered within 24 h, reaching the lag phase after 48 h. In addition, in vitro antibacterial test against *S. aureus* displayed complete inhibition of the pathogen, while in vivo experiments in mice treated with SFP/PVP/baicalein exhibited a significant acceleration of the wound closure process. SF was employed with hyaluronic acid to fabricate nanofibers by coaxial electrospinning [140], an innovative synthetic methodology able to produce nanofibers with sheath/core morphology, utilizing two needles that, coaxially placed, allowed to feed core and shell solutions throughout two different channels. Specifically, the device was structured by a shell of SF, while hyaluronic acid and olive leaf extract, a source of bioactives, formed the core. The analysis of the release profiles showed an almost complete delivery (>90%) in nine days, reaching the lag time after two weeks. Olive leaf extract-loaded nanofibers also revealed remarkable antibacterial features against *S. aureus* and *E. coli* bacteria. The same synthetic methodology was proposed to fabricate core-shell nanofibers from zein (core) and tragacanth gum (shell) [141] for the encapsulation of saffron extract [175,178]. Release values in the range 16.1–43.9% after 2 h were recorded in saliva, water, and in media, simulating gastric and intestinal fluids. Zein nanofiber mats loaded with ethanol propolis extracts were also effectively fabricated by the classic electrospinning method, and their antimicrobial activities were investigated against various microorganisms, highlighting that the nanofibers were able to mainly inhibit the growth of the Gram-positive species [142].

Finally, electrospun nanocomposite fibers were fabricated, employing soy protein isolate, PEO, and raspberry extract, a natural mixture containing high levels of anthocyanin, displaying a significant growth inhibition of *S. epidermidis* [173].

5. Nanoparticles as Carriers of Antimicrobial Natural Products

Several examples are present in the literature, describing the involvement of nanoparticles in chemical reactions to form new effective carriers to deliver antimicrobial agents from natural sources in order to eliminate pathogens without introducing chemical undesirable preservatives (Table 5) [179,180].

The different methodology can be involved in the fabrication of nanoparticles with suitable properties, including soft lithography, mechanical stretching, microfluidics, or self-assembly, using suitable starting materials, such as small molecules or polymeric structures. When loading bioactive molecules into nanoparticle carriers with the aim to control pathogens growth and/or to prevent infection, different physicochemical and mechanical parameters should be considered, including size, shape, surface, and interior properties (Figure 3).

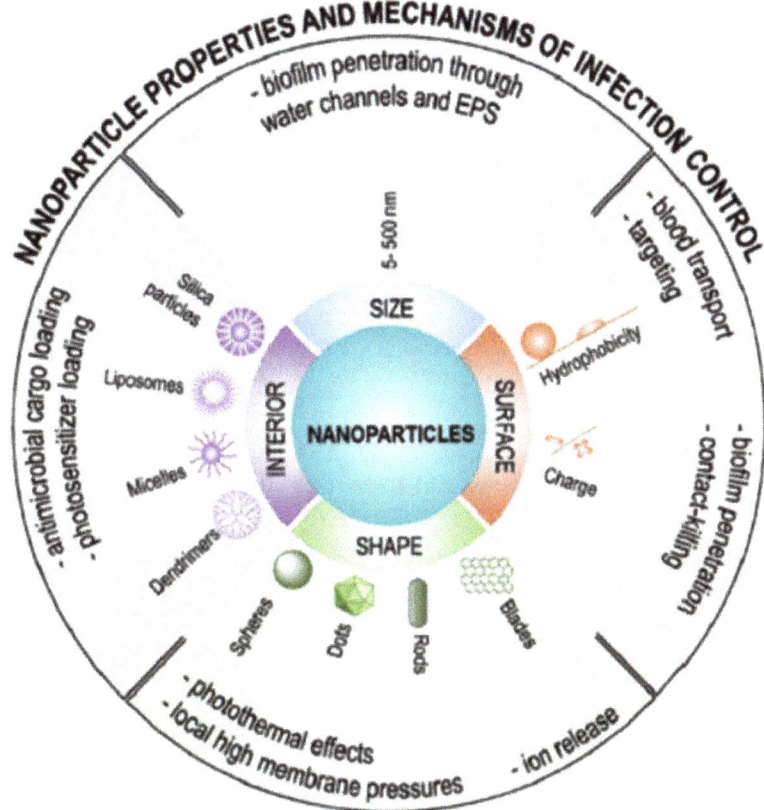

Figure 3. Size, shape, surface, and interior properties of nanoparticles important for their use in infection control. Reproduced with permission from [5], RSC, 2019.

Nanoparticles size plays a crucial role in their penetration into biofilm-bacteria, ensuring to overcome the inconvenience usually related to the multidrug-resistant strains. Ideal nanoparticle sizes to fight bacterial infections range between 5 and 500 nm. Generally, to improve the nanocarriers' efficiency, their size should not exceed the dimensions of water-filled channels into biofilms. In addition, nanoparticles sizes above 500 nm can be easily recognized by the immune system and eliminated from the bloodstream [5]. Surface properties should be also considered during nanoparticle design to ensure the inhibition of bacteria proliferation. Specifically, stealth transport through the bloodstream can be accomplished by decorating nanoparticles with suitable uncharged (polyethylene glycol) or zwitterionic hydrophilic polymers. Contact-killing capacity is strongly influenced by the nanoparticle shape that affects local adhesion forces and subsequently the extent of damage to the bacterial membrane [5]. In this regard, nano-blades or nano-knives by puncturing bacteria membranes determine the dispersion of intracellular components and cell death. Finally, the hydrophobic/hydrophilic balance into the interior of the nanoparticles should be designed to guarantee high loading capacity towards antimicrobial substances, avoiding the unnoticed loss of the cargo on their way to the infection site.

Cinnamon bark extract was embedded in PLGA/PVA nanoparticles synthesized by an emulsion evaporation method using different ratios of lactide/glycolide (65:35 and 50:50); TEM images revealed that nanoparticles were all spherical with a darker perimeter on the edge of the spheres attributed to the PVA. These products were able to gradually release active molecules and effectively inhibit *S. enterica* serovar Typhimurium and *L. monocytogenes* after 24 and 72 h at concentrations ranging from 224.42–549.23 µg/mL (Table 4) [181]. Acerola, guava, and passion fruit by-product extracts were also embedded in PLGA/PVA nanoparticles with a spherical shape and smooth surface. The antimicrobial performances against *L. monocytogenes* Scott A and *E. coli* K12 were concentration and time-dependent, with MIC values ranging from 200–1000 µg/mL, higher than the corresponding isolated extracts (from 500–3000 µg/mL) [182]. Passion fruit by-products (seed and cake) extracts were encapsulated into nanospheres synthesized by emulsion solvent evaporation method, involving different PLGA (lactide to glycolide ratios equal to 50:50 and 65:35) as organic phase and PVA aqueous solution (0.5 % *w/w*). The antimicrobial properties of the systems were evaluated against *E. coli* and *L. innocua*, and PLGA 65:35 particles showed a MIC value of 188 µg/mL against *L. innocua*, while the best PLGA against *E. coli* was PLGA 50:50 particle with a MIC of 226 µg/mL. In all the cases, the extracts were derived from cake extracts [183].

Similarly, PLGA/PVA nanoparticles (size range from 145–162 nm) were encapsulated with guabiroba extract (GE), a rich source of polyphenols and carotenoids. Release experiments, performed at 37°C and neutral pH, displayed an initial burst effect, more pronounced decreasing the lactide/glycolide ration in the PLGA chain, followed by a slower release rate of carotenoids. Nanoparticles based on PLGA 65:35 released 77% of the enclosed molecules after 6 h, while PLGA 50:50 displayed a marked burst effect (92% after 1 h). This behavior was a consequence of the highest lactide content able to delay the diffusion of the lipophilic carotenoids through the polymeric chains. Nanoparticles showed the growth inhibition of *L. innocua* within the concentration range tested (<1200 mg/mL), not displayed by the free extract [184]. The same authors improved the synthetic methodologies to achieve polymeric nanoparticles, proposing a modified emulsion-evaporation encapsulation method, allowing the synthesis of delivery devices able to preserve the extract's phenolic content for a prolonged time during release. In this study, GE showed improved antioxidant efficacy and an interesting MIC value of 2.251 µg/mL for PLGA 65:35 nanoparticles against *L. innocua* [185].

In the search for new antibacterial materials, silica mesoporous nanoparticles (SMN) have also attracted burgeoning attention due to high surface area, good biodegradability, high biocompatibility, tunable pore/particle size, and easy surface functionalization [186]. In addition, the presence of a significant porous structure allows designing high-performance devices to be applied as a carrier in the pharmaceutical and biomedical fields. Sol-gel chemistry is the synthetic strategy usually proposed to prepare SMN, mainly involving two reaction steps: (i) synthesis of silica precursor around a template by reactions of hydrolysis and condensation; (ii) removing of the template by solvent extraction and calcination [187]. The synthetic strategy deeply determined physicochemical and the morphological properties of the SMNs, such as size, porosity, and surface properties, as well as their cytotoxicity and biocompatibility, which represent important peculiarity to their employment in biological fluids. In this regard, SMNs are hydrolyzed to the nontoxic silicic acid, easily and safely excreted, and/or absorbed by the human body [188].

By using tetra-alkylammonium and pluronic surfactants with different molecular weights, it was possible to easily tune SMN pore sizes to better control loading capacity and cargo release rate. In addition, a relevant concentration of silanol groups on the SMNs surface permitted the preparation of hybrid inorganic/organic nanodevices, mainly through condensation reactions, grafting methodology, or direct incorporation of organic moieties into the silica wall [189].

MCM-41 represents a member of SMN with specific morphological and structural properties: uniform hexagonal array and channels with pores ranging from 2–50 nm [190].

This structure was proposed as a carrier of red propolis [191], showing remarkable antibacterial, antioxidant, and anticancer properties [192]. MCM-41 nanocarrier was fabricated by the co-condensation method using n-cetyl-n,n,n-trimethyl ammonium bromide as a template. In this view, different amounts of red propolis were embedded in silica mesoporous nanoparticles and tested against *S. aureus* at concentrations of 1050, 750, 500, 375, 225, and 150 µg/mL, finding an inhibition zone of approximately 19, 20, 21, 17, 16, and 17 mm in diameter, respectively.

Table 5. Synthetic polymers employed in the fabrication of nanoparticles for the delivery of antimicrobial natural extracts.

Nanoparticle	Incorporated Species	Antimicrobial Activity Against	Applications	Ref.
Poly(D,L-lactide-*co*-glycolide)/poly(vinyl alcohol)	Cinnamon bark extract	*Salmonella enterica* serovar Typhimurium, *Listeria monocytogenes*	Antimicrobial activity	[181]
Poly(D,L-lactide-*co*-glycolide)/poly(vinyl alcohol)	Acerola, guava, and passion fruit waste extracts	*L. monocytogenes* Scott A, *Escherichia coli* K12	Improvement of physical texture	[182]
Poly(D,L-lactide-*co*-glycolide)/poly(vinyl alcohol)	Passion fruit by-products	*E. coli*, *Listeria innocua*	Chemical disinfectants	[183]
Poly(D,L-lactide-*co*-glycolide)/poly(vinyl alcohol)	Guabiroba extract	*L. innocua*	Delivery systems	[184,185]
Silica mesoporous nanoparticles	Red propolis	*Staphylococcus aureus*	Antimicrobial activity	[191]
Silica mesoporous nanoparticles	*Salvia officinalis* L. and *Thymus serpyllum* L.	*S. enterica, Shigella flexneri* serotype 2b, *Enterococcus faecalis, E. coli, Pseudomonas aeruginosa, S. aureus, Streptococcus pneumoniae, Streptococcus pyogenes, Bacteroides fragilis, Candida albicans, Candida parapsilosis*	Antimicrobial activity	[193]

MCM-41 was also synthesized by the sol-gel method assisted by hydrothermal treatment and employing tetraethyl orthosilicate and n-cetyl-n,n,n-trimethyl ammonium bromide as silica source and template, respectively. Polyphenolic extracts of *Salvia officinalis* L. and *Thymus serpyllum* L. were encapsulated in these matrices and tested against *S. enterica, S. flexneri* serotype 2b, *E. faecalis, E. coli, P. aeruginosa, S. aureus, S. pneumoniae, S. pyogenes, B. fragilis, C. albicans*, and *C.n parapsilosis*, although showing milder improved antibacterial properties with respect to the parent extracts [193].

6. Conclusions and Future Perspectives

Nanotechnologies have been proposed as a valuable tool to overcome the problems frequently related to the employment of natural products with pharmacological activities. Indeed, most of the clinical trials involving natural products fail due to their poor water solubility, unsuitable molecular weight, and low lipophilicity, which produce unstable structures undergoing high metabolic rate and fast clearance. In addition, if the bioactive molecules are accumulated in non-targeted tissues and organs, significant side effects can be detected.

Currently, different studies proposed polymeric nanocarriers as favorable devices to increase bioavailability and activities of natural products, representing a plausible approach for the treatment of a variety of diseases. In particular, the perspectives of a multidisciplinary approach, expecting the combination between nanotechnology-based delivery systems and antimicrobial features from natural extracts, are promising in the infection control in order to produce multi-component devices able to avoid the multidrug-resistance, usually associated with the infections. Nanodevices, such as nanofibers or nanoparticles, were effectively proposed as carriers of extracts from plants, herbals, and agro-food by-products with remarkable antimicrobial properties.

Electrospun nanofibers, usually fabricated by single-fluid electrospinning, represent a valuable approach to produce high performing nanodevices. This goal was reached by employing both natural and synthetic polymers. However, the best results were recorded, fabricating blended macromolecular structures able to conjugate the feature of synthetic constituents (cheapness, mechanical resistance, and electrospinnability) with the highest biocompatibility of the natural polymers, reducing the adverse effects, potentially affecting the different biological compartments. In addition, the loading of several bioactive molecules within nanofibers required the optimization of different key factors, such as burst release reduction and/or low delivery efficiency. Recently, coaxial electrospinning was proposed as an innovative tool to fabricate core-shell nanostructures able to optimize the distribution of bioactive molecules according to the required function. In this way, the burst effect was highly reduced, and the antimicrobial effect against both Gram-positive and Gram-negative pathogens was recorded.

Alternatively, polymeric nanoparticles represent a valuable device with tailored physicochemical features to become a therapeutic revolution against human pathogens. They have shown to be biocompatible, non-toxic, safe, biodegradable, and easily eliminated, providing many advantages to release natural molecules with antimicrobial activity.

However, the transfer of these polymeric systems from the laboratory to practical healthcare applications remains a significant obstacle. In general, rigorous protocols of validation of in vitro and in vivo procedures are required to simplify translation from the bench to the clinical trials. Nowadays, some formulations are in clinical or preclinical stages in order to verify long-term toxicity, as well as degradation and metabolism. In the future, the clinical potential of these complex nanostructures should be deeply investigated, employing effective devices in the pharmaceutical and biomedical fields as delivery systems and/or tissue engineering scaffolds, useful to ensure infection control, to speed up skin regeneration, enhancing, in this way, patient's quality of life.

Similarly, the challenges for large scale fabrication necessitate novelty from engineers and chemists, and regulatory policies have to facilitate access to trials and patients. Thus, employing these nanocarriers in clinical practice remains challenging and will represent a major focus in the next decades.

Author Contributions: Conceptualization, U.G.S.; software, G.C.; validation, F.A. and D.R.; investigation, U.G.S. and F.A.; resources, D.R.; data curation, U.G.S.; writing-original draft preparation, U.G.S., G.C., F.A. and D.R.; writing-review and editing, U.G.S., F.A., A.F. and D.R.; All authors have read and agreed to the published version of the manuscript.

Funding: This research received no external funding.

Acknowledgments: Authors acknowledge Ministero dell'Istruzione, dell'Università e della Ricerca for the "Department of Excellence 2018–2022" grant (Italina Law n. 232/2016).

Conflicts of Interest: The authors declare no conflict of interest.

References

1. Sridhar, R.; Lakshminarayanan, R.; Madhaiyan, K.; Barathi, V.A.; Limh, K.H.C.; Ramakrishna, S. Electrosprayed nanoparticles and electrospun nanofibers based on natural materials: Applications in tissue regeneration, drug delivery and pharmaceuticals. *Chem. Soc. Rev.* **2015**, *44*, 790–814. [CrossRef]
2. Curcio, M.; Altimari, I.; Spizzirri, U.G.; Cirillo, G.; Vittorio, O.; Puoci, F.; Picci, N.; Iemma, F. Biodegradable gelatin-based nanospheres as pH-responsive drug delivery systems. *J. Nanoparticle Res.* **2013**, *15*. [CrossRef]
3. Cirillo, G.; Spataro, T.; Curcio, M.; Spizzirri, U.G.; Nicoletta, F.P.; Picci, N.; Iemma, F. Tunable thermo-responsive hydrogels: Synthesis, structural analysis and drug release studies. *Mater. Sci. Eng. C* **2015**, *48*, 499–510. [CrossRef]
4. Saka, R.; Chella, N. Nanotechnology for delivery of natural therapeutic substances: A review. *Environ. Chem. Lett.* **2020**. [CrossRef]
5. Liu, Y.; Shi, L.; Su, L.; Van der Mei, H.C.; Jutte, P.C.; Ren, Y.; Busscher, H.J. Nanotechnology-based antimicrobials and delivery systems for biofilm-infection control. *Chem. Soc. Rev.* **2019**, *48*, 428–446. [CrossRef]

6. Rahman, H.S.; Othman, H.H.; Hammadi, N.I.; Yeap, S.K.; Amin, K.M.; Samad, N.A.; Alitheen, N.B. Novel drug delivery systems for loading of natural plant extracts and their biomedical applications. *Int. J. Nanomed.* **2020**, *15*, 2439–2483. [CrossRef]
7. Sansone, F.; Mencherini, T.; Picerno, P.; Lauro, M.R.; Cerrato, M.; Aquino, R.P. Development of health products from natural sources. *Curr. Med. Chem.* **2019**, *26*, 4606–4630. [CrossRef] [PubMed]
8. Miguel, S.P.; Sequeira, R.S.; Moreira, A.F.; Cabral, C.S.D.; Mendonça, A.G.; Ferreira, P.; Correia, I.J. An overview of electrospun membranes loaded with bioactive molecules for improving the wound healing process. *Eur. J. Pharm. Biopharm.* **2019**, *139*, 1–22. [CrossRef] [PubMed]
9. Ambekar, R.S.; Kandasubramanian, B. Advancements in nanofibers for wound dressing: A review. *Eur. Polym. J.* **2019**, *117*, 304–336. [CrossRef]
10. Sabra, S.; Ragab, D.M.; Agwa, M.M.; Rohani, S. Recent advances in electrospun nanofibers for some biomedical applications. *Eur. J. Pharm. Sci.* **2020**, *144*, 105224. [CrossRef]
11. Sofi, H.S.; Rashid, R.; Amna, T.; Hamid, R.; Sheikh, F.A. Recent advances in formulating electrospun nanofiber membranes: Delivering active phytoconstituents. *J. Drug Deliv. Sci. Technol.* **2020**, *60*, 102038. [CrossRef]
12. Aiello, F.; Armentano, B.; Polerà, N.; Carullo, G.; Loizzo, M.R.; Bonesi, M.; Cappello, M.S.; Capobianco, L.; Tundis, R. From Vegetable Waste to New Agents for Potential Health Applications: Antioxidant Properties and Effects of Extracts, Fractions and Pinocembrin from Glycyrrhiza glabra L. Aerial Parts on Viability of Five Human Cancer Cell Lines. *J. Agric. Food Chem.* **2017**, *65*, 7944–7954. [CrossRef]
13. Aiello, F.; Carullo, G.; Badolato, M.; Brizzi, A. TRPV1-FAAH-COX: The couples game in pain treatment. *ChemMedChem* **2016**, *11*, 1686–1694. [CrossRef] [PubMed]
14. Tundis, R.; Frattaruolo, L.; Carullo, G.; Armentano, B.; Badolato, M.; Loizzo, M.R.; Aiello, F.; Cappello, A.R. An ancient remedial repurposing: Synthesis of new pinocembrin fatty acid acyl derivatives as potential antimicrobial/anti-inflammatory agents. *Nat. Prod. Res.* **2018**, *6419*, 1–7. [CrossRef] [PubMed]
15. Badolato, M.; Carullo, G.; Cione, E.; Aiello, F.; Caroleo, M.C. From the hive: Honey, a novel weapon against cancer. *Eur. J. Med. Chem.* **2017**, *142*, 290–299. [CrossRef]
16. Carullo, G.; Cappello, A.R.; Frattaruolo, L.; Badolato, M.; Armentano, B.; Aiello, F. Quercetin and derivatives: Useful tools in inflammation and pain management. *Future Med. Chem.* **2017**, *9*, 79–93. [CrossRef]
17. Carullo, G.; Aiello, F. Quercetin-3-oleate. *Molbank* **2018**, *2018*, M1006. [CrossRef]
18. Governa, P.; Carullo, G.; Biagi, M.; Rago, V.; Aiello, F. Evaluation of the in vitro wound-healing activity of calabrian honeys. *Antioxidants* **2019**, *8*, 36. [CrossRef]
19. Carullo, G.; Sciubba, F.; Governa, P.; Mazzotta, S.; Frattaruolo, L.; Grillo, G.; Cappello, A.R.; Cravotto, G.; Di Cocco, M.E.; Aiello, F. Mantonico and pecorello grape seed extracts: Chemical characterization and evaluation of in vitro wound-healing and anti-inflammatory activities. *Pharmaceuticals* **2020**, *13*, 97. [CrossRef] [PubMed]
20. Carullo, G.; Ahmed, A.; Fusi, F.; Sciubba, F.; Di Cocco, M.E.; Restuccia, D.; Spizzirri, U.G.; Saponara, S.; Aiello, F. Vasorelaxant Effects Induced by Red Wine and Pomace Extracts of Magliocco Dolce cv. *Pharmaceuticals* **2020**, *13*, 87. [CrossRef]
21. Carullo, G.; Durante, M.; Sciubba, F.; Restuccia, D.; Spizzirri, U.G.; Ahmed, A.; Di Cocco, M.E.; Saponara, S.; Aiello, F.; Fusi, F. Vasoactivity of Mantonico and Pecorello grape pomaces on rat aorta rings: An insight into nutraceutical development. *J. Funct. Foods* **2019**, *57*, 328–334. [CrossRef]
22. Spizzirri, U.G.; Carullo, G.; De Cicco, L.; Crispini, A.; Scarpelli, F.; Restuccia, D.; Aiello, F. Synthesis and characterization of a (+)-catechin and L-(+)-ascorbic acid cocrystal as a new functional ingredient for tea drinks. *Heliyon* **2019**, *5*, e02291. [CrossRef]
23. Restuccia, D.; Giorgi, G.; Gianfranco Spizzirri, U.; Sciubba, F.; Capuani, G.; Rago, V.; Carullo, G.; Aiello, F. Autochthonous white grape pomaces as bioactive source for functional jams. *Int. J. Food Sci. Technol.* **2019**, *54*, 1313–1320. [CrossRef]
24. Badolato, M.; Carullo, G.; Perri, M.; Cione, E.; Manetti, F.; Di Gioia, M.L.; Brizzi, A.; Caroleo, M.C.; Aiello, F. Quercetin/oleic acid-based G-protein-coupled receptor 40 ligands as new insulin secretion modulators. *Future Med. Chem.* **2017**, *9*, 1873–1885. [CrossRef]
25. Carullo, G.; Spizzirri, U.G.; Loizzo, M.R.; Leporini, M.; Sicari, V.; Aiello, F.; Restuccia, D. Valorization of red grape (Vitis vinifera cv. Sangiovese) pomace as functional food ingredient. *Ital. J. Food Sci.* **2020**, *32*, 367–385. [CrossRef]
26. Carullo, G.; Governa, P.; Spizzirri, U.G.; Biagi, M.; Sciubba, F.; Giorgi, G.; Loizzo, M.R.; Di Cocco, M.E.; Aiello, F.; Restuccia, D. Sangiovese cv pomace seeds extract-fortified kefir exerts anti-inflammatory activity in an in vitro model of intestinal epithelium using caco-2 cells. *Antioxidants* **2020**, *9*, 54. [CrossRef] [PubMed]
27. Mazzotta, S.; Carullo, G.; Schiano Moriello, A.; Amodeo, P.; Di Marzo, V.; Vega-Holm, M.; Vitale, R.M.; Aiello, F.; Brizzi, A.; De Petrocellis, L. Design, Synthesis and In Vitro Experimental Validation of Novel TRPV4 Antagonists Inspired by Labdane Diterpenes. *Mar. Drugs* **2020**, *18*, 519. [CrossRef]
28. Carullo, G.; Ahmed, A.; Trezza, A.; Spiga, O.; Brizzi, A.; Saponara, S.; Fusi, F.; Aiello, F. Design, synthesis and pharmacological evaluation of ester-based quercetin derivatives as selective vascular KCa1.1 channel stimulators. *Bioorg. Chem.* **2020**, *105*, 104404. [CrossRef]
29. Carullo, G.; Mazzotta, S.; Koch, A.; Hartmann, K.M.; Friedrich, O.; Gilbert, D.F.; Vega-Holm, M.; Schneider-Stock, R.; Aiello, F. New oleoyl hybrids of natural antioxidants: Synthesis and in vitro evaluation as inducers of apoptosis in colorectal cancer cells. *Antioxidants* **2020**, *9*, 1077. [CrossRef] [PubMed]

30. Fröhlich, T.; Ndreshkjana, B.; Muenzner, J.K.; Reiter, C.; Hofmeister, E.; Mederer, S.; Fatfat, M.; El-Baba, C.; Gali-Muhtasib, H.; Schneider-Stock, R.; et al. Synthesis of Novel Hybrids of Thymoquinone and Artemisinin with High Activity and Selectivity Against Colon Cancer. *ChemMedChem* **2017**, *12*, 226–234. [CrossRef]
31. Mazzotta, S.; Frattaruolo, L.; Brindisi, M.; Ulivieri, C.; Vanni, F.; Brizzi, A.; Carullo, G.; Cappello, A.R.; Aiello, F. 3-Amino-alkylated indoles: Unexplored green products acting as anti-inflammatory agents. *Future Med. Chem.* **2020**, *12*, 5–17. [CrossRef] [PubMed]
32. Mazzotta, S.; Cebrero-Cangueiro, T.; Frattaruolo, L.; Vega-Holm, M.; Carretero-Ledesma, M.; Sánchez-Céspedes, J.; Cappello, A.R.; Aiello, F.; Pachón, J.; Vega-Pérez, J.M.; et al. Exploration of piperazine-derived thioureas as antibacterial and anti-inflammatory agents. In vitro evaluation against clinical isolates of colistin-resistant Acinetobacter baumannii. *Bioorg. Med. Chem. Lett.* **2020**, *30*, 127411. [CrossRef]
33. Karra, S.; Sebii, H.; Jardak, M.; Bouaziz, M.A.; Attia, H.; Blecker, C.; Besbes, S. Male date palm flowers: Valuable nutritional food ingredients and alternative antioxidant source and antimicrobial agent. *S. Afr. J. Bot.* **2020**, *131*, 181–187. [CrossRef]
34. Sun, Z.L.; Liu, T.; Wang, S.Y.; Ji, X.Y.; Mu, Q. TLC-bioautography directed isolation of antibacterial compounds from active fractionation of Ferula ferulioides. *Nat. Prod. Res.* **2019**, *33*, 1761–1764. [CrossRef] [PubMed]
35. Mohotti, S.; Rajendran, S.; Muhammad, T.; Strömstedt, A.A.; Adhikari, A.; Burman, R.; de Silva, E.D.; Göransson, U.; Hettiarachchi, C.M.; Gunasekera, S. Screening for bioactive secondary metabolites in Sri Lankan medicinal plants by microfractionation and targeted isolation of antimicrobial flavonoids from Derris scandens. *J. Ethnopharmacol.* **2020**, *246*, 112158. [CrossRef] [PubMed]
36. Değirmenci, H.; Erkurt, H. Relationship between volatile components, antimicrobial and antioxidant properties of the essential oil, hydrosol and extracts of Citrus aurantium L. flowers. *J. Infect. Public Health* **2020**, *13*, 58–67. [CrossRef]
37. Shafiei, Z.; Rahim, Z.H.A.; Philip, K.; Thurairajah, N.; Yaacob, H. Potential effects of Psidium sp., Mangifera sp., Mentha sp. and its mixture (PEM) in reducing bacterial populations in biofilms, adherence and acid production of S. sanguinis and S. mutans. *Arch. Oral Biol.* **2020**, *109*, 104554. [CrossRef] [PubMed]
38. Abdel Bar, F.M.; Elsbaey, M.; Taha, N.; Elgaml, A.; Abdel-Fattah, G.M. Phytochemical, antimicrobial and antiquorum-sensing studies of pulicaria undulata L.: A revision on the structure on 1β,2α,3β,19α,23-pentahydroxy-urs-12-en-28-oic acid. *Nat. Prod. Res.* **2020**, *34*, 804–809. [CrossRef] [PubMed]
39. Barek, S.; Rahmoun, N.M.; Aissaoui, M.; El Haci, I.A.; Bensouici, C.; Choukchou-Braham, E.N. Phenolic Contents, Antioxidant, and Antibacterial Activities of the Algerian Genista saharae Solvent Extracts. *J. Herbs Spices Med. Plants* **2020**, *26*, 1–13. [CrossRef]
40. Frankova, A.; Vistejnova, L.; Merinas-Amo, T.; Leheckova, Z.; Doskocil, I.; Wong Soon, J.; Kudera, T.; Laupua, F.; Alonso-Moraga, A.; Kokoska, L. In vitro antibacterial activity of extracts from Samoan medicinal plants and their effect on proliferation and migration of human fibroblasts. *J. Ethnopharmacol.* **2021**, *264*, 113220. [CrossRef]
41. Ranadive, K.R.; Belsare, M.H.; Deokule, S.S.; Jagtap, N.V.; Jadhav, H.K.; Vaidya, J.G. Glimpses of antimicrobial activity of fungi from World. *J. New Biol. Reports* **2013**, *2*, 142–162.
42. Zhang, W.; Wang, J.; Chen, Y.; Zheng, H.; Xie, B.; Sun, Z. Flavonoid compounds and antibacterial mechanisms of different parts of white guava (Psidium guajava L. cv. Pearl). *Nat. Prod. Res.* **2020**, *34*, 1621–1625. [CrossRef] [PubMed]
43. Rosa, D.; Halim, Y.; Kam, N.; Sugata, M.; Samantha, A. Antibacterial Activity of Polyscias Scutellaria Fosberg Against *Acinetobacter* sp. *Asian J. Pharm. Clin. Res.* **2019**, *12*, 516. [CrossRef]
44. Terán Baptista, Z.P.; de los Angeles Gómez, A.; Kritsanida, M.; Grougnet, R.; Mandova, T.; Aredes Fernandez, P.A.; Sampietro, D.A. Antibacterial activity of native plants from Northwest Argentina against phytopathogenic bacteria. *Nat. Prod. Res.* **2020**, *34*, 1782–1785. [CrossRef]
45. Souissi, M.; Azelmat, J.; Chaieb, K.; Grenier, D. Antibacterial and anti-inflammatory activities of cardamom (*Elettaria cardamomum*) extracts: Potential therapeutic benefits for periodontal infections. *Anaerobe* **2020**, *61*, 102089. [CrossRef] [PubMed]
46. Fournomiti, M.; Kimbaris, A.; Mantzourani, I.; Plessas, S.; Theodoridou, I.; Papaemmanouil, V.; Kapsiotis, I.; Panopoulou, M.; Stavropoulou, E.; Bezirtzoglou, E.E.; et al. Antimicrobial activity of essential oils of cultivated oregano (*Origanum vulgare*), sage (*Salvia officinalis*), and thyme (*Thymus vulgaris*) against clinical isolates of Escherichia coli, Klebsiella oxytoca, and Klebsiella pneumoniae. *Microb. Ecol. Health Dis.* **2015**, *26*. [CrossRef]
47. Dechayont, B.; Phuaklee, P.; Chunthorng-Orn, J.; Poomirat, S.; Juckmeta, T.; Phumlek, K.; Mokmued, K.; Ouncharoen, K. Antimicrobial, Anti-inflammatory, and Antioxidant Activities of the Wood of Myristica fragrans. *J. Herbs Spices Med. Plants* **2020**, *26*, 49–60. [CrossRef]
48. De Araújo, K.M.; De Lima, A.; Silva, J.D.N.; Rodrigues, L.L.; Amorim, A.G.N.; Quelemes, P.V.; Dos Santos, R.C.; Rocha, J.A.; De Andrades, É.O.; Leite, J.R.S.A.; et al. Identification of phenolic compounds and evaluation of antioxidant and antimicrobial properties of Euphorbia tirucalli L. *Antioxidants* **2014**, *3*, 159–175. [CrossRef]
49. Tan, J.B.L.; Yap, W.J.; Tan, S.Y.; Lim, Y.Y.; Lee, S.M. Antioxidant content, antioxidant activity, and antibacterial activity of five plants from the commelinaceae family. *Antioxidants* **2014**, *3*, 758–769. [CrossRef]
50. Ahmed, D.; Khan, M.M.; Saeed, R. Comparative analysis of phenolics, flavonoids, and antioxidant and antibacterial potential of methanolic, hexanic and aqueous extracts from Adiantum caudatum leaves. *Antioxidants* **2015**, *4*, 394–409. [CrossRef]
51. Park, C.H.; Yeo, H.J.; Baskar, T.B.; Park, Y.E.; Park, J.S.; Lee, S.Y.; Park, S.U. In vitro antioxidant and antimicrobial properties of flower, leaf, and stem extracts of Korean mint. *Antioxidants* **2019**, *8*, 75. [CrossRef]
52. Karpiński, T.M.; Adamczak, A. Fucoxanthin—An antibacterial carotenoid. *Antioxidants* **2019**, *8*, 239. [CrossRef]

53. Tanase, C.; Mocan, A.; Coșarcă, S.; Gavan, A.; Nicolescu, A.; Gheldiu, A.M.; Vodnar, D.C.; Muntean, D.L.; Crișan, O. Biological and chemical insights of beech (*Fagus sylvatica* l.) bark: A source of bioactive compounds with functional properties. *Antioxidants* **2019**, *8*, 417. [CrossRef]
54. Tian, H.L.; Zhan, P.; Li, K.X. Analysis of components and study on antioxidant and antimicrobial activities of oil in apple seeds. *Int. J. Food Sci. Nutr.* **2010**, *61*, 395–403. [CrossRef] [PubMed]
55. Szabo, K.; Diaconeasa, Z.; Cătoi, A.F.; Vodnar, D.C. Screening of ten tomato varieties processing waste for bioactive components and their related antioxidant and antimicrobial activities. *Antioxidants* **2019**, *8*, 292. [CrossRef] [PubMed]
56. Chiboub, W.; Sassi, A.B.; Amina, C.M.h.; Souilem, F.; El Ayeb, A.; Djlassi, B.; Ascrizzi, R.; Flamini, G.; Harzallah-Skhiri, F. Valorization of the Green Waste from Two Varieties of Fennel and Carrot Cultivated in Tunisia by Identification of the Phytochemical Profile and Evaluation of the Antimicrobial Activities of Their Essentials Oils. *Chem. Biodivers.* **2019**, *16*. [CrossRef] [PubMed]
57. Chanda, P.; Mitra, S.; Sen, S.K.; Bhavana, S. Exploration of Betel Leaf Waste for Its Antibacterial Activity. *Bioscan* **2013**, *8*, 611–615.
58. Leouifoudi, I.; Harnafi, H.; Zyad, A. Olive Mill Waste Extracts: Polyphenols Content, Antioxidant, and Antimicrobial Activities. *Adv. Pharmacol. Sci.* **2015**, *2015*. [CrossRef]
59. Olabanji, I.O.; Ajayi, S.O.; Akinkunmi, E.O.; Kilanko, O.; Adefemi, G.O. Physicochemical and in vitro antimicrobial activity of the oils and soap of the seed and peel of Citrus sinensis. *Afr. J. Microbiol. Res.* **2016**, *10*, 245–253. [CrossRef]
60. Geraci, A.; Di Stefano, V.; Di Martino, E.; Schillaci, D.; Schicchi, R. Essential oil components of orange peels and antimicrobial activity. *Nat. Prod. Res.* **2017**, *31*, 653–659. [CrossRef] [PubMed]
61. Kulastic Jassy, A.; Dillwyn, S.; Pragalyaashree, M.M.; Tiroutchelvame, D. Evaluation of antibacterial and antioxidant properties of different varieties of grape seeds(*Vitis vinifera* L.). *Int. J. Sci. Technol. Res.* **2020**, *9*, 4116–4120.
62. Cheng, V.J.; Bekhit, A.E.D.A.; McConnell, M.; Mros, S.; Zhao, J. Effect of extraction solvent, waste fraction and grape variety on the antimicrobial and antioxidant activities of extracts from wine residue from cool climate. *Food Chem.* **2012**, *134*, 474–482. [CrossRef]
63. Vasileva, I.; Denkova, R.; Chochkov, R.; Teneva, D.; Denkova, Z.; Dessev, T.; Denev, P.; Slavov, A. Effect of lavender (*Lavandula angustifolia*) and melissa (*Melissa officinalis*) waste on quality and shelf life of bread. *Food Chem.* **2018**, *253*, 13–21. [CrossRef] [PubMed]
64. Adan, A.A.; Ojwang, R.A.; Muge, E.K.; Mwanza, B.K.; Nyaboga, E.N. Phytochemical composition and essential mineral profile, antioxidant and antimicrobial potential of unutilized parts of jackfruit. *Food Res.* **2020**, *4*, 1125–1134. [CrossRef]
65. Mutua, J.K.; Imathiu, S.; Owino, W. Evaluation of the proximate composition, antioxidant potential, and antimicrobial activity of mango seed kernel extracts. *Food Sci. Nutr.* **2017**, *5*, 349–357. [CrossRef]
66. Garzón, G.A.; Soto, C.Y.; López-R, M.; Riedl, K.M.; Browmiller, C.R.; Howard, L. Phenolic profile, in vitro antimicrobial activity and antioxidant capacity of Vaccinium meridionale swartz pomace. *Heliyon* **2020**, *6*. [CrossRef]
67. Fernández-Agulló, A.; Pereira, E.; Freire, M.S.; Valentão, P.; Andrade, P.B.; González-álvarez, J.; Pereira, J.A. Influence of solvent on the antioxidant and antimicrobial properties of walnut (*Juglans regia* L.) green husk extracts. *Ind. Crops Prod.* **2013**, *42*, 126–132. [CrossRef]
68. Do Prado, A.C.P.; da Silva, H.S.; da Silveira, S.M.; Barreto, P.L.M.; Vieira, C.R.W.; Maraschin, M.; Ferreira, S.R.S.; Block, J.M. Effect of the extraction process on the phenolic compounds profile and the antioxidant and antimicrobial activity of extracts of pecan nut [Carya illinoinensis (Wangenh) C. Koch] shell. *Ind. Crops Prod.* **2014**, *52*, 552–561. [CrossRef]
69. Kallel, F.; Driss, D.; Chaari, F.; Belghith, L.; Bouaziz, F.; Ghorbel, R.; Chaabouni, S.E. Garlic (*Allium sativum* L.) husk waste as a potential source of phenolic compounds: Influence of extracting solvents on its antimicrobial and antioxidant properties. *Ind. Crops Prod.* **2014**, *62*, 34–41. [CrossRef]
70. Palakawong, C.; Sophanodora, P.; Toivonen, P.; Delaquis, P. Optimized extraction and characterization of antimicrobial phenolic compounds from mangosteen (*Garcinia mangostana* L.) cultivation and processing waste. *J. Sci. Food Agric.* **2013**, *93*, 3792–3800. [CrossRef]
71. Guo, C.; Shan, Y.; Yang, Z.; Zhang, L.; Ling, W.; Liang, Y.; Ouyang, Z.; Zhong, B.; Zhang, J. Chemical composition, antioxidant, antibacterial, and tyrosinase inhibition activity of extracts from Newhall navel orange (Citrus sinensis Osbeck cv. Newhall) peel. *J. Sci. Food Agric.* **2020**, *100*, 2664–2674. [CrossRef] [PubMed]
72. Foujdar, R.; Bera, M.B.; Chopra, H.K. Optimization of process variables of probe ultrasonic-assisted extraction of phenolic compounds from the peel of Punica granatum Var. Bhagwa and it's chemical and bioactivity characterization. *J. Food Process. Preserv.* **2020**, *44*, 1–16. [CrossRef]
73. Socaci, S.A.; Fărcaș, A.C.; Diaconeasa, Z.M.; Vodnar, D.C.; Rusu, B.; Tofană, M. Influence of the extraction solvent on phenolic content, antioxidant, antimicrobial and antimutagenic activities of brewers' spent grain. *J. Cereal Sci.* **2018**, *80*, 180–187. [CrossRef]
74. Ade-Ajayi, a.F.; Hammuel, C.; Ezeayanaso, C.; Ogabiela, E.E.; Udiba, U.U.; Anyim, B.; Olabanji, O. Preliminary phytochemical and antimicrobial screening of Agave sisalana Perrine juice (waste). *J. Environ. Chem. Ecotoxicol.* **2011**, *3*, 180–183.
75. Saleem, M.; Saeed, M.T. Potential application of waste fruit peels (orange, yellow lemon and banana) as wide range natural antimicrobial agent. *J. King Saud Univ. Sci.* **2020**, *32*, 805–810. [CrossRef]
76. Martin, J.G.P.; Porto, E.; Corrêa, C.B.; Alencar, S.M.D.; Gloria, E.M.D.; Ribeiro, I.S.; Cabral, L.M.D.A. Antimicrobial potential and chemical composition of agro-industrial wastes. *J. Nat. Prod.* **2012**, *5*, 27–36.

77. El-hawary, S.S.; Rabeh, M.A. Mangifera indica peels: A common waste product with impressive immunostimulant, anticancer and antimicrobial potency. *J. Nat. Sci. Res.* **2014**, *4*, 102–115.
78. Conceição, N.; Albuquerque, B.R.; Pereira, C.; Corrêa, R.C.G.; Lopes, C.B.; Calhelha, R.C.; Alves, M.J.; Barros, L.; Ferreira, I.C.F.R. By-products of camu-camu [Myrciaria dubia (Kunth) McVaugh] as promising sources of bioactive high added-value food ingredients: Functionalization of yogurts. *Molecules* **2020**, *25*, 70. [CrossRef]
79. Silvan, J.M.; Pinto-Bustillos, M.A.; Vásquez-Ponce, P.; Prodanov, M.; Martinez-Rodriguez, A.J. Olive mill wastewater as a potential source of antibacterial and anti-inflammatory compounds against the food-borne pathogen Campylobacter. *Innov. Food Sci. Emerg. Technol.* **2019**, *51*, 177–185. [CrossRef]
80. Moreira, M.D.; Melo, M.M.; Coimbra, J.M.; Reis, K.C.d.; Schwan, R.F.; Silva, C.F. Solid coffee waste as alternative to produce carotenoids with antioxidant and antimicrobial activities. *Waste Manag.* **2018**, *82*, 93–99. [CrossRef]
81. Juncos Bombin, A.D.; Dunne, N.J.; McCarthy, H.O. Electrospinning of natural polymers for the production of nanofibres for wound healing applications. *Mater. Sci. Eng. C* **2020**, *114*, 110994. [CrossRef]
82. Nazarnezhad, S.; Baino, F.; Kim, H.W.; Webster, T.J.; Kargozar, S. Electrospun Nanofibers for Improved Angiogenesis: Promises for Tissue Engineering Applications. *Nanomaterials* **2020**, *10*, 1609. [CrossRef] [PubMed]
83. Croitoru, A.M.; Ficai, D.; Ficai, A.; Mihailescu, N.; Andronescu, E.; Turculet, C.F. Nanostructured fibers containing natural or synthetic bioactive compounds in wound dressing applications. *Materials* **2020**, *13*, 2407. [CrossRef]
84. Kim, J.I.; Pant, H.R.; Sim, H.J.; Lee, K.M.; Kim, C.S. Electrospun propolis/polyurethane composite nanofibers for biomedical applications. *Mater. Sci. Eng. C* **2014**, *44*, 52–57. [CrossRef]
85. Ma, X.; Wu, G.; Dai, F.; Li, D.; Li, H.; Zhang, L.; Deng, H. Chitosan/polydopamine layer by layer self-assembled silk fibroin nanofibers for biomedical applications. *Carbohydr. Polym.* **2021**, *251*, 117058. [CrossRef] [PubMed]
86. Soltani, S.; Khanian, N.; Choong, T.S.Y.; Rashid, U. Recent progress in the design and synthesis of nanofibers with diverse synthetic methodologies: Characterization and potential applications. *New J. Chem.* **2020**, *44*, 9581–9606. [CrossRef]
87. Ibrahim, H.M.; Klingner, A. A review on electrospun polymeric nanofibers: Production parameters and potential applications. *Polym. Test.* **2020**, *90*, 106647. [CrossRef]
88. Parham, S.; Kharazi, A.Z.; Bakhsheshi-Rad, H.R.; Ghayour, H.; Ismail, A.F.; Nur, H.; Berto, F. Electrospun Nano-fibers for biomedical and tissue engineering applications: A comprehensive review. *Materials* **2020**, *13*, 2153. [CrossRef]
89. Kurakula, M.; Koteswara Rao, G.S.N. Moving polyvinyl pyrrolidone electrospun nanofibers and bioprinted scaffolds toward multidisciplinary biomedical applications. *Eur. Polym. J.* **2020**, *136*. [CrossRef]
90. Padil, V.V.T.; Cheong, J.Y.; AkshayKumar, A.K.; Makvandi, P.; Zare, E.N.; Torres-Mendieta, R.; Wacławek, S.; Černík, M.; Kim, I.D.; Varma, R.S. Electrospun fibers based on carbohydrate gum polymers and their multifaceted applications. *Carbohydr. Polym.* **2020**, *247*, 116705. [CrossRef] [PubMed]
91. Garg, T.; Rath, G.; Goyal, A.K. Biomaterials-based nanofiber scaffold: Targeted and controlled carrier for cell and drug delivery. *J. Drug Target.* **2015**, *23*, 202–221. [CrossRef]
92. Fayemi, O.E.; Ekennia, A.C.; Katata-Seru, L.; Ebokaiwe, A.P.; Ijomone, O.M.; Onwudiwe, D.C.; Ebenso, E.E. Antimicrobial and Wound Healing Properties of Polyacrylonitrile-Moringa Extract Nanofibers. *ACS Omega* **2018**, *3*, 4791–4797. [CrossRef]
93. Yadav, R.; Balasubramanian, K. Polyacrylonitrile/Syzygium aromaticum hierarchical hydrophilic nanocomposite as a carrier for antibacterial drug delivery systems. *RSC Adv.* **2015**, *5*, 3291–3298. [CrossRef]
94. Balasubramanian, K.; Kodam, K.M. Encapsulation of therapeutic lavender oil in an electrolyte assisted polyacrylonitrile nanofibres for antibacterial applications. *RSC Adv.* **2014**, *4*, 54892–54901. [CrossRef]
95. Zhang, W.; Huang, C.; Kusmartseva, O.; Thomas, N.L.; Mele, E. Electrospinning of polylactic acid fibres containing tea tree and manuka oil. *React. Funct. Polym.* **2017**, *117*, 106–111. [CrossRef]
96. Al-Youssef, H.M.; Amina, M.; Hassan, S.; Amna, T.; Jeong, J.W.; Nam, K.T.; Kim, H.Y. Herbal drug loaded poly(D,L-lactide-co-glycolide) ultrafine fibers: Interaction with pathogenic bacteria. *Macromol. Res.* **2013**, *21*, 589–598. [CrossRef]
97. Garcia-Orue, I.; Gainza, G.; Gutierrez, F.B.; Aguirre, J.J.; Evora, C.; Pedraz, J.L.; Hernandez, R.M.; Delgado, A.; Igartua, M. Novel nanofibrous dressings containing rhEGF and Aloe vera for wound healing applications. *Int. J. Pharm.* **2017**, *523*, 556–566. [CrossRef]
98. Namboodiri, A.G.; Parameswaran, R. Fibro-porous polycaprolactone membrane containing extracts of Biophytum sensitivum: A prospective antibacterial wound dressing. *J. Appl. Polym. Sci.* **2013**, *129*, 2280–2286. [CrossRef]
99. Ramalingam, R.; Dhand, C.; Leung, C.M.; Ong, S.T.; Annamalai, S.K.; Kamruddin, M.; Verma, N.K.; Ramakrishna, S.; Lakshminarayanan, R.; Arunachalam, K.D. Antimicrobial properties and biocompatibility of electrospun poly-ε-caprolactone fibrous mats containing Gymnema sylvestre leaf extract. *Mater. Sci. Eng. C* **2019**, *98*, 503–514. [CrossRef]
100. Ravichandran, S.; Radhakrishnan, J.; Jayabal, P.; Venkatasubbu, G.D. Antibacterial screening studies of electrospun Polycaprolactone nano fibrous mat containing Clerodendrum phlomidis leaves extract. *Appl. Surf. Sci.* **2019**, *484*, 676–687. [CrossRef]
101. Ghaseminezhad, K.; Zare, M.; Lashkarara, S.; Yousefzadeh, M.; Aghazadeh Mohandesi, J. Fabrication of althea officinalis loaded electrospun nanofibrous scaffold for potential application of skin tissue engineering. *J. Appl. Polym. Sci.* **2020**, *137*, 1–9. [CrossRef]
102. Figueroa-Lopez, K.J.; Castro-Mayorga, J.L.; Andrade-Mahecha, M.M.; Cabedo, L.; Lagaron, J.M. Antibacterial and barrier properties of gelatin coated by electrospun polycaprolactone ultrathin fibers containing black pepper oleoresin of interest in active food biopackaging applications. *Nanomaterials* **2018**, *8*, 199. [CrossRef]

103. Suganya, S.; Venugopal, J.; Ramakrishna, S.; Lakshmi, B.S.; Dev, V.R.G. Naturally derived biofunctional nanofibrous scaffold for skin tissue regeneration. *Int. J. Biol. Macromol.* **2014**, *68*, 135–143. [CrossRef]
104. Urena-Saborio, H.; Rodríguez, G.; Madrigal-Carballo, S.; Gunasekaran, S. Characterization and applications of silver nanoparticles-decorated electrospun nanofibers loaded with polyphenolic extract from rambutan (*Nepelium lappaceum*). *Materialia* **2020**, *11*, 100687. [CrossRef]
105. Unnithan, A.R.; Pichiah, P.B.T.; Gnanasekaran, G.; Seenivasan, K.; Barakat, N.A.M.; Cha, Y.S.; Jung, C.H.; Shanmugam, A.; Kim, H.Y. Emu oil-based electrospun nanofibrous scaffolds for wound skin tissue engineering. *Colloids Surf. A Physicochem. Eng. Asp.* **2012**, *415*, 454–460. [CrossRef]
106. Avci, H.; Gergeroglu, H. Synergistic effects of plant extracts and polymers on structural and antibacterial properties for wound healing. *Polym. Bull.* **2019**, *76*, 3709–3731. [CrossRef]
107. Canbay-Gokce, E.; Akgul, Y.; Gokce, A.Y.; Tasdelen-Yucedag, C.; Kilic, A.; Hassanin, A. Characterization of solution blown thermoplastic polyurethane nanofibers modified with Syzygium aromaticum extract. *J. Text. Inst.* **2020**, *111*, 10–15. [CrossRef]
108. Kim, J.h.; Lee, H.; Lee, J.; Kim, I.S. Preparation and characterization of Juniperus chinensis extract-loaded polyurethane nanofiber laminate with polyurethane resin on polyethylene terephthalate fabric. *Polym. Bull.* **2020**, *77*, 919–928. [CrossRef]
109. Almasian, A.; Najafi, F.; Eftekhari, M.; Ardekani, M.R.S.; Sharifzadeh, M.; Khanavi, M. Polyurethane/carboxymethylcellulose nanofibers containing Malva sylvestris extract for healing diabetic wounds: Preparation, characterization, in vitro and in vivo studies. *Mater. Sci. Eng. C* **2020**, *114*. [CrossRef] [PubMed]
110. Avci, H.; Monticello, R.; Kotek, R. Preparation of antibacterial PVA and PEO nanofibers containing Lawsonia Inermis (henna) leaf extracts. *J. Biomater. Sci. Polym. Ed.* **2013**, *24*, 1815–1830. [CrossRef]
111. Ganesan, P.; Pradeepa, P. Development and characterization of nanofibrous mat from PVA/Tridax Procumbens (TP) leaves extracts. *Wound Med.* **2017**, *19*, 15–22. [CrossRef]
112. Yang, S.B.; Kim, E.H.; Kim, S.H.; Kim, Y.H.; Oh, W.; Lee, J.T.; Jang, Y.A.; Sabina, Y.; Ji, B.C.; Yeum, J.H. Electrospinning fabrication of poly(Vinyl alcohol)/coptis chinensis extract nanofibers for antimicrobial exploits. *Nanomaterials* **2018**, *8*, 734. [CrossRef] [PubMed]
113. Zeyohanness, S.S.; Abd Hamid, H.; Zulkifli, F.H. Poly(vinyl alcohol) electrospun nanofibers containing antimicrobial Rhodomyrtus tomentosa extract. *J. Bioact. Compat. Polym.* **2018**, *33*, 585–596. [CrossRef]
114. Jeong, J.; Lee, S. Electrospun poly(vinyl alcohol) nanofibrous membranes containing Coptidis Rhizoma extracts for potential biomedical applications. *Text. Res. J.* **2019**, *89*, 3506–3518. [CrossRef]
115. Costa, L.M.M.; de Olyveira, G.M.; Cherian, B.M.; Leão, A.L.; de Souza, S.F.; Ferreira, M. Bionanocomposites from electrospun PVA/pineapple nanofibers/Stryphnodendron adstringens bark extract for medical applications. *Ind. Crops Prod.* **2013**, *41*, 198–202. [CrossRef]
116. Jenifer, P.; Kalachaveedu, M.; Viswanathan, A.; Gnanamani, A. Mubeena Fabricated approach for an effective wound dressing material based on a natural gum impregnated with Acalypha indica extract. *J. Bioact. Compat. Polym.* **2018**, *33*, 612–628. [CrossRef]
117. Rafiq, M.; Hussain, T.; Abid, S.; Nazir, A.; Masood, R. Development of sodium alginate/PVA antibacterial nanofibers by the incorporation of essential oils. *Mater. Res. Express* **2018**, *5*. [CrossRef]
118. Choi, J.; Yang, B.J.; Bae, G.N.; Jung, J.H. Herbal Extract Incorporated Nanofiber Fabricated by an Electrospinning Technique and its Application to Antimicrobial Air Filtration. *ACS Appl. Mater. Interfaces* **2015**, *7*, 25313–25320. [CrossRef] [PubMed]
119. Kesici Güler, H.; Cengiz Çallıoğlu, F.; Sesli Çetin, E. Antibacterial PVP/cinnamon essential oil nanofibers by emulsion electrospinning. *J. Text. Inst.* **2019**, *110*, 302–310. [CrossRef]
120. Liakos, I.; Rizzello, L.; Hajiali, H.; Brunetti, V.; Carzino, R.; Pompa, P.P.; Athanassiou, A.; Mele, E. Fibrous wound dressings encapsulating essential oils as natural antimicrobial agents. *J. Mater. Chem. B* **2015**, *3*, 1583–1589. [CrossRef]
121. Liakos, I.L.; Holban, A.M.; Carzino, R.; Lauciello, S.; Grumezescu, A.M. Electrospun fiber pads of cellulose acetate and essential oils with antimicrobial activity. *Nanomaterials* **2017**, *7*, 84. [CrossRef] [PubMed]
122. Peršin, Z.; Ravber, M.; Stana Kleinschek, K.; Knez, Ž.; Škerget, M.; Kurečič, M. Bio-nanofibrous mats as potential delivering systems of natural substances. *Text. Res. J.* **2017**, *87*, 444–459. [CrossRef]
123. Ahmadi, R.; Ghanbarzadeh, B.; Ayaseh, A.; Kafil, H.S.; Özyurt, H.; Katourani, A.; Ostadrahimi, A. The antimicrobial bio-nanocomposite containing non-hydrolyzed cellulose nanofiber (CNF) and Miswak (*Salvadora persica* L.) extract. *Carbohydr. Polym.* **2019**, *214*, 15–25. [CrossRef]
124. Yadav, C.; Maji, P.K. Synergistic effect of cellulose nanofibres and bio- extracts for fabricating high strength sodium alginate based composite bio-sponges with antibacterial properties. *Carbohydr. Polym.* **2019**, *203*, 396–408. [CrossRef] [PubMed]
125. Cui, H.; Zhang, C.; Li, C.; Lin, L. Preparation and antibacterial activity of Litsea cubeba essential oil/dandelion polysaccharide nanofiber. *Ind. Crops Prod.* **2019**, *140*, 111739. [CrossRef]
126. Charernsriwilaiwat, N.; Rojanarata, T.; Ngawhirunpat, T.; Sukma, M.; Opanasopit, P. Electrospun chitosan-based nanofiber mats loaded with Garcinia mangostana extracts. *Int. J. Pharm.* **2013**, *452*, 333–343. [CrossRef] [PubMed]
127. Kegere, J.; Ouf, A.; Siam, R.; Mamdouh, W. Fabrication of Poly(vinyl alcohol)/Chitosan/Bidens pilosa Composite Electrospun Nanofibers with Enhanced Antibacterial Activities. *ACS Omega* **2019**, *4*, 8778–8785. [CrossRef]
128. Sarhan, W.A.; Azzazy, H.M.E. High concentration honey chitosan electrospun nanofibers: Biocompatibility and antibacterial effects. *Carbohydr. Polym.* **2015**, *122*, 135–143. [CrossRef]

129. Sarhan, W.A.; Azzazy, H.M.E.; El-Sherbiny, I.M. The effect of increasing honey concentration on the properties of the honey/polyvinyl alcohol/chitosan nanofibers. *Mater. Sci. Eng. C* **2016**, *67*, 276–284. [CrossRef]
130. Sarhan, W.A.; Azzazy, H.M.E.; El-Sherbiny, I.M. Honey/Chitosan Nanofiber Wound Dressing Enriched with Allium sativum and Cleome droserifolia: Enhanced Antimicrobial and Wound Healing Activity. *ACS Appl. Mater. Interfaces* **2016**, *8*, 6379–6390. [CrossRef]
131. Rieger, K.A.; Schiffman, J.D. Electrospinning an essential oil: Cinnamaldehyde enhances the antimicrobial efficacy of chitosan/poly(ethylene oxide) nanofibers. *Carbohydr. Polym.* **2014**, *113*, 561–568. [CrossRef] [PubMed]
132. Sadri, M.; Arab-Sorkhi, S.; Vatani, H.; Bagheri-Pebdeni, A. New wound dressing polymeric nanofiber containing green tea extract prepared by electrospinning method. *Fibers Polym.* **2015**, *16*, 1742–1750. [CrossRef]
133. Kwak, H.W.; Kang, M.J.; Bae, J.H.; Hur, S.B.; Kim, I.S.; Park, Y.H.; Lee, K.H. Fabrication of Phaeodactylum tricornutum extract-loaded gelatin nanofibrous mats exhibiting antimicrobial activity. *Int. J. Biol. Macromol.* **2014**, *63*, 198–204. [CrossRef] [PubMed]
134. Yao, C.H.; Yeh, J.Y.; Chen, Y.S.; Li, M.H.; Huang, C.H. Wound-healing effect of electrospun gelatin nanofibres containing Centella asiatica extract in a rat model. *J. Tissue Eng. Regen. Med.* **2017**, *11*, 905–915. [CrossRef]
135. Chiu, C.; Nootem, J.; Santiwat, T.; Srisuwannaket, C. Curcuma comosa Roxb. Extract in Electrospun. *Fibers* **2019**, *7*, 76. [CrossRef]
136. Barnthip, N.; Paosoi, J.; Pinyakong, O. Concentration effect of Chromolaena odorata (Siam weed) crude extract on size and properties of gelatin nanofibers fabricated by electrospinning process. *J. Ind. Text.* **2020**, 1–12. [CrossRef]
137. Baghersad, S.; Bahrami, S.H.; Ranjbar, M.; Reza, M.; Mojtahedi, M.; Brouki, P. Development of biodegradable electrospun gelatin/aloe-vera/poly (ε-caprolactone) hybrid nano fi brous sca ff old for application as skin substitutes. *Mater. Sci. Eng. C* **2018**, *93*, 367–379.
138. Yang, X.; Fan, L.; Ma, L.; Wang, Y.; Lin, S.; Yu, F.; Pan, X.; Luo, G.; Zhang, D.; Wang, H. Green electrospun Manuka honey/silk fibroin fibrous matrices as potential wound dressing. *Mater. Des.* **2017**, *119*, 76–84. [CrossRef]
139. Chan, W.P.; Huang, K.C.; Bai, M.Y. Silk fibroin protein-based nonwoven mats incorporating baicalein Chinese herbal extract: Preparation, characterizations, and in vivo evaluation. *J. Biomed. Mater. Res. Part B Appl. Biomater.* **2017**, *105*, 420–430. [CrossRef]
140. Doğan, G.; Başal, G.; Bayraktar, O.; Ozyildiz, F.; Uzel, A.; Erdoğan, I. Bioactive Sheath/Core nanofibers containing olive leaf extract. *Microsc. Res. Tech.* **2016**, *79*, 38–49. [CrossRef]
141. Dehcheshmeh, M.A.; Fathi, M. Production of core-shell nanofibers from zein and tragacanth for encapsulation of saffron extract. *Int. J. Biol. Macromol.* **2019**, *122*, 272–279. [CrossRef] [PubMed]
142. Moradkhannejhad, L.; Abdouss, M.; Nikfarjam, N.; Mazinani, S.; Heydari, V. Electrospinning of zein/propolis nanofibers; antimicrobial properties and morphology investigation. *J. Mater. Sci. Mater. Med.* **2018**, *29*. [CrossRef]
143. Wang, S.; Marcone, M.F.; Barbut, S.; Lim, L.T. Electrospun soy protein isolate-based fiber fortified with anthocyanin-rich red raspberry (*Rubus strigosus*) extracts. *Food Res. Int.* **2013**, *52*, 467–472. [CrossRef]
144. Selvam, A.K.; Nallathambi, G. Polyacrylonitrile/silver nanoparticle electrospun nanocomposite matrix for bacterial filtration. *Fibers Polym.* **2015**, *16*, 1327–1335. [CrossRef]
145. Aslan, S.; Loebick, C.Z.; Kang, S.; Elimelech, M.; Pfefferle, L.D.; Van Tassel, P.R. Antimicrobial biomaterials based on carbon nanotubes dispersed in poly(lactic-co-glycolic acid). *Nanoscale* **2010**, *2*, 1789–1794. [CrossRef]
146. Govardhan Singh, R.S.; Negi, P.S.; Radha, C. Phenolic composition, antioxidant and antimicrobial activities of free and bound phenolic extracts of Moringa oleifera seed flour. *J. Funct. Foods* **2013**, *5*, 1883–1891. [CrossRef]
147. Matan, N.; Rimkeeree, H.; Mawson, A.J.; Chompreeda, P.; Haruthaithanasan, V.; Parker, M. Antimicrobial activity of cinnamon and clove oils under modified atmosphere conditions. *Int. J. Food Microbiol.* **2006**, *107*, 180–185. [CrossRef] [PubMed]
148. Divakara Shetty, S.; Shetty, N. Investigation of mechanical properties and applications of polylactic acids—A review. *Mater. Res. Express* **2019**, *6*. [CrossRef]
149. Santoro, M.; Shah, S.R.; Walker, J.L.; Mikos, A.G. Poly(lactic acid) nanofibrous scaffolds for tissue engineering. *Adv. Drug Deliv. Rev.* **2016**, *107*, 206–212. [CrossRef] [PubMed]
150. Otto, M. Staphylococcus epidermidis—The "accidental" pathogen. *Nat. Rev. Microbiol.* **2009**, *7*, 555–567. [CrossRef]
151. Killeen, D.P.; Larsen, L.; Dayan, F.E.; Gordon, K.C.; Perry, N.B.; Van Klink, J.W. Nortriketones: Antimicrobial Trimethylated Acylphloroglucinols from Mānuka (*Leptospermum scoparium*). *J. Nat. Prod.* **2016**, *79*, 564–569. [CrossRef]
152. Imran Ul-Haq, M.; Lai, B.F.L.; Chapanian, R.; Kizhakkedathu, J.N. Influence of architecture of high molecular weight linear and branched polyglycerols on their biocompatibility and biodistribution. *Biomaterials* **2012**, *33*, 9135–9147. [CrossRef]
153. Perumal, G.; Pappuru, S.; Chakraborty, D.; Maya Nandkumar, A.; Chand, D.K.; Doble, M. Synthesis and characterization of curcumin loaded PLA—Hyperbranched polyglycerol electrospun blend for wound dressing applications. *Mater. Sci. Eng. C* **2017**, *76*, 1196–1204. [CrossRef] [PubMed]
154. Keat, C.L.; Aziz, A.; Eid, A.M.; Elmarzugi, N.A. Biosynthesis of nanoparticles and silver nanoparticles. *Bioresour. Bioprocess.* **2015**, *2*. [CrossRef]
155. Sheikh, F.A.; Barakat, N.A.M.; Kanjwal, M.A.; Chaudhari, A.A.; Jung, I.H.; Lee, J.H.; Kim, H.Y. Electrospun antimicrobial polyurethane nanofibers containing silver nanoparticles for biotechnological applications. *Macromol. Res.* **2009**, *17*, 688–696. [CrossRef]
156. Xu, Y.; Luo, L.; Chen, B.; Fu, Y. Recent development of chemical components in propolis. *Front. Biol. China* **2009**, *4*, 385–391. [CrossRef]

157. Koski, A.; Yim, K.; Shivkumar, S. Effect of molecular weight on fibrous PVA produced by electrospinning. *Mater. Lett.* **2004**, *58*, 493–497. [CrossRef]
158. Calixto, J.B. Efficacy, safety, quality control, marketing and regulatory guidelines for herbal medicines (phytotherapeutic agents). *Braz. J. Med. Biol. Res.* **2000**, *33*, 179–189. [CrossRef] [PubMed]
159. Wang, L.; Chang, M.W.; Ahmad, Z.; Zheng, H.; Li, J.S. Mass and controlled fabrication of aligned PVP fibers for matrix type antibiotic drug delivery systems. *Chem. Eng. J.* **2017**, *307*, 661–669. [CrossRef]
160. Zhang, L.; Menkhaus, T.J.; Fong, H. Fabrication and bioseparation studies of adsorptive membranes/felts made from electrospun cellulose acetate nanofibers. *J. Memb. Sci.* **2008**, *319*, 176–184. [CrossRef]
161. Fan, L.; Peng, K.; Li, M.; Wang, L.; Wang, T. Preparation and properties of carboxymethyl κ-carrageenan/alginate blend fibers. *J. Biomater. Sci. Polym. Ed.* **2013**, *24*, 1099–1111. [CrossRef] [PubMed]
162. Lisnyak, Y.V.; Martynov, A.V.; Baumer, V.N.; Shishkin, O.V.; Gubskaya, A.V. Crystal and molecular structure of β-cyclodextrin inclusion complex with succinic acid. *J. Incl. Phenom. Macrocycl. Chem.* **2007**, *58*, 367–375. [CrossRef]
163. Lin, L.; Zhu, Y.; Li, C.; Liu, L.; Surendhiran, D.; Cui, H. Antibacterial activity of PEO nanofibers incorporating polysaccharide from dandelion and its derivative. *Carbohydr. Polym.* **2018**, *198*, 225–232. [CrossRef] [PubMed]
164. Jayakumar, R.; Prabaharan, M.; Sudheesh Kumar, P.T.; Nair, S.V.; Tamura, H. Biomaterials based on chitin and chitosan in wound dressing applications. *Biotechnol. Adv.* **2011**, *29*, 322–337. [CrossRef] [PubMed]
165. Cirillo, G.; Curcio, M.; Spizzirri, U.G.; Vittorio, O.; Valli, E.; Farfalla, A.; Leggio, A.; Nicoletta, F.P.; Iemma, F. Chitosan–Quercetin Bioconjugate as Multi-Functional Component of Antioxidants and Dual-Responsive Hydrogel Networks. *Macromol. Mater. Eng.* **2019**, *304*, 1–12. [CrossRef]
166. Li, C.W.; Fu, R.Q.; Yu, C.P.; Li, Z.H.; Guan, H.Y.; Hu, D.Q.; Zhao, D.H.; Lu, L.C. Silver nanoparticle/chitosan oligosaccharide/poly(vinyl alcohol) nanofibers as wound dressings: A preclinical study. *Int. J. Nanomed.* **2013**, *8*, 4131–4145. [CrossRef]
167. Jana, S.; Florczyk, S.J.; Leung, M.; Zhang, M. High-strength pristine porous chitosan scaffolds for tissue engineering. *J. Mater. Chem.* **2012**, *22*, 6291–6299. [CrossRef]
168. Su, P.; Wang, C.; Yang, X.; Chen, X.; Gao, C.; Feng, X.X.; Chen, J.Y.; Ye, J.; Gou, Z. Electrospinning of chitosan nanofibers: The favorable effect of metal ions. *Carbohydr. Polym.* **2011**, *84*, 239–246. [CrossRef]
169. Yan, E.; Fan, S.; Li, X.; Wang, C.; Sun, Z.; Ni, L.; Zhang, D. Electrospun polyvinyl alcohol/chitosan composite nanofibers involving Au nanoparticles and their in vitro release properties. *Mater. Sci. Eng. C* **2013**, *33*, 461–465. [CrossRef]
170. Chomnawang, M.T.; Surassmo, S.; Wongsariya, K.; Bunyapraphatsara, N. Antibacterial Activity of Thai Medicinal Plants against Methicillin-resistant Staphylococcus aureus. *Fitoterapia* **2009**, *80*, 102–104. [CrossRef]
171. Mandal, M.D.; Mandal, S. Honey: Its medicinal property and antibacterial activity. *Asian Pac. J. Trop. Biomed.* **2011**, *1*, 154–160. [CrossRef]
172. Wang, P.; He, J.H. Electrospun polyvinyl alcohol-honey nanofibers. *Therm. Sci.* **2013**, *17*, 1549–1550. [CrossRef]
173. Taokaew, S.; Seetabhawang, S.; Siripong, P.; Phisalaphong, M. Biosynthesis and characterization of nanocellulose-gelatin films. *Materials* **2013**, *6*, 782–794. [CrossRef]
174. Desbois, A.P.; Walton, M.; Smith, V.J. Differential antibacterial activities of fusiform and oval morphotypes of phaeodactylum tricornutum (bacillariophyceae). *J. Mar. Biol. Assoc. UK* **2010**, *90*, 769–774. [CrossRef]
175. Yao, Z.C.; Zhang, C.; Ahmad, Z.; Huang, J.; Li, J.S.; Chang, M.W. Designer fibers from 2D to 3D—Simultaneous and controlled engineering of morphology, shape and size. *Chem. Eng. J.* **2018**, *334*, 89–98. [CrossRef]
176. Calamak, S.; Aksoy, E.A.; Ertas, N.; Erdogdu, C.; Sagiroglu, M.; Ulubayram, K. Ag/silk fibroin nanofibers: Effect of fibroin morphology on Ag+ release and antibacterial activity. *Eur. Polym. J.* **2015**, *67*, 99–112. [CrossRef]
177. Cooper, R.A.; Jenkins, L.; Henriques, A.F.M.; Duggan, R.S.; Burton, N.F. Absence of bacterial resistance to medical-grade manuka honey. *Eur. J. Clin. Microbiol. Infect. Dis.* **2010**, *29*, 1237–1241. [CrossRef]
178. Hashemi, S.M.B.; Jafarpour, D. The efficacy of edible film from Konjac glucomannan and saffron petal extract to improve shelf life of fresh-cut cucumber. *Food Sci. Nutr.* **2020**, *8*, 3128–3137. [CrossRef]
179. Manuel Franco, C.; Vázquez, B.I. Natural compounds as antimicrobial agents. *Antibiotics* **2020**, *9*, 217. [CrossRef]
180. Sanna, V.; Lubinu, G.; Madau, P.; Pala, N.; Nurra, S.; Mariani, A.; Sechi, M. Polymeric nanoparticles encapsulating white tea extract for nutraceutical application. *J. Agric. Food Chem.* **2015**, *63*, 2026–2032. [CrossRef] [PubMed]
181. Hill, L.E.; Taylor, T.M.; Gomes, C. Antimicrobial Efficacy of Poly (DL-lactide-co-glycolide) (PLGA) Nanoparticles with Entrapped Cinnamon Bark Extract against Listeria monocytogenes and Salmonella typhimurium. *J. Food Sci.* **2013**, *78*. [CrossRef]
182. Silva, L.M.; Hill, L.E.; Figueiredo, E.; Gomes, C.L. Delivery of phytochemicals of tropical fruit by-products using poly (dl-lactide-co-glycolide) (PLGA) nanoparticles: Synthesis, characterization, and antimicrobial activity. *Food Chem.* **2014**, *165*, 362–370. [CrossRef]
183. Oliveira, D.A.; Angonese, M.; Ferreira, S.R.S.; Gomes, C.L. Nanoencapsulation of passion fruit by-products extracts for enhanced antimicrobial activity. *Food Bioprod. Process.* **2017**, *104*, 137–146. [CrossRef]
184. Pereira, M.C.; Hill, L.E.; Zambiazi, R.C.; Mertens-Talcott, S.; Talcott, S.; Gomes, C.L. Nanoencapsulation of hydrophobic phytochemicals using poly (dl-lactide-co-glycolide) (PLGA) for antioxidant and antimicrobial delivery applications: Guabiroba fruit (Campomanesia xanthocarpa O. Berg) study. *LWT Food Sci. Technol.* **2015**, *63*, 100–107. [CrossRef]

185. Pereira, M.C.; Oliveira, D.A.; Hill, L.E.; Zambiazi, R.C.; Borges, C.D.; Vizzotto, M.; Mertens-Talcott, S.; Talcott, S.; Gomes, C.L. Effect of nanoencapsulation using PLGA on antioxidant and antimicrobial activities of guabiroba fruit phenolic extract. *Food Chem.* **2018**, *240*, 396–404. [CrossRef]
186. Bernardos, A.; Piacenza, E.; Sancenón, F.; Hamidi, M.; Maleki, A.; Turner, R.J.; Martínez-Máñez, R. Mesoporous Silica-Based Materials with Bactericidal Properties. *Small* **2019**, *15*, 1–34. [CrossRef] [PubMed]
187. Asefa, T.; Tao, Z. Biocompatibility of Mesoporous Silica Nanoparticles. *Chem. Res. Toxicol.* **2012**, *25*, 2265–2284. [CrossRef] [PubMed]
188. Croissant, J.G.; Fatieiev, Y.; Khashab, N.M. Degradability and Clearance of Silicon, Organosilica, Silsesquioxane, Silica Mixed Oxide, and Mesoporous Silica Nanoparticles. *Adv. Mater.* **2017**, *29*, 1604634. [CrossRef]
189. Wu, S.-H.; Mou, C.-Y.; Lin, H.-P. Synthesis of Mesoporous Silica Nanoparticles. *Chem. Soc. Rev.* **2013**, *42*, 3862–3875. [CrossRef]
190. Slowing, I.I.; Vivero-Escoto, J.L.; Trewyn, B.G.; Lin, V.S.Y. Mesoporous silica nanoparticles: Structural design and applications. *J. Mater. Chem.* **2010**, *20*, 7924–7937. [CrossRef]
191. Laís, L.F.; Teles da Silva, L.V.d.A.; do Nascimento, T.G.; de Almeida, L.M.; Calumby, R.J.N.; Nunes, Á.M.; de Magalhães Oliveira, L.M.T.; da Silva Fonseca, E.J. Antioxidant and antimicrobial activity of red propolis embedded mesoporous silica nanoparticles. *Drug Dev. Ind. Pharm.* **2020**, *46*, 1199–1208. [CrossRef]
192. Righi, A.A.; Alves, T.R.; Negri, G.; Marques, L.M.; Breyer, H.; Salatino, A. Brazilian red propolis: Unreported substances, antioxidant and antibacterial activities. *J. Sci. Food Agric.* **2011**, *91*, 2363–2370. [CrossRef] [PubMed]
193. Brezoiu, A.M.; Prundeanu, M.; Berger, D.; Deaconu, M.; Matei, C.; Oprea, O.; Vasile, E.; Negreanu-Pîrjol, T.; Muntean, D.; Danciu, C. Properties of salvia offcinalis l. And thymus serpyllum l. extracts free and embedded into mesopores of silica and titania nanomaterials. *Nanomaterials* **2020**, *10*, 820. [CrossRef] [PubMed]

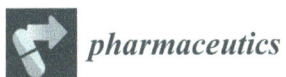

Review

Bromelain and Nisin: The Natural Antimicrobials with High Potential in Biomedicine

Urška Jančič [1] and Selestina Gorgieva [1,2,*]

1. Institute of Engineering Materials and Design, Faculty of Mechanical Engineering, University of Maribor, Smetanova ulica 17, 2000 Maribor, Slovenia; urska.jancic@um.si
2. Institute of Automation, Faculty of Electrical Engineering and Computer Science, University of Maribor, Koroška cesta 46, 2000 Maribor, Slovenia
* Correspondence: selestina.gorgieva@um.si; Tel.: +386-2-220-7740

Abstract: Infectious diseases along with various cancer types are among the most significant public health problems and the leading cause of death worldwide. The situation has become even more complex with the rapid development of multidrug-resistant microorganisms. New drugs are urgently needed to curb the increasing spread of diseases in humans and livestock. Promising candidates are natural antimicrobial peptides produced by bacteria, and therapeutic enzymes, extracted from medicinal plants. This review highlights the structure and properties of plant origin bromelain and antimicrobial peptide nisin, along with their mechanism of action, the immobilization strategies, and recent applications in the field of biomedicine. Future perspectives towards the commercialization of new biomedical products, including these important bioactive compounds, have been highlighted.

Keywords: bromelain; nisin; bioactivity; antimicrobial agent; biomedicine; carrier

Citation: Jančič, U.; Gorgieva, S. Bromelain and Nisin: The Natural Antimicrobials with High Potential in Biomedicine. *Pharmaceutics* **2022**, *14*, 76. https://doi.org/10.3390/pharmaceutics14010076

Academic Editor: Umile Gianfranco Spizzirri

Received: 22 November 2021
Accepted: 23 December 2021
Published: 29 December 2021

Publisher's Note: MDPI stays neutral with regard to jurisdictional claims in published maps and institutional affiliations.

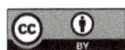

Copyright: © 2021 by the authors. Licensee MDPI, Basel, Switzerland. This article is an open access article distributed under the terms and conditions of the Creative Commons Attribution (CC BY) license (https://creativecommons.org/licenses/by/4.0/).

1. Introduction

One of the tremendous burdens on human health worldwide is infectious diseases [1], where antibiotics act as first-line therapy in treating infections caused by bacteria. Still, their widespread use, over-utilization and improper consumption in humans and animals cause an increase in the number of resistant bacterial strains. Furthermore, one pathogen organism is gaining resistance to more than one antibiotic, leading to the development of multidrug resistance strains for various species, such as *Staphylococcus aureus* (*S. aureus*), *Pseudomonas aeruginosa* (*P. aeruginosa*), *Salmonella* spp., *Enterococcus faecium* (*E. faecium*), *Campylobacter*, *Neisseria gonorrhoeae* (*N. gonorrhoeae*), *Streptococcus pneumonia* (*S. pneumonia*) [2], etc. Consequently, the cost of hospitalization and healthcare, together with morbidity and death are increasing [3]. According to World Health Organization and Organisation for Economic Co-operation and Development at least 700,000 patients die every year from infections caused by resistant microorganisms [2] and approximately 2.4 million people in Europe, North America, and Australia are expected to die due to diseases caused by drug-resistant pathogens over the next 30 years, which means $3.5 billion in economic cost per year [4]. Furthermore, multidrug resistance of cancer cells against conventional chemotherapeutic agents [5] is another problem that needs to be solved. Therefore, it is necessary to search for innovative alternative therapies and new drug candidates [6]. Various studies exhibit promising results when natural antimicrobial peptides and proteins are used as therapeutics [7], especially since their conjunction with conventional chemotherapeutic agents promotes effectiveness, decreases antibiotics use and possibly reduces instances of chemotherapy resistance [8].

This review gives a comprehensive overview on two compounds obtained from two different natural sources, i.e., nisin as a bacterial origin representative and bromelain as a plant origin representative. With nearly 50 years of safe usage in the food industry, and very little evidence of cross-resistance compared with that of conventional antibiotics [7,8], non-toxicity and low immunogenicity [9], researchers have begun to explore the nisin, an antimicrobial peptide with a broad-spectrum of antibacterial activity [6] as a potential alternative agent for infectious diseases [7]. On the other hand, the demand for medicinal plants with therapeutic agents has been rising [10] as natural plant products are increasingly recognized as non-toxic, side-effect free, readily available and affordable [1]. Among them, pineapple has been identified to possess valuable qualities for medical purposes, especially its proteolytic enzyme bromelain due to its antimicrobial, anti-inflammatory, antithrombotic, fibrinolytic and anti-cancer functions [11]. The present review comprehensively discusses the structure, isolation and suggested bioactivity mechanisms, as well as immobilization strategies and application of nisin and bromelain in the last 10 years. Published reports were collected using the Web of Science and Scopus databases, with search terms "bromelain", "nisin", "bioactive", "antimicrobial", "anticancer", "anti-inflammatory", "toxicity", "immobilization", "adsorption", "encapsulation", "entrapment" and "carrier". Our aim is to emphasize the importance and relevance of these bioactive compounds, where the researchers and relevant stakeholders may gain the latest fundamental knowledge to explore the new possibility of bromelain- or nisin-based products in biomedicine and pharmacy. Moreover, giving comprehensive information for two different origin bioactive compounds can allow direct comparison of their ultimate properties and action, giving the ease of selecting the suitable candidate for a particular biomedical application. Relating to this, we also point to very limited clinical trials (and even fewer approved products) involving bromelain and nisin, as contradictory to the potential they hold in this segment. As a hypothetically written, future perspective, the possibility to combine both bioactive components in an attempt to merge and even boost their multiple bioactivities, utilising diverse immobilization routes, have been brought forward.

2. Bromelain

2.1. Structural and Biological Properties

Bromelain is a protein purified from a crude aqueous extract of pineapples (*Bromeliaceae* family) [1]. Pineapple is a common name of *Ananas comosus*, also known as *Ananassa sativa*, *A. sativus*, *Bromelia ananas* or *B. comosa*, grown in several (sub)tropical countries such as Costa Rica, Philippines, Brazil, Thailand, China, Indonesia, India, Malaysia, Hawaii and Kenya [1,12]. In the pineapple plant, bromelain acts as a defensive protein; it protects the pineapple throughout the development, maturation and ripening process [13,14].

Bromelain was identified for the first time in 1891 by Vicente Marcano, a Venezuelan chemist, while its isolation and analysis started in 1894. However, its commercial production began in 1957 with Heinecke's discovery that the pineapple fruit contains less bromelain than the pineapple stem [15], making a waste by-product stem bromelain more commercialized [13].

Bromelain belongs to the class of proteases also known as proteinases or peptidases, a group of enzymes that catalyzes proteolytic reactions where the breakdown of proteins into smaller polypeptides or single amino acids occurs [13,16,17]. More specifically, it is classified as cysteine proteinase (EC 3.4.22, CP, also known as thiol proteinase) due to the cysteine thiol in its active site [1,13]. Crude bromelain (crude extract of the pineapple) contains various cysteine endopeptidases and other components, including phosphatases, glucosidase, peroxidases, cellulases, glycoproteins, carbohydrates, ribonucleases, protease inhibitors and organically bound calcium [1,12,15]. Among them, the specific activity of proteases is the highest, e.g., the specific activity of protease, peroxidase, acid phosphatase, alkaline phosphatase and amylase studied in the crude bromelain extracted from pineapple crown leaf was 45 U/mg, 2.19 U/mg, 1.12 U/mg, 0.98 U/mg, 0.65 U/mg, respectively [18]. At least four evolutionarily and structurally related cysteine endopeptidases can be synthesized from crude bromelain: stem bromelain (EC 3.4.22.32), fruit bromelain (EC 3.4.22.33), ananain (EC 3.4.22.31) and comosain (Table 1) [1,13,15]. Stem bromelain is the major protease present in the stem of the pineapple plant, and fruit bromelain is the major protease in the pineapple fruit [1,19]. Ananain and comosain were detected only in minor quantities in stem pineapple [1]. All the endopeptidases of the pineapple plant have generally been referred to as "the bromelains" and the name "bromelain" was originally used to describe any protease of the *Bromeliaceae* family [15].

All four cysteine endopeptidases possess distinguished physicochemical properties, as summarized in Table 1. Fruit bromelain is an acidic protein, unlike stem bromelain, which is alkaline (isoelectric point 4.6 and ≥9.5, respectively). Generally, the molecular weight of stem and fruit bromelain is from 23.8 to 37.0 kDa and 23.0 to 32.5 kDa, respectively. This heterogeneity in molecular weight may be due to heterogeneity of the amino acid sequence and the glycosylation pattern [20], both being a consequence of the formation of various forms of bromelain isolated from crude bromelain [21]. Furthermore, different purification methods and several purification steps could also contribute to molecular weight heterogeneity. The optimum temperature range for stem bromelain is between 40 and 60 °C (37–70 °C for fruit bromelain) and its optimum pH range is 4–8 (3–8 for fruit bromelain) [1,13,15,22–24]. However, its activity is no longer susceptible to the effect of the pH once it is combined with a substrate [1]. Bromelain preferentially cleaves glycyl, alanyl and leucyl peptide bonds [25]. Its activity can be determined using different substrates, including casein [16,26–28], gelatin [1], azocasein [19,29], azoalbumin, hemoglobin, sodium caseinate [23,30], and synthetic peptide substrates (Nα-CBZ-ʟ-Lysine p- nitrophenyl ester, Z-Arg-Arg-pNa, Bz-Phe-Val-Arg-pNA, H-Val-Ala-pNA, Suc-Ala-Ala-Val-pNA, Suc-Ala-Pro-Leu-Phe-pNA, Suc-Phe-Leu-Phe-pNA, Z-Phe-Arg-pNA and Z-Phe-pNA) [31,32]. The value of Michaelis–Menten constant (K_m) vary significantly when different substrates (azoalbumin, azocasein, sodium caseinate, casein and hemoglobin) are used for fruit bromelain activity determination, being the lowest (0.026 mM) for azoalbumin and the highest (0.165 mM) for hemoglobin [33]. The most suitable substrate for the fruit bromelain activity is azocasein, followed by azoalbumin, casein, sodium caseinate and hemoglobin according to the enzyme catalytic power parameter (V_{max}/K_m ratio), being 0.104, 0.096, 0.022, 0.020 and 0.014, respectively [33]. Bromelain inactivation rate follows first-order kinetics at 55 °C and 60 °C, but not above 70 °C, while its thermal deactivation is entirely irreversible and follows a two-stage mechanism, including the formulation of an intermediate between native and denatured states [15]. Bromelain retains more than 50% of its original proteolytic activity after 30 min incubation at 60 °C, from 9% to 22% after 15 min incubation at 70 °C, and becomes utterly inactive when heated for 10 min at 100 °C [34]. Aqueous proteolytic activity of bromelain decreases rapidly at 21 °C, while its concentrated forms (>50 mg/mL) are stable for one week at room temperature and can be repeatedly frozen and thawed [35].

Table 1. Physiochemical properties of cysteine endopeptidases derived from pineapple plants [1,13,15,22–24].

	Stem Bromelain	Fruit Bromelain	Ananain	Comosain
Source	Pineapple stem	Pineapple fruit	Pineapple stem	Pineapple stem
Molecular weight [kDa]	23.8–37.0	23.0–32.5	23.4–25.0	24.4–24.5
Isoelectric point	≥9.5	4.6	>10	>10
Amino acid sequence	212, 291, 285	326, 351	216	186
Optimum T [°C]	40–60	37–70	/	/
Optimum pH	4–8	3–8	/	/
Presence of Glycoproteins	Yes	Yes/No	No	Yes

The activation energy of bromelain is 41.7 kcal/mol [23], and same can be activated by many chemical agents, including calcium chloride, cysteine, sodium cyanide, bisulfate salt, hydrogen sulfide, sodium sulfide and benzoate [13,36,37]. Stem bromelain is reversibly inhibited during reaction with organic mercury, ions of mercury and tetrathionate. Its irreversible inhibition occurs by reacting with *N*-ethylmaleimide, *N*-(4-dimethyl-

3,5-dinitrophenyl) maleimide, monoiodoacetic acid and 1,3-dibromine acetone due to alkylation of the thiol group, an essential group for the activity of the enzyme [15].

Until now, several different (fruits or stem) bromelain amino acids sequences have been deposited in the National Center for Biotechnology Information (NCBI) Genbank database with around 90–100% similarity. Alanine, glycine and serine are the most abundant amino acids in stem and fruit bromelains, while histidine is present in the lowest amount [13]. Bromelain amino acid sequence is highly similar to papain, actinidin, proteinase Ω and chymopapain [24]. A single polypeptide chain constitutes the primary structure of bromelain with amino acids folded into two structure domains: α-helix domain (domain cathepsin propeptide inhibitor—I29) and antiparallel β-sheet domain (domain peptidase C1) (Figure 1). Mainly, the I29 domains are located between amino acids number 1 and 100 of the N-terminal sites. The structure domains are stabilized by disulfide bridges and numerous hydrogen bonds. Stem bromelain differs from the fruit bromelain in the number of polar amino acids (arginine and lysine), and acidic amino acids (aspartate and glutamate). The stem bromelain contains more polar amino acids, and the fruit bromelain has more acidic amino acids, leading to a difference in isoelectric point (4.6 and ≥9.5 for fruit and stem bromelain, respectively). The active site is located on the surface molecules between domains and the proposed catalytic residues for the modeled BAA21848 structure is composed of three amino acids Cys-121, His-254 and Asn-275; for CAA08861 structure Cys-147, His-281 and Asn-302 are proposed, which fall into approximately the exact locations as in papain catalytic residues (Cys-25, His-159 and Asn-175) [13,38].

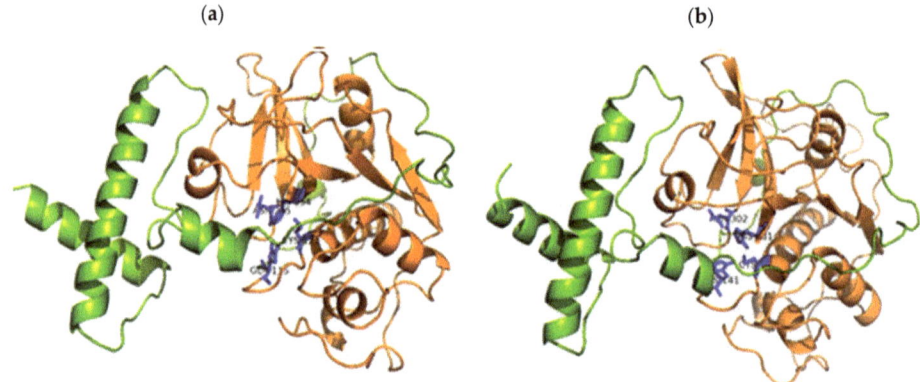

Figure 1. Model domain organisation of (**a**) fruit bromelain (sequences with the accession number of BAA21848 in the NCBI Genbank database and 352 amino acids) and (**b**) stem bromelain (sequences with the accession number of CAA08861 in the NCBI Genbank database and 357 amino acids). α-helix domain (domain I29 at the N-terminal region) is colored in green, β-sheet domain (domain peptidase C1 at the C-terminal region) is colored in orange. The catalytic amino acids of both models are represented as sticks (Reproduced with permission from [13], Elsevier, Amsterdam, The Netherlands, 2018).

2.2. *Isolation, Extraction and Purification*

Bromelain can be isolated from all parts of the pineapple plant (stem, core, peel, crown and leaves), which affect the concentration and composition. The stem and pineapple fruit allow the production of high amounts of bromelain, while the pineapple core, peel and leaves contain smaller quantities, yet, together with pineapple stem and crown, they represent up to 50% (*w/w*) of the total pineapple waste [16], making extraction of bromelain from pineapple waste economically and environmental attractive [28]. Consequently, the most commercially available bromelain is usually obtained from pineapple stem, which is also therapeutically more effective and shows higher proteolytic activity than fruit bromelain [17].

Numerous strategies have been developed for the extraction and purification of bromelain. The bromelain production process consists of several sequential steps, as depicted in Figure 2. Fresh pineapple stem parts or any other parts of the pineapple are washed, cut into small pieces, crushed in an industrial blender to disrupt the plant cells and separate the enzyme from the cells, filtered to remove the fibrous material and centrifugated to remove insoluble materials [1,38–40]. The obtained supernatant is called crude extract and is further purified as impurities and by-products (e.g., proteins, pigments, polysaccharides) can react with bromelain and inhibit its activity [17]. Purification can be done using chromatographic processes (among them ion-exchange chromatography with prior precipitation by adding ammonium sulfate is the most relevant, a two-phase aqueous system (e.g., PEG/K_2SO_4, PEG/$MgSO_4$, PEG/poly(acrylic acid), PEG/$(NH_4)_2SO_4$) or a reverse micellar system [1,17,41], the selection primarily depends on the application. Purification can also be performed by membrane-based processes (microfiltration, ultrafiltration) [40] or precipitation, followed by centrifugation and solubilization in phosphate buffer [38]. The residual specific activity of crude pineapple extract purified by fractionation using ammonium sulfate at 20–50% saturation level is 70 U/mg with the total activity of 167.3 U, total protein content of 2.39 mg and the purity level of 5.3 fold compared to the crude enzyme extract [16]. When acetone (50–80% saturation) was used as fractionating agent, the residual specific activity of bromelain fraction was 19.7 U/mg [16]. The crude bromelain of pineapple fruit purified by high-speed counter-current chromatography coupled with the reverse micelle solvent system yielded 3.01 g of bromelain from 5.00 g crude extract in 200 min [42]. The choice of a purification method determines the purity of the enzyme and the enzyme production cost [40]. Commercially available bromelain is produced by a lengthy and costly purification method that yields bromelain in varying degrees of purity [32]. The purification steps correspond to 70–90% of the total production costs [38], implying the need to develop innovative, cost-efficient methods for pure bromelain production in fewer steps [39].

Isolation of bromelain from pineapple fruit and its various parts is not the only way to obtain bromelain; researchers are also trying to clone the bromelain gene in multiple hosts, such as *E. coli* BL21-AI [32,43,44], *E. coli* BL21-CodonPlus(DE3) [45], *E. coli* BL21 DE3pLysS [14], *Pichia pastori* [46] and Chinese cabbage (*Brassica rapa*) [47], leading to recombinant bromelain—an intracellular enzyme abundant in the cytoplasm of the host cell, meaning that the host cell wall needs to be disrupted using homogenization, chemical lysis, sonication with lysozyme or freeze-thawing to release the bromelain [44]. Amid et al. [32] reported about higher specific activity of recombinant bromelain (1.231 U/mg) in comparison to commercial bromelain (0.846 U/mg) when the release of p-nitrophenol from a synthetic substrate Nα-CBZ-ʟ-Lysine p-nitrophenyl ester was monitored. The recombinant bromelain obtained in a single step immobilized metal affinity chromatography was purified 41-fold and showed optimum activity at pH 4.6 and 45 °C [32]. In contrast, George and co-workers [14] reported a higher protease activity of native bromelain obtained from Sigma (a purified form of crude stem bromelain) in comparison to recombinant bromelain when casein was used as a substrate. Crude bromelain showed even higher proteolytic activity than native bromelain due to its composition of a mixture of protease complexes which can cleave substrate even more effectively. However, the effectiveness of the extraction of the (recombinant) bromelain and its residual activity are related to the choice of buffer, presence of chelating agents (ethylenediaminetetraacetic acid (EDTA), cyclohexane-1,2-diaminoetetraacetic acid (CDTA), hydroxyethyl ethylenediamine triacetic acid (HEDTA)), reducing agents and protease inhibitors [44].

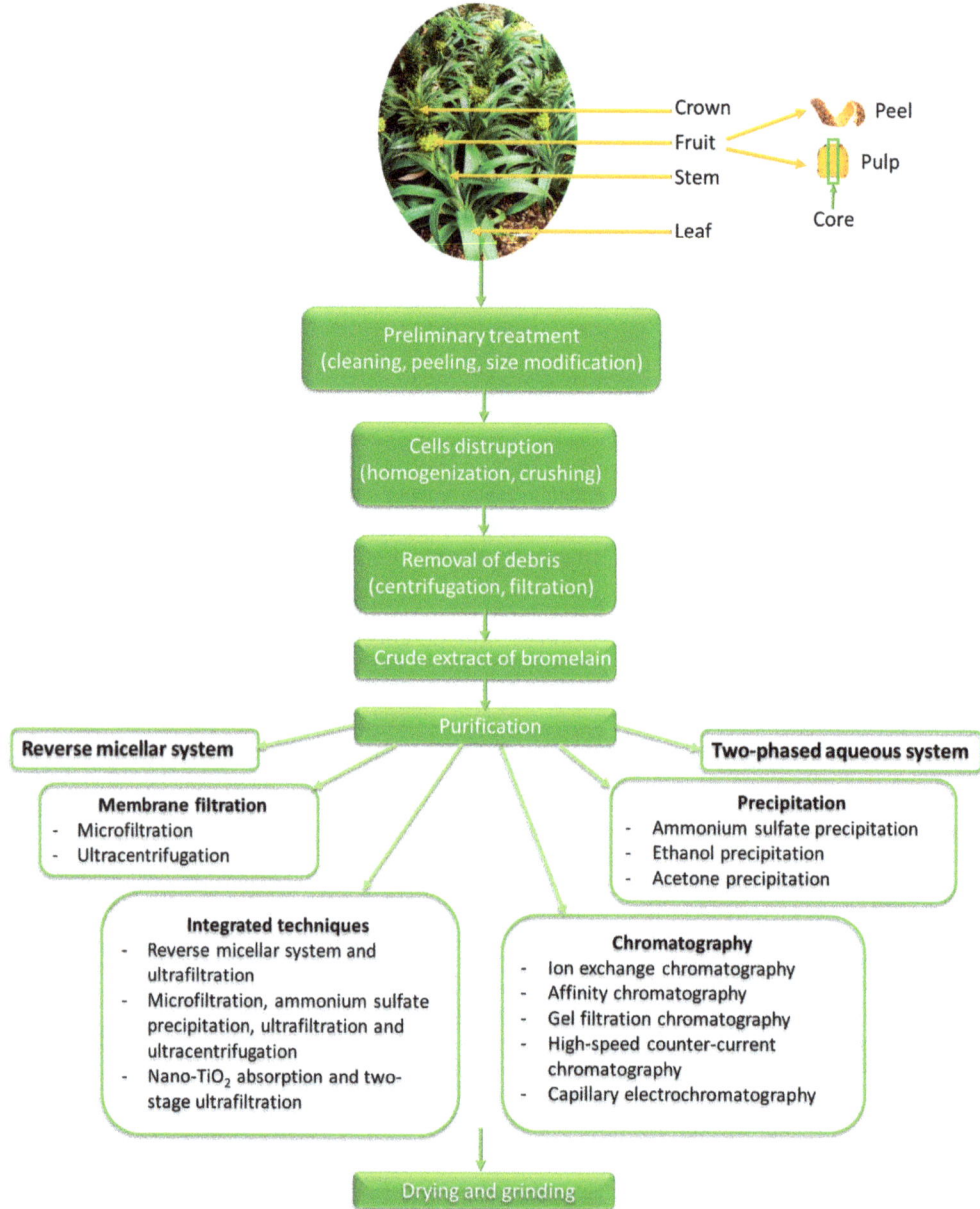

Figure 2. Scheme of a typical bromelain production.

2.3. Bioactivity

Bromelain has been a valuable compound in traditional medicine in Southeast Asia, Kenya, India, and China for a long time [28,48] due to its numerous therapeutic effects (Figure 3), including antimicrobial [16,49,50], anti-inflammatory [30,51], anticoagulant [52], anticancer [53,54], antiplaque [55,56], and antiulcer properties [50]. Furthermore, it is also beneficial for wound healing [57–60], dermatological disorders [19], post-surgery recovery, enhanced antibiotic absorption [1], treatment of osteoarthritis [61], sinusitis and diarrhea [17]. Recently, bromelain is suggested as an antiviral agent against COVID-19 due to the inhibition of different versions of SARS-CoV-2 [62]. Some of its therapeutic mechanisms are discussed below.

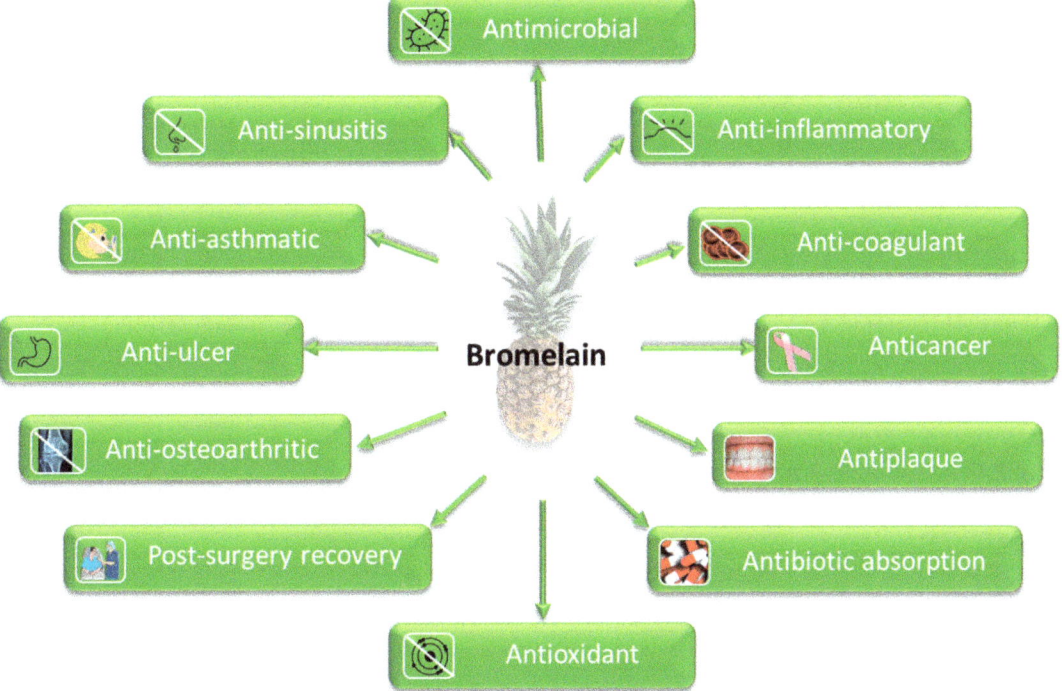

Figure 3. Overview of the bromelain bioactivity.

The mechanism behind the antimicrobial activity of bromelain is not well known, yet, is believed that bromelain may hinder bacterial growth by hydrolyzing some peptide bonds in the bacterial cell wall [14]. When bromelain digests the surface proteins, the cell wall is damaged, allowing the cell to leak, swell, and open [1]. Bromelain also inhibits the growth of some bacteria by preventing bacterial adhesion to specific glycoprotein receptors on the surface [1,48]. Furthermore, bromelain inhibits enterotoxin production of *Escherichia coli* (*E. coli*) and prevents diarrhea caused by *E. coli* [17]. Bromelain shows antimicrobial activity against both Gram-positive and Gram-negative bacteria, including *E. coli*, *Aggregatibacter actinomycetemcomitans* (*A. actinomycetemcomitans*), *Porphyromonas gingivalis* (*P. gingivalis*), *Streptococcus mutans* (*S. mutans*) [56], *Bacillus subtilis* (*B. subtilis*), (*S. aureus*), *Pseudomonas aeruginosa* (*P. aeruginosa*), *Proteus* spp., *Acinetobacter* spp., ... [1,63]. Additionally, synergistic use of bromelain and antibiotics increases the antibacterial effect due to increased absorption of antibiotics induced by bromelain, leading to better drug distribution in the microbes [1,17]. Bromelain has also been reported to act as an inhibitor of fungal pathogens [39,64].

Inflammation is the body's attempt to protect itself [28]. It is a complex biological mechanism primarily regulated by the disruption of tissue homeostasis [17]. Most often, non-steroidal anti-inflammatory drugs are prescribed to combat the classic signs of inflammation (heat, pain, redness and swelling), leading to severe damage to the gastrointestinal tract and numerous side effects. In such cases, the bromelain can be used as an alternative [28] due to its anti-inflammatory activity mediated by (Figure 4):

- increased serum fibrinolytic activity, reduced plasma fibrinogen levels and decreased bradykinin levels (resulting in reduced vascular permeability), thereby reducing edema and pain;
- modulating the formation of pro-inflammatory prostaglandins (by lowering levels of prostaglandin E2 (PGE2) and thromboxane A2 (TXA-2)), enhancing the anti-inflammatory mediators and the levels of prostaglandin I2 (PGI-2);
- modulating specific immune cell surface adhesion molecules—acting on the migration of neutrophils to inflammation sites [28,61,65].

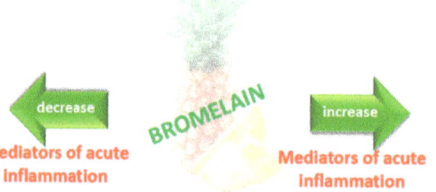
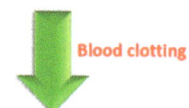

- **Bradykinin** (vascular permeability, pain)
- **TXA-2** (vasoconstriction, platelet aggregation)
- **PGE-2** (vasodilation)

Mediators of acute inflammation

Mediators of acute inflammation

- **TNF** (leukocytes adhesion)
- **IL-1** (leukocytes adhesion)
- **PGI-2** (vasodilation, platelet aggregation)

Blood clotting

- **Degradation of fibrin**
- **Prothrombin reduction**
- **Prekallikrein reduction**

Figure 4. Anti-inflammatory and anticoagulant mechanisms of action of bromelain (Adapted with permission from [65], MDPI, Basel, Switzerland, 2021).

Because of these actions, bromelain is potentially effective in several conditions and diseases associated with inflammation, including rheumatoid arthritis, osteoarthritis, cardiovascular diseases, skin wounds and burns, perioperative sports injuries and chronic rhinosinusitis [65]. Furthermore, inflammation is also associated with cancer; suppressing chronic inflammation may inhibit cancer progression due to reduced PGE-2 and prostaglandin-endoperoxide synthase 2 (COX-2) after bromelain administration [17]. The anti-inflammatory effect of bromelain is also the most traditional and established one [17].

Bromelain affects blood clotting by increasing the fibrinolytic capacity of serum and inhibiting the synthesis of the blood-clotting protein fibrin (Figure 4). It also decreases prekallikrein—a proenzyme that must be converted to kallikrein to help in coagulation. Consequently, it inhibits the generation of bradykinin, leading to pain and edema reduction, and increased circulation on the side of the injury [17,28,39].

The molecular mechanisms of bromelain's anticancer activity are also not fully understood [11]. However, some research has suggested that the bromelain anticancer mechanism is mainly attributed to its protease components and proteolysis [11,35]. One of the described anti-tumor mechanisms of bromelain includes induced differentiation of leukemic cells, leading to apoptosis of tumor cells [1]. Bromelain inhibits the growth of cancer cells by increasing the expression of two activators of apoptosis in mouse skin—p53 and Bax [66]. It also decreases the activity of cell survival regulators such as Akt and Erk, promoting apoptotic cell death in tumors. Expression of promoters of cancer progression—nuclear factor kappa B (NF-κB) and Cox-2 are also inhibited by bromelain in mouse papillomas and models of skin tumorigenesis [1,11].

Bromelain is well tolerated and considered a safe nutraceutical with no serious adverse effects [30,65]. It has already received FDA approval for clinical use as an orally administered anti-inflammatory and anticoagulant therapeutic [52]. Its oral administration is well tolerated even in high doses (up to 3 g/day) for prolonged therapy periods, even up to several years [11]. It has a very low level of toxicity [48]. The lethal dose (LD50) for intraperitoneal administration is 37 mg/kg and 85 mg/kg for mice and rabbits, respectively, and 30 mg/kg and 20 mg/kg for intravenous administration [65], with no immediate toxic reactions [25]. Daily oral administration of 500 mg/kg of bromelain did not provoke any alteration in food intake, growth, histology of the heart, kidney and spleen, or hematological parameters in rats [25]. After daily bromelain administration up to 750 mg/kg no toxicity was observed in dogs after 6 months [17]. No relevant side effects have been observed in humans at doses of up to 2000 mg/kg, even with prolonged oral administration [65]. However, clinical trials have reported some side effects, mainly gastrointestinal (i.e., diarrhea, nausea and flatulence), headache, tiredness, dry mouth, allergic reactions, and bleeding risk, especially in individuals treated with other anticoagulant drugs [17,61,65].

2.4. Immobilization Strategies

One of the issues related to enzymes (such as bromelain) utilization is a decline of their activity with time or after processing. Indeed, enzymes, isolated from their natural environments, are susceptible to process conditions, such as pH, temperature, strong acids and bases, and non-aqueous solvents, which may affect their activity [67], health benefits and pharmaceutical applicability [68]. A promising strategy to secure their efficiency is immobilization [69], which requires selecting supporting material (inorganic components, synthetic polymers or natural polymers) with suitable surface chemistry for controlled enzymatic attachment. The next step is optimizing the immobilization process towards desired immobilization yield, activity retention of even amplification, stability and reusability [69] (Figure 5). Successful immobilization requires thorough knowledge and control of the interactions between the carrier and the enzyme [70]. The choice of immobilization method and carrier depends on the nature of the immobilized compound and the goal of immobilization (resistance against high temperature, pH, controlling the release, preventing negative interactions . . .) [71].

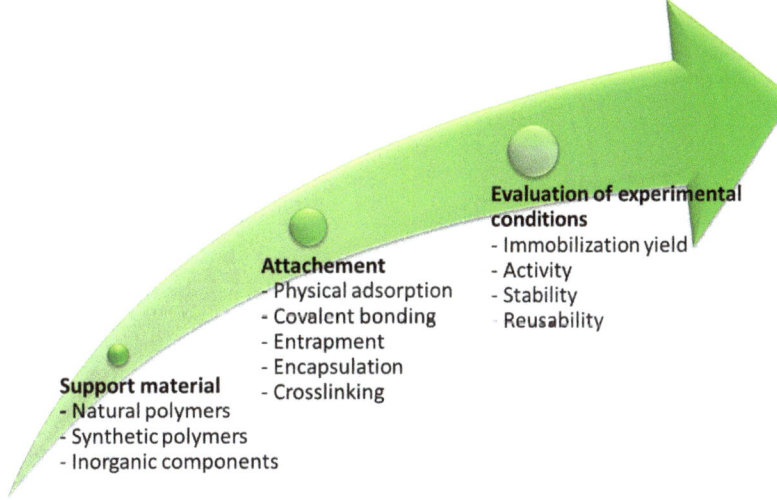

Figure 5. Steps for immobilization of bioactive enzymes.

Immobilization methods and carriers utilized for immobilization of bromelain in the last 10 years are summarized in Table 2 and Figure 6. Bromelain has been combined mostly with nanoparticles, hydrogels, fibers and matrices with the aim to improve the properties of the final formulation [29]. Baker and co-workers [72] encapsulated bromelain in silica nanosphere aggregates, using sodium metasilicate as a silica precursor and ethyleneamines (diethylenetriamine (DETA), triethylenetetramine (TETA), tetraethylenepentamine (TEPA), and pentaethylenehexamine (PEHA)) of different chain lengths as initiators. They found out that increased loading mass of bromelain resulted in the increased activity of bromelain, being 61.7% when 10 mg of bromelain was encapsulated in silica and only 12.1% when 2 mg of bromelain was used. The encapsulation also increases the thermostability with maximum activity at 40 °C for free bromelain and at 50 °C for encapsulated bromelain. At 70 °C free bromelain lost its activity while encapsulated bromelain retained approximately 30% of its activity [72]. Chitosan-methyl cellulose hydrogel [73], freeze-dried chitosan nanoparticles [29], chitosan microspheres [74], poly(lactide-co-glycolic) acid nanoparticles [75] and katira gum nanoparticles [76] have also been studied for encapsulation of bromelain, showing various immobilization yield and bromelain activity. Esti et al. [77] covalently immobilized stem bromelain on chitosan beads by direct mechanism, involving the bromelain carboxyl groups of Asp or Glu residues and the amino groups of the chitosan. Ataied et al. [78] studied bacterial nanocellulose as a support material for physical adsorption of bromelain and reported about 9-times increased antimicrobial activity of adsorbed bromelain. Holyavka et al. [70] also used the adsorption method for immobilization of cysteine proteases onto chitosan and observed significant loss of the bromelain catalytic activity due to: (a) nonspecific binding, (b) structural changes of bromelain upon interaction with the carrier, and (c) diffusional and steric limitations, leading to impeded access of the active bromelain center [70]. All the studies clearly show the influence of the carrier and immobilization method on bromelain's immobilization yield, residual activity, and thermal stability. By choosing a suitable carrier and immobilization method, it is possible to significantly reduce the influence of the carrier on the structural and functional properties of the bromelain [70], enhance its stability and activity upon exposure to a wide range of pH and high temperatures and improve its antimicrobial and anti-inflammatory activity. However, there is not yet a standard, highly efficient immobilization approach for bromelain delivery [29].

Table 2. Review of bromelain immobilization methods.

Immobilization Method	Carrier/Support Material	Crosslinking Agent or Initiator	Outcomes	References
Covalent immobilization	APTES–modified mesoporous silica nanoparticles (MSN)	1-ethyl-(3-dimethylaminopropyl) carbodiimide/N-hydroxysuccinimide (EDC/NHS)	- Enhanced diffusion of MSN within the tumor extracellular matrix	[52]
	Chitosan beads (Chitopearl BCW-3010)	/	- 22% immobilization yield - Higher resistance to the SO_2, skin and seed tannins	[77]
	Lyocell fibres	Epichlorohydrin + glutaraldehyde (GA), EDC, and APTES + GA	- 88.14% activity yield of immobilized bromelain at pH 7 - High stability of immobilized bromelain at pH range 6–8 - pH 7 is ideal for immobilization	[79]
	Chitosan–cobalt–magnetite nanoparticle	GA	- 77% immobilization binding - 85 ± 2% of the initial catalytic activity retained - 50% of the initial catalytic activity after the fifth use	[80]
	Chitosan—clay (montmorillonites/bentonites or sepiolite) nanocompositefilm	GA	- Increased immobilization yield, decreased catalytic activity of the immobilized bromelain	[81]

Table 2. Cont.

Immobilization Method	Carrier/Support Material	Crosslinking Agent or Initiator	Outcomes	References
Adsorption	Chitosan matrix	/	- Increased stability of bromelain concerning UV irradiation in comparison with free enzymes - Chitosan matrix acts as photoprotector	[82]
	Chitosan colloidal particles	/	- Destruction of a part of the helical structure - Decreased catalytic activity of bromelain	[70]
	Magnetic carbon nanotubes	/	- Adsorption followed second-order kinetics - Bromelain (c = 100 µg/mL) alone and in combination with nanotubes efficiently inhibited the HT-29 colorectal cancerous cells	[66]
	Ag nanoparticles	/	- Spontaneous interaction of AgNP with bromelain - Main forces are electrostatic and hydrophobic interactions - Adsorption follows pseudo-second-order kinetics	[83]
	Magnetic nanoparticles with chitosan and reactive red 120 (Red 120-CS-MNP)	/	- Red 120-CS-MNP are suitable carrier - Adsorption isotherm fitted the Freundlich model well	[84]
	Spores of the probiotic *Bacillus*	/	- Improved stability and activity of the bromelain upon exposure to a wide range of pH and high temperatures	[85]
	Bacterial nanocellulose	/	- Improved antimicrobial activity	[78]
Entrapment	N-isopropylacrylamide (PNIPAAm) hydrogels	/	- New release system evolving hydrogels and bromelain for wound healing	[86]
	Alginate—arabic gum hydrogels	/	- 19% of bromelain was incorporated, 227% swelling ratio of final hydrogel	[87]

Table 2. Cont.

Immobilization Method	Carrier/Support Material	Crosslinking Agent or Initiator	Outcomes	References
Encapsulation	Silica nanoparticles	DETA, TETA, TEPA, or PEHA	- Increased thermal stability	[72]
	Chitosan—methyl cellulose hydrogel	GA	- Bromelain as a drug for digestion problem	[73]
	Freeze-dried chitosan nanoparticles	Sodium tripolyphosphate	- 85.1 ± 1% encapsulation efficiency - Chitosan-bromelain-nanoparticles presented 4.9 U/mL of enzymatic activity (104.7% of free bromelain activity) - Freeze-dried chitosan-bromelain-nanoparticles improve bromelain and nanoparticle stability (maltose as lyoprotectant)	[29]
	Katira gum nanoparticles	/	- Enhanced anti-inflammatory activity of bromelain against carrageenan	[76]
	Glutaraldehyde crosslinked chitosan microspheres	/	- 84.75% encapsulation efficiency	[74]
	Poly(lactide-co-glycolic) acid nanoparticles	/	- 48 ± 4.81% entrapment efficiency - Enhanced antitumor effect	[75]
	Poly(lactide-co-glycolic) acid nanoparticles	/	- Oral administration of encapsulated nanoparticles reduced the tumor burden of Ehrlich ascites carcinoma in mice and increased their life-span (160.0 ± 5.8%) when compared with free bromelain (24 ± 3.2%) - Enhanced anti-carcinogenic potential upon oral administration	[53]
	Eudragit L 100 nanoparticles	/	- 85.42 ± 5.34% entrapment efficiency - Lyophilized formulation ensured 2-year shelf-life at room temperature - Oral bromelain delivery in inflammatory conditions	[88]
	Nanostructured lipid carrier (lecithin-steric acid-Span-80) emulsified with PVA solution		- ~77% entrapment efficiency - Diminished of paw edema, joint stiffness, mechanical allodynia, tissue damage - Alleviation of oxidative stress and immunological markers - Application in rheumatoid arthritis	[89]

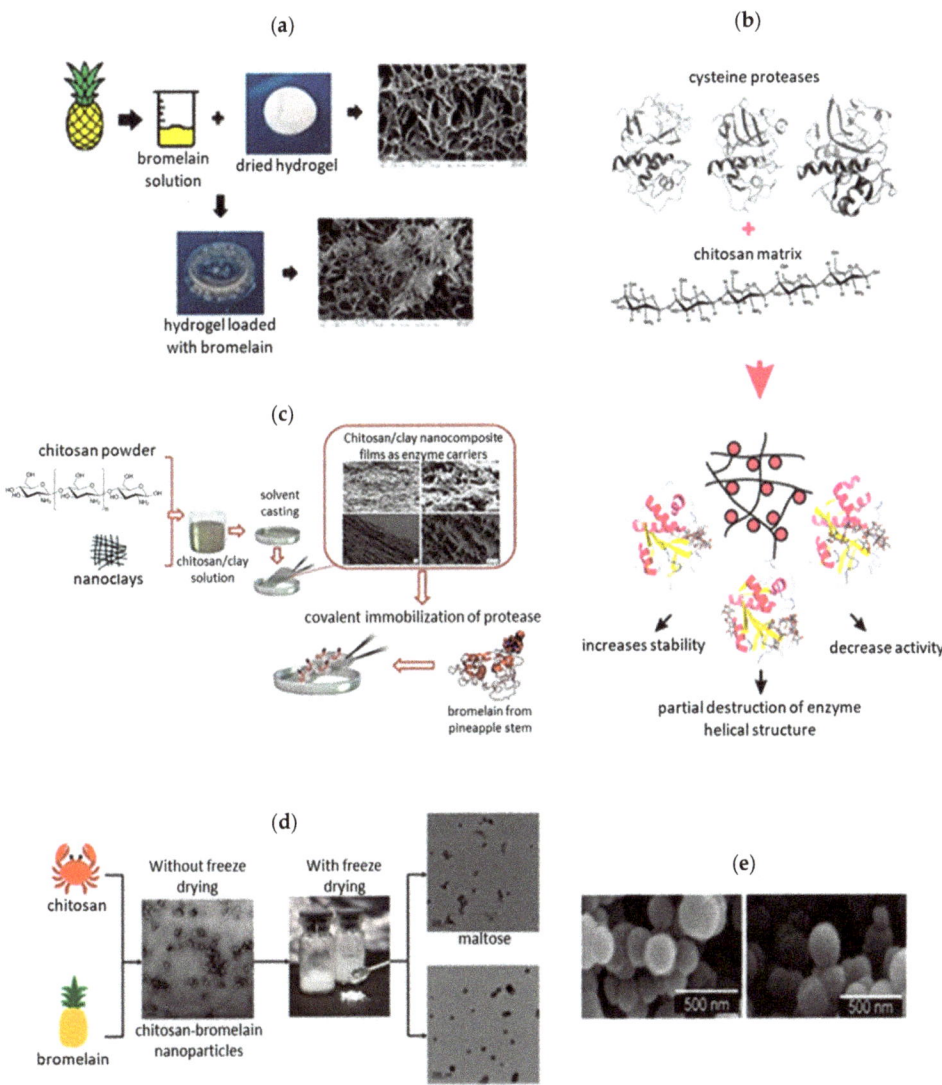

Figure 6. Schematic illustration and SEM micrographs of immobilization methods of bromelain: (**a**) entrapment into hydrogels (Reproduced with permission from [86], Elsevier, Amsterdam, The Netherlands, 2018); (**b**) adsorption onto chitosan matrix (Reproduced with permission from [70], Elsevier, Amsterdam, The Netherlands, 2021); (**c**) covalent immobilization (Reproduced with permission from [81], Elsevier, Amsterdam, The Netherlands, 2018); (**d**) entrapment into nanoparticles (Reproduced with permission from [29], Elsevier, Amsterdam, The Netherlands, 2021); (**e**) SEM micrographs of encapsulated silica nanoparticles formed without bromelain (left) and with bromelain (right) (Reproduced with permission from [72], John Wiley and Sons, Hoboken, NJ, USA, 2014).

2.5. Applications

Bromelain finds widespread applications in several areas, including medicine, health, food, and cosmetics [15]. In the food industry, it is used for meat tenderization [90–92] (together with papain representing 95% of the enzymes used to tenderize meat in the

USA [32]), baking process [93], protein hydrolysate production [94], as a food supplement [95–97] and as an anti-browning agent in fruit juices [98]. Furthermore, bromelain also shows antimicrobial activity against *Alicyclobacillus acidoterrestris* (*A. acidoterrestris*), Gram-positive bacteria often related to the deterioration of acidic products (citrus juices, iced tea, isotonic drinks and tomato extract) [99]. Still, its main application continues to be in the pharmaceutical industry [24].

Several experimental data and clinical studies showed better burns and wound healing under the influence of bromelain due to its proteolytic, anti-inflammatory, antibacterial, and anti-edematogenic effects [58,59,73,86,100–102]. Recently, Chen et al. demonstrated reduced inflammation and improved wound healing rate in a rat model when treated with bromelain-immobilized electrospun poly(ε-caprolactone) fibres [100]. These fibres also effectively prevented wound infections due to their antibacterial activity against Gram-positive bacteria *S. aureus*, dominant in the initial stage of chronic wound formation, and Gram-negative bacteria *E. coli* [100]. Aichele et al. confirmed the effect of bromelain on myofibroblast reduction, resulting in attenuated fibrotic development [58]. Topical application of bromelain is effective in the eschar removal (debridement) of uncomplicated gunshot wounds when used as an adjunct to a simple wound incision and simplifies the conventional wound excision treatment [103]. Bromelain treatment has a characteristic of attacking mainly necrotic tissue, while healthy tissue seems unaffected [58]. One example is bromelain-based enzymatic debridement product NexoBrid (produced by MediWound Ltd., Yavne, Israel), which reduced infection, blood loss, length of hospital stays, and the need for skin grafting in treating deep partial and full-thickness burns due to early non-surgical eschar removal without harming surrounding viable tissue (Figure 7) [59,101,104,105]. The NexoBrid, a topically-applied concentrate of proteolytic enzymes enriched in bromelain, was clinically approved in 2012 by the European Medicines Agency (EMA) to remove dead tissue in severe skin burns, and until now is the only clinical-approved application of bromelain [106]. Moreover, EscharEx (MediWound Ltd., Yavne, Israel) is another bromelain-based enzymatic debridement currently in development for chronic wounds [107,108]. Several researchers have also incorporated bromelain into various hydrogels [73,86,87,102] to create a dressing that ensures a moist environment around the wound and provides a barrier against infection [87].

Bromelain has clinical potential for the treatment of skin problems such as acne owing to its antimicrobial activity against microbial flora that is often associated with acne infection, including *P. acne*, *S. aureus*, *C. diphtheria* and *E. coli*, among which *S. aureus* was the most susceptible organism to the action of bromelain extracts, followed by *P. acne* [16,19].

In addition, bromelain can be used to inhibit the growth of bacteria that causes dental caries due to the intense antimicrobial activity against *P. gingivalis* (diameter of clear zone of 21 mm) [56]. The minimum inhibitory concentration (MIC) of bromelain against microorganisms associated with periodontal diseases was also determined by Praveen and co-workers, being 2 mg/mL, 4.15 mg/mL, 16.6 mg/mL and 31.25 mg/mL for *S. mutans*, *P. gingivalis*, *A. actinomycetemcomitans* and *Enterococcus fecalis* (*E. fecalis*), respectively [50]. The minimum bactericidal concentration (MBC) of crude bromelain of pineapple fruit to multidrug-resistance Gram-negative *P. aeruginosa* is 0.75 g/mL [109]. *P. aeruginosa* is a leading cause of nosocomial infections, responsible for 10% of hospital-acquired infections [109]. Crude bromelain, extracted from pineapple fruit, exhibited a 12 mm zone of inhibition against *Streptococcus pneumoniae* (*S. pneumoniae*), *P. aeruginosa* and *S. aureus* at a concentration of 1.0 g/mL [63]. Crude bromelain extracted from pineapple crown leaf (aqueous extract of pineapple crown leaf) showed 70–95% inhibition of microbial growth with MIC range of 1.65–4.95 mg/mL against laboratory strain *Saccharomyces cerevisiae* (*S. cerevisiae*) and *E. coli* XL1 blue, type strain *S. aureus*, drug-resistant strain *E. coli* DH5α pet16b Amp^r and two pathogenic strain *B. subtilis* and *Candida albicans* (*C. albicans*) [18]. It is also hypothesized that bromelain inhibits the development and progression of periodontitis through the elimination of important cell surface molecules (CD25) in leucocytes (proteolytic activity of bromelain), decreased growth of periodontal microorganisms (anti-adhesion property), reduced migration of neutrophils to periodontal sites (the hyperactivity of the neutrophils leads to damage of the periodontium), downregulating of inflammatory mediators (COX-2, tumor necrosis factor (TNF)), decreased osteoclastogenesis process with reduction in alveolar bone loss (Figure 8a,b) [110,111]. A clinical study conducted by Odresi et al. confirmed the anti-edematous action of bromelain in third molar surgery. The group treated with bromelain showed a reduced inflammatory response compared to the control group [112].

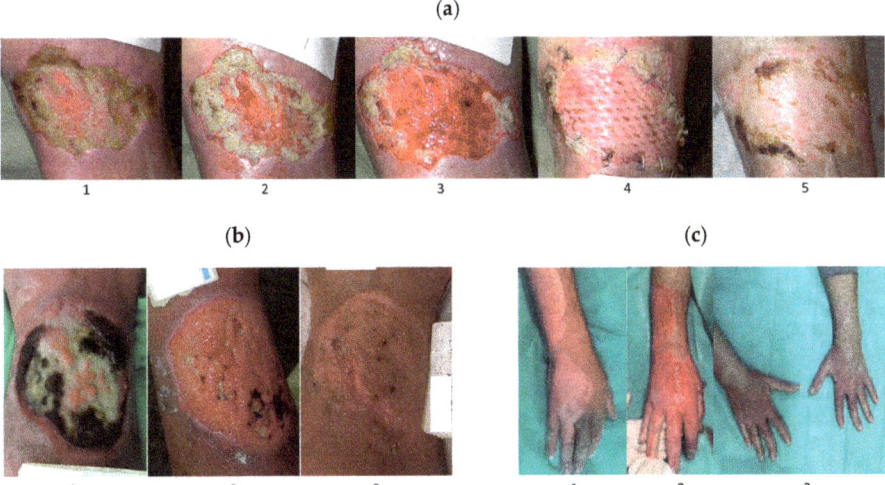

Figure 7. Bromelain-based treatment (BBT): (a) venous insufficiency ulcer; 1—pre-existing for 5 months, 2—after first BBT 4-h application, 3—after fourth BBT 4-h application (16 h total exposure to bromelain-based debridement), 4—one week post-split-thickness skin grafting, 5—seven weeks post-split-thickness skin grafting (Adapted with permission from [108], John Wiley and Sons, Hoboken, NJ, USA, 2018); (b) large venous leg ulcers; 1—venous leg ulcer pre-existing 10 weeks, 2—after 7 BBT, and 3—two months after split-thickness skin grafting (Reproduced with permission from [107], John Wiley and Sons, Hoboken, NJ, USA, 2021); (c) hand burn; 1—before BBT, 2—after BBT, 3—outcome 38 days post-burn (Reproduced with permission from [104], Baoshideng Publishing Group Inc., Pleasanton, CA, USA, 2017).

The anticarcinogenic effect of bromelain has been investigated through in vitro studies involving various cancer cell lines [66]. It can inhibit the growth and proliferation of mouse breast carcinoma 4T1, human breast adenocarcinoma GI-101A and MCF7, human prostate carcinoma PC3 and human gastric carcinoma AGS in a dose-dependent manner [43,113–115]. Bromelain concentration >75 µg/mL remarkably decreased cell viability in MCF7, PC3 and AGS human cell lines as a single therapy [113]. Moreover, it is also effective as an anticancer agent against cell lines of melanoma (A375), epidermoid carcinoma (A431) [116], gastric carcinoma (KATO-III and MKN45) [117], colorectal cancer (human colon adenocarcinoma (Caco-2)) [118], ovarian cancer (A2780), colon cancer (HT29) [119], lung cancer [120], pancreatic [121] and liver cancer (hepatocellular carcinoma HepG2) [10]. The absorption and efficiency of chemotherapy drugs (5-fluorouracil, vincristine, cisplatin, idarubicin, doxorubicin), antibiotics (amoxicillin and tetracycline) or blood pressure medication (captopril and lisinopril) [17,122–124] can be potentiated when combined with oral, subcutaneous or intramuscular administration of bromelain [17]. Higashi et al. [121] investigated whether bromelain could be used to degrade the barrier of dense extracellular matrix (ECM), a characteristic inhibitor of penetration of anticancer drugs in the treatment of pancreatic cancer. Due to the short half-life of the bromelain in the blood, they prepared reversibly PEGylated bromelain using "self-assembly PEGylation retaining activity (SPRA)" technology, thus retaining high bromelain activity and causing ECM degradation and increase of anticancer drugs in tumor tissue of pancreatic cancer (Figure 8c) [121]. Encapsulated bromelain also enables slow delivery, thus being favorable for cancer treatment [66].

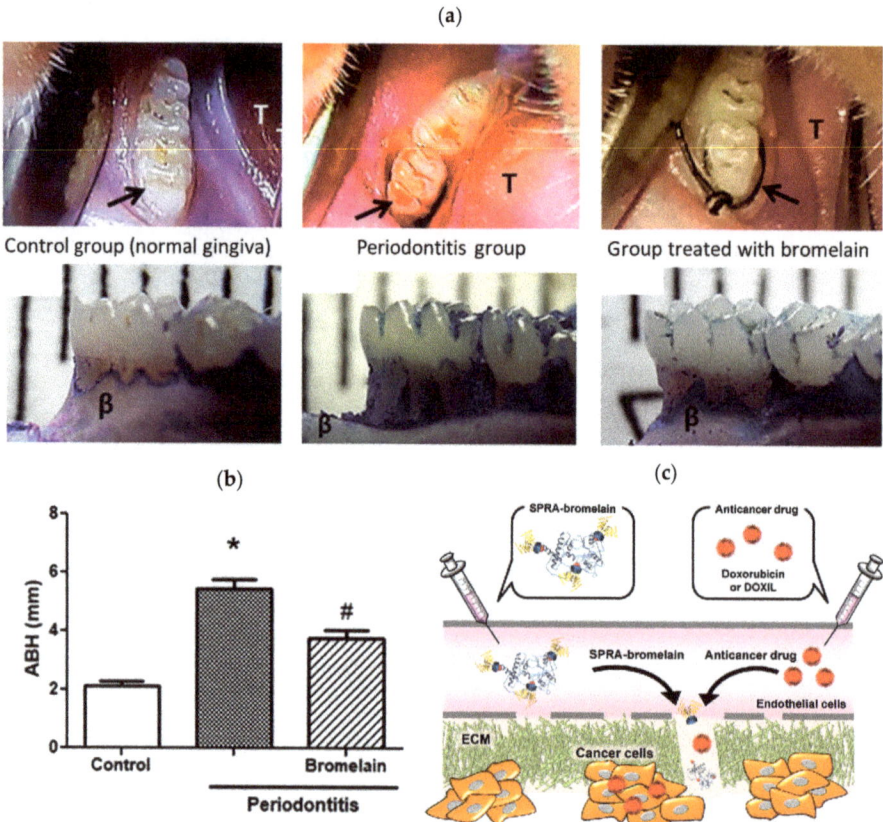

Figure 8. (a) Comparison of the control group (normal gingiva), periodontitis group and group treated with bromelain 15 mg/kg (arrow shows the first molar and the letter T shows the tongue). Group treated with bromelain indicates improvement of gingival papilla staining, reduction in edema, absence of bleeding and moderate bone loss (Reproduced with permission from [111], John Wiley and Sons, Hoboken, NJ, USA, 2020); (b) morphometric analyses of alveolar bone height; * $p < 0.05$ indicates the Periodontitis groups versus the Control group and # $p < 0.05$ indicates the Periodontitis groups versus the Bromelain group (Reproduced with permission from [111], John Wiley and Sons, Hoboken, NJ, USA, 2020); (c) the scheme of the SPRA-bromelain suggested a mechanism of ECM-degradation in pancreatic cancer (Reproduced with permission from [121], ACS Publications, Washington, DC, USA, 2020).

Bromelain effectively reduces the risk of clots-associated problems, including stroke or heart attack [15,17,25] due to the breaking down of the blood-clotting protein fibrin [125]. Bromelain has been shown to be effective in treating rheumatoid arthritis [86], exercise-induced muscle injuries [125] and edema caused by post-surgical trauma [19]. It was also used in treating patients with osteoarthritis, where it worked similarly to diclofenac treatments [126]. In combination with *Boswellia serrata* (*B. serrata*), bromelain improved the quality of life of patients suffering from different forms of osteoarthritis [96].

3. Nisin
3.1. Structural and Biological Properties

Antimicrobial peptides (AMPs) are cationic, hydrophobic or amphipathic natural antibiotics, consisting of amino acid residues of varying lengths (up to 100) in a linear or cyclic arrangement [127], derived from bacteria, insects, plants, birds, amphibians, fish, and mammals [128–130]. AMPs have attracted much attention because of their potent antibacterial activity against a broad spectrum of microorganisms, multiple modes of action, a low bacterial resistance rate, ability to destroy target cells rapidly and low cytotoxicity [127,131–134], therefore showing potential to overcome the growing problems of antibiotic resistance [135,136]. An example of AMPs is also an odorless, colorless, tasteless substance—nisin [131]. It is a cationic, amphiphilic, antimicrobial polypeptide [137,138], ribosomally synthesized and posttranslationally modified to its biologically active form [139]. It is a member of bacteriocins, classified as a Type A (I) lantibiotic [140], identified in 1928 in fermented milk cultures [6]. It contains the hydrophobic residues at the N—terminus and hydrophilic residues at the C—terminus (Figure 9a) [138], five thioether rings and four amino acids, usually not found in nature: lanthionine (Lan), β-methyl lanthionine (MeLan), and two dehydrated amino acids—dehydroalanine (Dha) and dehydrobutyrine (Dhb) (Figure 9b,c) [141,142]. These amino acids result from posttranslational modification of serine, threonine, and cysteine [143]. Moreover, the thioether rings give nisin unique properties, including nanomolar antimicrobial activity, resistance against proteolytic degradation and high heat stability [135]. The first two thioethers rings can bind lipid II, the flexible hinge region together with the last two thioethers rings can flip into the membrane and create a pore [3]. Unmodified prenisin contains 57 amino acids: the first 23 from the leader peptide and the last 34 residues from the core peptide [144]. The leader peptide renders the propeptide inactive and must be cleaved for a nisin to gain antimicrobial activity [142]. Therefore, active nisin consists of only 34 amino acids [3].

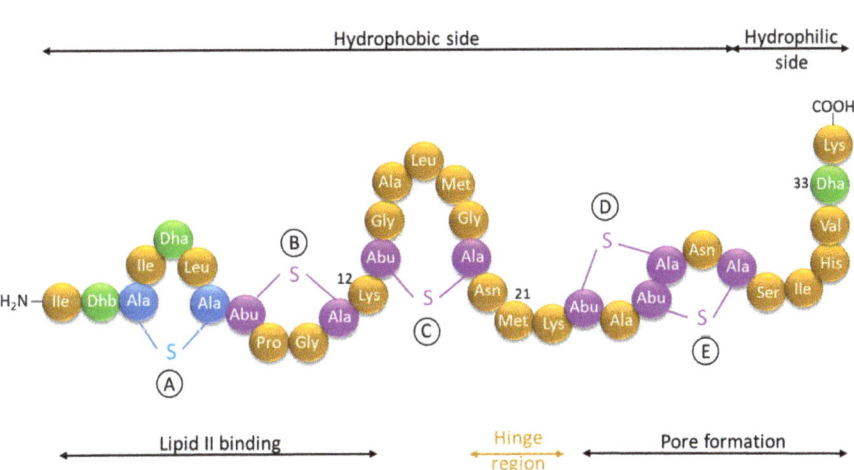

Figure 9. Cont.

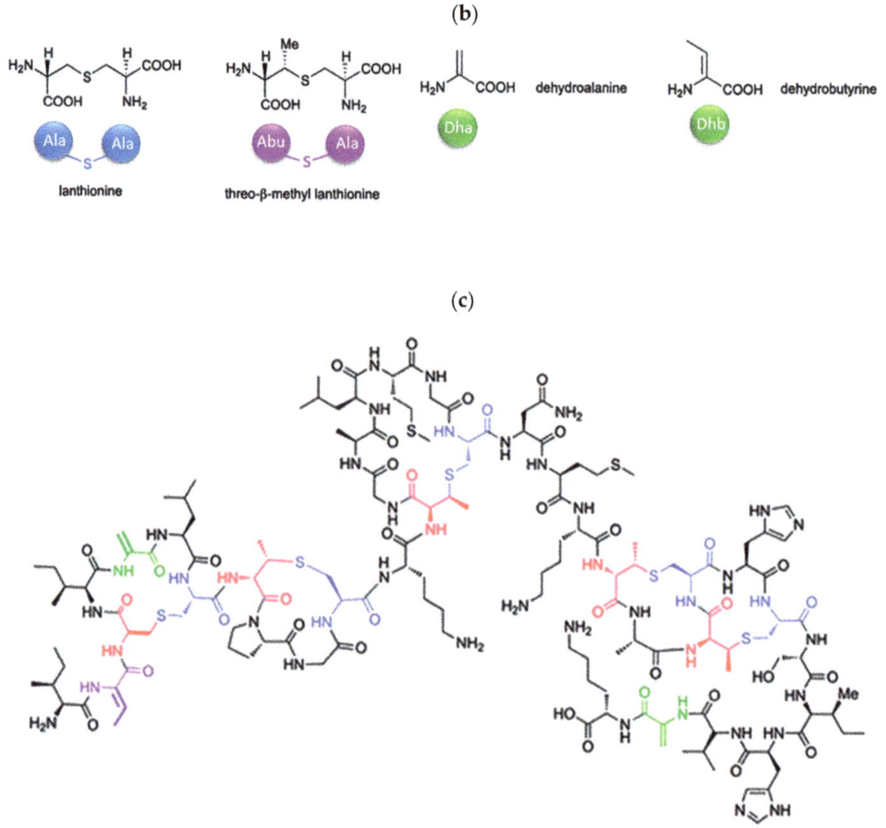

Figure 9. (a) Primary structure of nisin Z with highlighted residues involved in crucial aspects of the antimicrobial activity (Adapted with permission from [145], Elsevier, Amsterdam, The Netherlands, 2018); (b) chemical formula of dehydroalanine (Dha), dehydrobutyrine (Dhb), lanthionine (Lan), and β-methyl lanthionine (MeLan) (Adapted with permission from [145], Elsevier, Amsterdam, The Netherlands, 2018); (c) chemical structure of nisin A (Reproduced with permission from [146], RSC, Cambridge, UK, 2012).

Nisin is mainly produced by Gram-positive bacteria that include *Lactococcus* and *Streptococcus* species [7] (e.g., *Lactococcus lactis* (*L. lactis*) [137], *Streptococcus hyointestinalis* (*S. hyointestinalis*) [147], ...). Various production strains also lead to different naturally occurring variants of nisin (nisin A, nisin Z, nisin F, ...). The molecular weight of nisin depends on the production strain; usually, it is between 3.0 and 3.5 kDa [147]. This polypeptide has an amphipathic property [140], is cationic at neutral pH and has an isoelectric point above 8.5 [148]. Nisin has no absorbance at 280 nm due to the absence of aromatic amino acids [149].

Nisin has been approved by the Joint Food and Agriculture Organization World Health Organization (FAO/WHO, 1969), the US Food and Drug Administration (FDA, 1988) [7], the European Food Safety Authority (acceptable uptake of 0.13 mg/kg/day/person [150]) and the Food Standards Australia New Zealand [151]. It was generally regarded as safe (GRAS) [151,152]. So far, it is the only bacteriocin in the market allowed to be used as a food additive [153].

3.2. Isolation

Since the first discovery of nisin (nisin A) in fermented milk cultures, several natural and bioengineered variants of nisin have been identified [7,147], which differ in their structure and properties (solubility, chemical reactivity, and spectra) [154]. Up to now, there are eleven reported natural occurring nisin analogues: nisin A, nisin Z, nisin F, nisin Q, nisin H, nisin O A1-A3, nisin O A4, nisin U, nisin U2, nisin P, nisin J (Table 3), isolated from various bacterial genera such as *Lactococcus, Streptococcus, Staphylococcus,* and *Blautia*, located in dairy products, human gastrointestinal tract, bovine mammary secretions, human skin microflora, porcine intestine, an alimentary tract of ruminants, fish gut and river water in Japan [7,155]. Nisin analogues from the same genera are more like each other than analogues from different genera. Nisin A and nisin Z are both isolated from *L. lactis*, found in dairy products, and differ only in one amino acid at position 27; histidine (His) in nisin A is substituted with asparagine (Asp) in nisin Z (Table 3, highlighted in yellow). This substitution mainly affects the solubility of the polypeptide. It causes nisin Z to be more soluble at neutral pH than nisin A due to a more polar side chain of the Asp in comparison to His at neutral pH; it has minimal effect on antimicrobial activity, resistance to pH changes, sensitivity to proteolytic enzymes and thermal stability [149,155]. Nisin F differs from nisin A due to Asp and valine (Val) at positions 27 and 30. Nisin Q differs in comparison to nisin A in three amino acids at four positions: valine (Val, in position 15 and 30), leucine (Leu, in position 21), and asparagine (Asp, in position 27) [155]. Nisin O (A1-A3 and A4), nisin U and U2, and nisin P are shorter than previously described nisin analogues; they contain 33, 32, and 31 amino acids, respectively. With 35 amino acids, nisin J is the longest natural nisin analogue identified to date [147].

Table 3. Primary structures of nisin natural analogues. The changes in amino acids compared to nisin A are highlighted in yellow (not valid for Nisin J).

	Natural nisin analogues represented with a primary structure (Reproduced with permission from [147,155], ASM Journals, Washington, USA, 2020 and Springer Nature, London, UK, 2020)	Production strain [7,155]	Molecular weight [Da] [147]
Nisin A		*Lactococcus lactis* (dairy products)	3354
Nisin Z		*Lactococcus lactis* NIZO 22,186 (dairy products)	3331
Nisin F		*Lactococcus lactis* F10 (fish gut)	3315

Table 3. Cont.

Natural nisin analogues represented with a primary structure (Reproduced with permission from [147,155], ASM Journals, Washington, USA, 2020 and Springer Nature, London, UK, 2020)		Production strain [7,155]	Molecular weight [Da] [147]
Nisin Q		Lactococcus lactis 61–14 (Japanese river water)	3327
Nisin H		Streptococcus hyointestinalis (porcine intestine)	3453
Nisin O A1-A3		Blautia obeum A2–162 (human gastrointestinal tract)	3546
Nisin O A4		Blautia obeum A2–162 (human gastrointestinal tract)	3259
Nisin U		Streptococcus uberis 42 (bovine mammary secretions)	3029
Nisin U2		Streptococcus uberis D536 (bovine mammary secretions)	3015
Nisin P		Streptococcus gallolyticus subsp. Pasteurianus (alimentary tract of ruminants)	2989
Nisin J		Staphylococcus capitis APC 2923 (human skin)	3458

Aside from natural nisin analogues, the bioengineered forms of nisin have been developed in the last twenty years by genetic modification tools [156], with an attempt to alter the solubility, stability and efficiency of nisin. A large number of generated bioengineered forms of nisin revealed that modifying amino acids at the hinge-region (three amino acids asparagine-methionine-lysine at position 20–21–22 in the center of the peptide, Figure 9a) and at position 29, respectively, displayed an essential role in enhancing activity against Gram-negative bacteria, and both Gram-positive and Gram-negative pathogens [7,156]. Nisin A K22T, A N20P, A M21V, A K22S, A S29A, A S29D, A S29E, A S29G, Z N20K and Z M21K are some genetically modified nisin derivatives with changes in those positions and more significant activity against foodborne and clinical pathogens [6,7,156]. The names indicate the substitution position and the replaced amino acid; for example, nisin A K22T means that the amino acid sequence is the same as in Nisin A, the only difference is at position 22, where lysine (K) is substituted with threonine (T). Nisin derivative Z N20K and Z M21K showed enhanced activity against Gram-negative bacteria, including *Shigella*, *Pseudomonas* and *Salmonella* species, and displayed more significant thermal stability and solubility at neutral or alkaline pH [7]. Nisin A K22T exhibit enhanced activity against human and bovine pathogen *Streptococcus agalactiae* (*S. agalactiae*). Nisin A M21V showed enhanced antimicrobial activity against medically significant pathogens, including heterogenous Vancomycin intermediate *S. aureus* (hVISA), methicillin-resistant *S. aureus* (MRSA), *Clostridium difficile* (*C. difficile*), *S. agalactiae* and *Listeria monocytogenes* (*L. monocytogenes*). The S29G and S29A nisin variants showed enhanced activity against Gram-positive and Gram-negative pathogens, differentiating them from all nisin derivatives generated to date [156].

3.3. Bioactivity

Nisin is known for its broad-spectrum of antibacterial activity against a wide range of Gram-positive bacteria [7,140], even better than conventional antibiotics [157], due to its stability at a higher temperature, tolerance to low pH, and dual-mode of antimicrobial activity [6]. The latter includes binding of nisin molecule to an essential precursor for bacterial wall biosynthesis (the lipid II) through electrostatic interaction between the positively charged nisin and the negatively charged membrane phospholipids. This results in the formation of the complex within the bacterial cell membrane, which creates 2 nm wide pores, thus preventing the growth of the peptidoglycan network and increased membrane permeability, leading to leakage of essential cellular components, and eventually to cell death (Figure 10) [71,139,149,158,159].

Nisin is active against a wide variety of Gram-positive *Lactococcus*, *Enterococcus*, *Streptococcus*, *Staphylococcus*, *Listeria* and *Micrococcus* bacterial strains, as well as the vegetative forms and outgrowing spores of *Bacillus* and *Clostridium* species [138,142,158]. The Gram-negative bacteria (e.g., *E. coli*) are usually resistant to nisin due to their outer lipopolysaccharide membranes, which act as a barrier/shield and impede its access to the cytoplasmic membrane [160,161]. Additionally, nisin shows no inhibitory activity against yeast cells, filamentous fungi and viruses [149]. However, many studies [6,7,142,156,158,160,162–164] demonstrate that bioengineered variants of nisin, high purity nisin, nisin-antibiotics, nisin-chelating agents (e.g., EDTA), nisin-inorganic nanoparticles (silver, gold, magnesium oxide, ...) or other outer membrane destabilizing component/processes (e.g., heat treatment, freezing) could also be effective against Gram-negative bacteria.

Required nisin concentration for efficient bacteria inhibition depends on several parameters, such as pH, heat treatment intensity, storage time and storage conditions. Aqueous solubility and structural stability of nisin are also pH dependent. The antimicrobial activity, solubility, and thermal stability of nisin are higher at acidic pH and deactivate under alkaline conditions due to irreversible structural changes of the nisin molecule. Nisin has higher antimicrobial activity in a liquid medium than a solid medium. Nisin is highly stable at low temperatures (e.g., during freezing), but undergoes a loss of activity during long-time heating. Proteolytic enzymes such as pancreatin, α-chymotrypsin and ficin can inactivate nisin due to their ability to break down the peptide chain of nisin. Other enzymes such as trypsin, pepsin and carboxypeptidase have no significant effect on its antimicrobial effect. The antimicrobial activity of nisin is also inhibited by the titanium dioxide and sodium metabisulphite due to the oxidation of disulfide bridges in the nisin molecule [149,165].

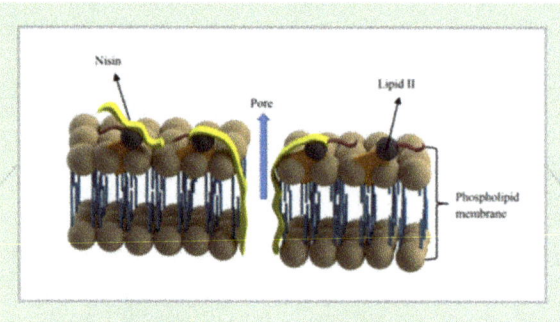

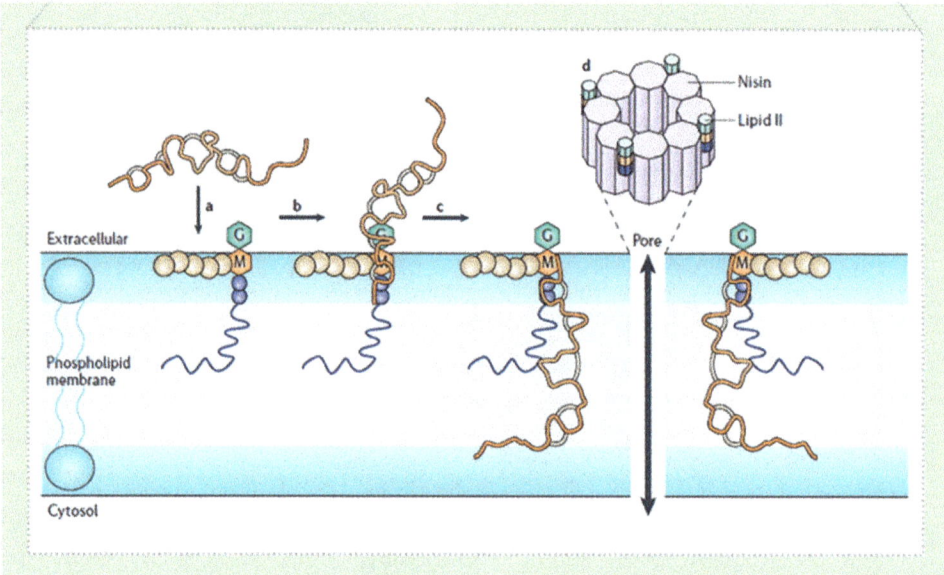

Figure 10. Schematic representation of the bactericidal mechanism of nisin: (**a**) nisin reaches the bacterial membrane; (**b**) adsorption of nisin to docking molecule (lipid II) via electrostatic interactions; (**c**) stable transmembrane orientation of nisin (cationic region of nisin interact with the negatively charged phospholipid heads, while the hydrophobic region of nisin interacts with the membrane core); (**d**) assembly of nisin-lipid II pore complex (consisting of 4 lipids II and 8 nisin molecules) (Reproduced with permission from [71,149], Elsevier, Amsterdam, The Netherlands, 2019 and Taylor & Francis, Abingdon, UK, 2016).

3.4. Immobilization Strategies

Various immobilization methods have been developed to protect nisin from environmental stresses, degradation by biological fluids or biocomponents (i.e., proteolytic enzymes) or deactivation under alkaline conditions [4,165], including covalent immobilization, encapsulation, entrapment, adsorption and co-culture fermentation, summarized in Table 4 and Figure 11. Most of the reported strategies for nisin immobilization required special pre-treatment of used support material/carrier, chemical modifications, crosslinking agents (carbodiimide/N-hydroxysuccinimide (EDC/NHS), hexamethylene diisocyanate, glutaraldehyde, ...) or a variety of other spacer molecules to obtain a composite with optimal, target-directed antimicrobial action against pathogenic bacteria [4,9,161]. In recent years, great emphasis has been placed on developing innovative nano-engineered approaches and nanostructured materials with enhanced antimicrobial activity in comparison to free nisin, including lipid-based nanoencapsulated nanoparticles (nanoliposomes, nanoemulsions, nanomicelles, solid lipid nanoparticles and nanostructured lipid carriers, Figure 12a), polymeric-based nanoencapsulated nanoparticles (nanocapsule and nanosphere, Figure 12b) and nanofibers [71,166]. Natural and synthetic materials studied as carrier or support material for immobilization of nisin includes liposomes [164,167], silica xerogels [168], polystyrene sheets [138], polyethylene oxide brush layer [169], soy lecithin liposomes [170], bacterial cellulose nanocrystals [151], chitosan nanoparticles [171], alginate beads [172] or a mixture of pectin-chitosan microcapsules [165], alginate-starch microcapsules [173], alginate-pectin microbeads [174] or chitosan-alginate microparticles [175],... having antimicrobial activity against various Gram-positive and Gram-negative bacteria (Table 4).

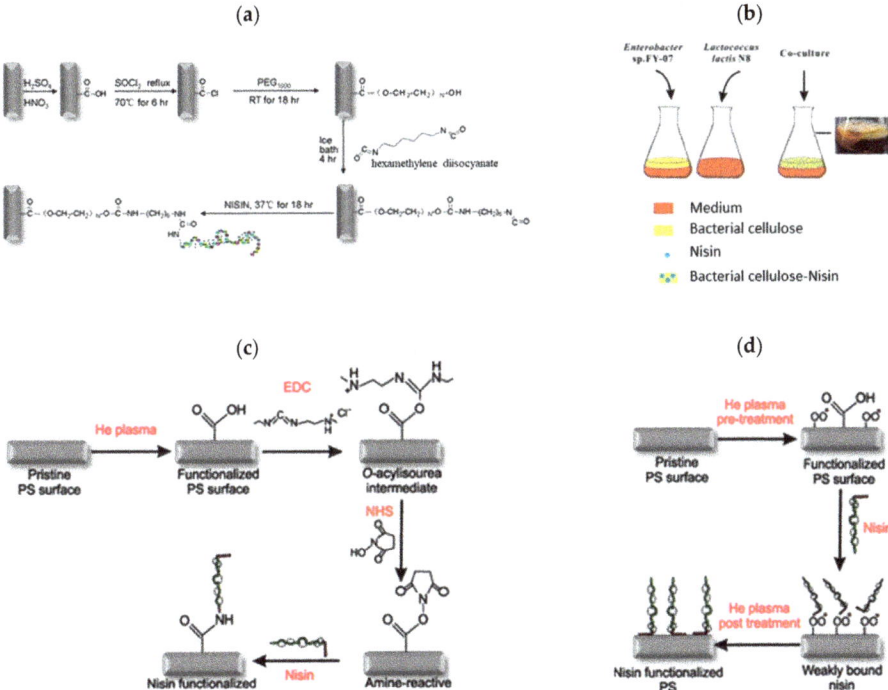

Figure 11. *Cont.*

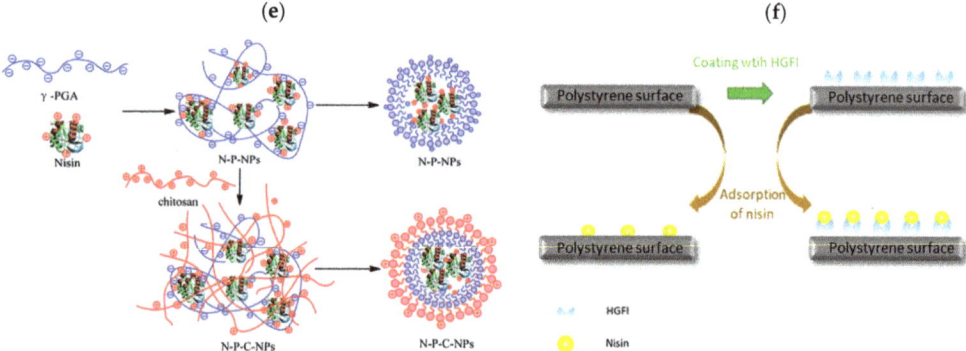

Figure 11. Schematic illustration of immobilization methods of nisin: (**a**) covalent immobilization onto multi-walled carbon nanotubes with PEG_{1000} as a linker and hexamethylene diisocyanate as a crosslinking agent (Adopted with permission from [176], RSC, 2011); (**b**) co-culture fermentation of nisin-producing (*Lactococcus lactis* N8) and bacterial cellulose-producing (*Enterobacter* sp. FY-07) bacteria (Adopted with permission from [153], Elsevier, Amsterdam, The Netherlands, 2021); (**c**) covalent immobilization onto plasma-treated, EDC/NHS ester functionalized polystyrene sheets (Adopted with permission from [138], RSC, 2017); (**d**) covalent immobilization onto plasma-treated polystyrene sheets (Adopted with permission from [138], RSC, 2017); (**e**) nisin loaded chitosan-poly-γ-glutamic acid nanoparticles (encapsulation) (Reproduced with permission from [179], RSC, Cambridge, UK, 2016); (**f**) adsorption of nisin on blank and HGFI-coated polystyrene surface together with antimicrobial activity of both surfaces (Adopted with permission from [9], Elsevier, Amsterdam, The Netherlands, 2021).

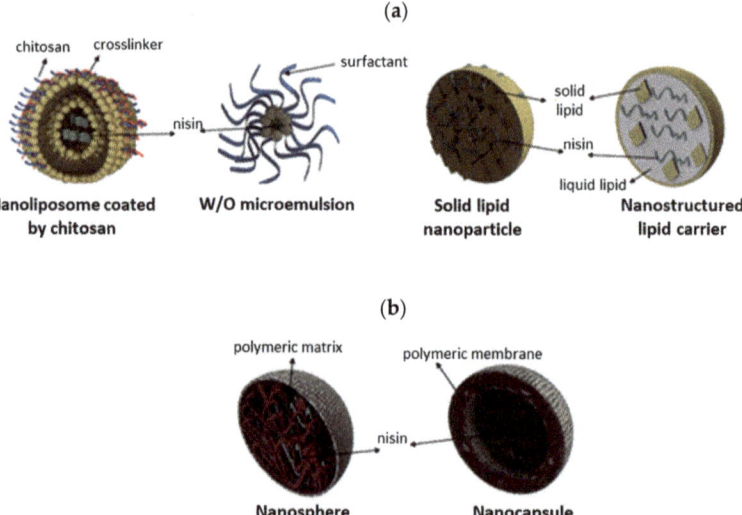

Figure 12. Scheme of (**a**) lipid-based nanoparticles and (**b**) biopolymeric nanoparticles for encapsulation of nisin (Adopted with permission from [71], Elsevier, Amsterdam, The Netherlands, 2019).

Table 4. Immobilization methods of nisin and antimicrobial activity against Gram-positive and Gram-negative bacteria.

Immobilization Method	Carrier/Support Material	Crosslinking Agent or Initiator	Antimicrobial Property against	References
Covalent immobilization	Multi-walled carbon nanotubes grafted with poly(ethylene glycol) (PEG$_{1000}$)	Hexamethylene diisocyanate	E. coli, P. aeruginosa, S. aureus, B. subtilis	[176]
	Polystyrene (PS) sheets	Atmospheric-pressure plasma	Gram-positive S. aureus and L. monocytogenes	[138]
	Poly(vinyl alcohol) films	Glutaric acid	Gram-positive S. aureus and Gram-negative E. coli	[177]
	Sodium alginate/gelatin wet-spun porous fibers	GA	S. aureus	[4]
	N-succinyl chitosan films	EDC	S. aureus, E. coli, S. enteritidis, Pseudomonas tolaasii (P. tolaasii)	[178]
Encapsulation	Silica xerogel	/	B. cereus, L. monocytogenes, S. aureus, E. coli, S. enterica	[168]
	Bacterial cellulose nanocrystals	/	L. rhamnosus LBM1	[151]
	Chitosan nanoparticles	/	E. coli and S. aureus	[171]
	Ca-alginate microparticles	/	Brochothrix thermosphacta (B. thermosphacta) 7R1	[172]
	Pectin-chitosan microcapsules	/	S. aureus, weak bactericidal effect on E. coli under acidic conditions	[165]
	Alginate-starch microcapsules	/	Pediococcus acidilactici (P. acidilactici) UL5	[173]
	Chitosan-alginate microparticles	/	N/A	[175]
	Chitosan-poly-γ-glutamic acid nanoparticles	/	E. coli and L. monocytogenes	[179]
	Phosphatidylcholine liposomes containing chitosan or chondroitin sulfate	/	L. monocytogenes	[180]
	Soybean lecithin or Phospholipon® liposomes	/	L. monocytogenes, Clostridium perfringens (C. perfringens) and Bacillus cereus (B. cereus)	[181]
Co-encapsulation	Phosphatidylcholine (PC) nanoliposomes coated with pectin or polygalacturonic acid	/	L. monocytogens, Salmonella Enteritidis (S. Enteritidis)	[167]
	Phosphatidylcholine (PC) nanoliposomes	/	L. monocytogenes, S. Enteritidis, E. coli and S. aureus	[164]

Table 4. *Cont.*

Immobilization Method	Carrier/Support Material	Crosslinking Agent or Initiator	Antimicrobial Property against	References
Adsorption	Low density polyethylene films treated with acrylic acid	/	*Listeria innocua* (*L. innocua*)	[182]
	Montmorillonite suspension	/	*E. faecium* C1	[183]
	Polyethylene oxide brush layers	/	N/A	[169]
	HGFI (class I hydrophobin)-coated polystyrene films	/	*S. aureus*	[9]
	ZnAl layered double hydroxides nanohybrids	/	N/A	[184]
Co-culture fermentation	None		*S. aureus*, *E. coli*	[153]
Entrapment	Polyethylene oxide brush layer	/	*Pediococcus pentosaceous* (*P. pentosaceous*)	[185]
	PET (polyethylene terephthalate) woven fabrics with thin alginate coating	/	*S. aureus*	[186]
	Poly-ethylene-co-vinyl acetate films	/	*Staphylococcus epidermidis* (*S. epidermidis*) ATCC 35984, *S. aureus* 815 and *L. monocytogenes* ATCC 7644	[187]
	Guar gum gel (biogel)	/	Canine oral enterococci collection (including *E. faecalis* and *E. faecium*)	[188]

However, different hydrophilic/hydrophobic surface properties of these carriers affect the orientation of the nisin (Figure 13). It is proposed that the hydrophobic region of the nisin binds to the hydrophobic surface, leading to the reduced number of hydrophobic regions available to interact with the bacterial cell membrane. Similarly, the hydrophilic region of nisin binds to the hydrophilic surface, allowing the hydrophobic region to interact with the bacterial cell membrane [138]. Furthermore, nisin reacts with EDC/NHS functionalized surface through its amine group at the N-terminus, which could cause inefficient adsorption to the carrier due to steric barriers of the hydrophobic region [138].

3.5. Applications

Nisin's properties, such as inhibitory efficiency against a wide range of microorganisms, low probability of developing microbial resistance, no effect on the normal microbiota of the intestine, non-toxicity, colourless and tasteless, enable its use in both the biomedicine and food industry [137,189], especially in the second segment, where use as food bio preservative is already much exhausted [190]. Nisin is used to preserve pasteurized milk, aged cheeses, canned soups, juice, meat and vegetables [71,149]. It shows a better choice for prolonging the shelf life of meat (Tan sheep meat) in comparison to preservative potassium sorbate due to reduced nutrient loss [191]. Furthermore, it can be combined with other pasteurization preservation treatments to increase inhibition effectiveness against heat-resistant spore-former and extend the food shelf life [149]. As a food additive, it is assigned as E234 [149] and has been approved for use in over 60 countries around the world as a natural agent to prevent food spoilage due to its low toxicity or non-toxicity, high efficiency [153], thermal stability, and colourless and tasteless properties [157]. Saini et al. [150] studied covalent immobilization of nisin on the surface of TEMPO-oxidized CNF and thus developed antimicrobial films, which could be used as active food packaging. Nisin was also studied to develop impedimetric label-free biosensors for bacterial contamination detection of *Salmonella* spp. [192].

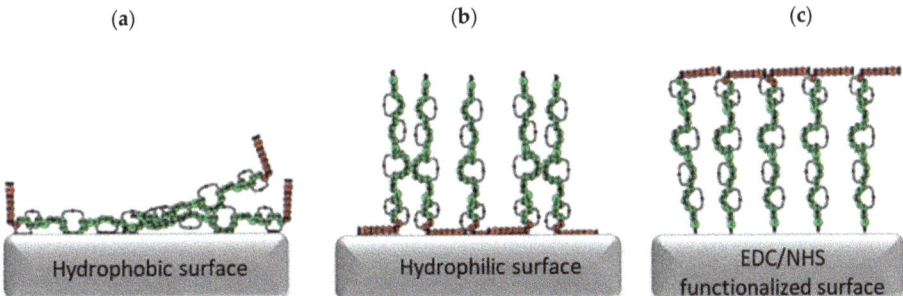

Figure 13. Proposed orientation of nisin on (**a**) hydrophobic surface, (**b**) hydrophilic surface and (**c**) with EDC/NHS functionalized surface (Adopted with permission from [138], RSC, 2017).

In light of biomedical potential, the nisin already demonstrates promising results as an alternative to traditional antimicrobial therapeutics due to its activity against specific (antibiotic-resistant bacterial) pathogens and disease conditions, particularly concerning mastitis in lactating women and dairy cows (inhibition of *S. aureus* and *S. epidermidis* [193–198]), respiratory infections (inhibition of *S. aureus* [199]) and skin infections, e.g., atopic dermatitis [200] and MRSA skin infections (inhibition of *S. aureus*) [147,201–204]. It can be used either as a single agent or in combination with other agents [7,157,189,201,205]. Furthermore, it showed potential in oral diseases, such as caries and periodontal diseases, due to inhibition of oral bacteria, including *Streptococcus sanguinis* (*S. sanguinis*), *Streptococcus sobrinus* (*S. sobrinus*), *Streptococcus gordonii* (*S. gordonii*), *P. gingivalis*, *Prevotella intermedia* (*P. intermedia*), *A. actinomycetemcomitans* and *Treponema denticola* (*T. denticola*) [140,206,207]. Shin and co-workers [140] studied nisin's antimicrobial efficiency against the formation of saliva-derived multi-species oral biofilms. They reported on reduced biofilm biomass in a dose-dependent manner (Figure 14); no apoptotic changes of human oral cells were observed at nisin concentration <200 µg/mL [140]. Nisin also has the potential to control periodontal disease in dogs [208].

Additionally, nisin has been studied as a possible anticancer agent due to the multidrug resistance of cancer cells and drastic side effects of traditional chemotherapeutics [209,210]. Hosseini and co-workers reported a significant decrease in the growth rate of SW480 colorectal cancer cell line after being treated with nisin [211]. Similar conclusions are reported by Tavakoli et al. [212]. Nisin also showed a significant efficiency as an adjuvant to conventional chemotherapeutic agents. Preet et al. studied synergism between doxorubicin, a chemotherapeutic drug traditionally used to treat breast cancer, lymphoma, bladder cancer, acute lymphocytic leukemia [8], and nisin against skin carcinogenesis [209]. They reported on augmented anticancer activities when both these agents were used in conjunction with each other [209]. Rana and colleagues studied the possible use of a 5-fluorouracil-nisin combination as a topically applied chemotherapeutic drug against skin cancer [210]. They observed faster clearance of tumors and a reduced dose of 5-fluorouracil when a 5-fluorouracil-nisin combination was used [210]. Joo et al. reported on increased cell apoptosis and decreased cell proliferation at head and neck squamous cell carcinoma by nisin treatment [159]. Furthermore, nisin A has been demonstrated to have a potential for treating nonhealing wounds, as it increases the mobility of skin cells, dampens the effect of lipopolysaccharide and proinflammatory cytokines, and decreases bacterial load in the wound [157].

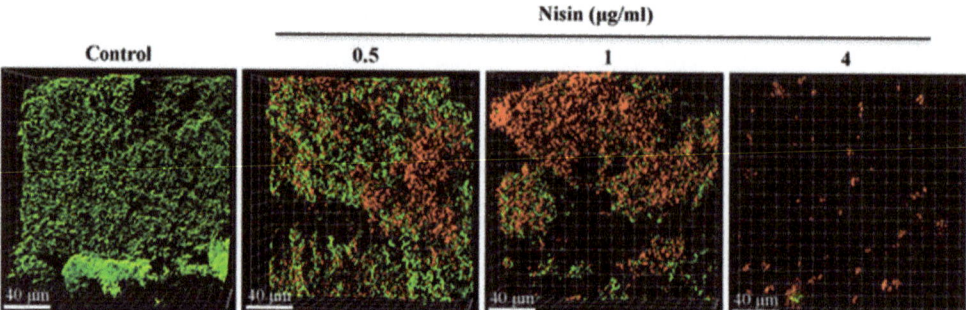

Figure 14. Confocal microscopy images of the influence of nisin concentration on oral biofilm formation under the controlled microfluidic model system. A green signal indicates viable live cells (Syto 9) and a red signal indicates damaged/dead cells (propidium iodide). No biofilm was observed at a nisin concentration of 4 µg/mL (Reproduced with permission from [140], Meta UCL, 2015).

4. Combination of Bioactive Compounds

Simultaneous use of (bio)active agents is common practice to collect multiple activities and even augment their efficiency to a higher level than their simple sum. The use of enzymatic mixtures, comprising enzymes with wide diversity in the reactions they are catalyzing, is one frequent case of simultaneous use of multiple bioactive compounds. Moreover, the "crude enzymatic cocktails" (as crude bromelain itself) are more frequently present in nature than a single, specific type. Aside from simple mixtures, more than one enzyme's co-immobilization was found very efficient in terms of product yield and thermal stability increment, as present in the triple enzyme system [213]. Another example is antibiotics, where the combined therapy utilizing more than one antibiotic at the time is practiced in particular cases in order to broaden the antibacterial spectrum, to treat the polymicrobial infections, to obtain synergistic effect bringing higher efficiency at lower doses and finally, to tackle the emergence of bacterial resistance [214].

The bacteriocin nisin offers a range of advantageous features that include protease and heat stability; its efficacy can be further boosted via combination with other antimicrobials or membrane-active substances. Nisin demonstrates synergistic activity with the antibiotics colistin and clarithromycin against *P. aeruginosa* [215] with ramoplanin and other-β-lactam antibiotics against many strains of MRSA and VRE [216] with penicillin, streptomycin, chloramphenicol and rifampicin against *Pseudomonas fluorescens* [217]. Combinations of derivatives nisin V + penicillin or nisin I4V + chloramphenicol had an enhanced inhibitory effect against *S. aureus* SA113 and *S. pseudintermedius* DSM21284, respectively, compared to the equivalent nisin A + antibiotic combinations or when each antimicrobial was administered alone [218].

Reported studies demonstrate that such mixtures boost the antimicrobial action, but the same does not introduce new bioactive functions. One-pot (co-immobilisation, simultaneous immobilisation), or successive immobilization of bioactive compounds, together with diverse immobilisation strategies, all together present modalities to be used in obtaining a multi-active system including different types of bioactive compounds. Such an example is a two-step polydopamine-based surface modification strategy, used to co-immobilize an antimicrobial peptide Palm and an enzyme targeting an important component of biofilm matrix (DNase I). This immobilization approach imparted polydimethylsiloxane surfaces with both anti-adhesive and antimicrobial properties against the adhesion of relevant bacteria as single and dual-species, with excellent stability and biocompatible and anti-biofilm properties, holding, therefore, great potential in the development of catheters able to prevent the catheter-associated infections [219].

To date, the co-immobilization of bromelain and nisin as proteolytic enzymes and protease-resistant antimicrobial peptide, respectively, has not been trialled. Aside from obstacles anticipated to such an experimental design, the potential success may offer a merge of an extensive portfolio of bioactive functions brought by both components. Both components are complementary in many terms, including the type of bacteria they are acting against, i.e., Gram-positive for nisin and Gram-negative for bromelain.

5. Conclusions and Prospects

Bromelain and nisin are undoubtedly among more perspective, natural bioactive components with outstanding potential in biomedicine due to diverse therapeutic benefits, demonstrated by several research groups in the recent decade. In vitro studies of bromelain and nisin show their potential in human medicine and healthcare, in the treatment of skin infections, caries, periodontal diseases, and many other conditions. Importantly, the bromelain shows promise within several in vitro studies involving cancer cell lines, yet, the clinical trials in this segment are in a premature stage, with only two examples at the moment (one for treatment of solid tumors in advanced stage of lung, breast, colon, ovary, cervix, uterus, prostatic, and liver and second for treatment of Pseudomyxoma Peritonei, Peritoneal Cancer, Mucinous Adenocarcinoma and Mucinous Tumor) [220]. The plant extract bromelain interacts with several biological processes that lead to its multi-action bioactivity, including antimicrobial, anti-inflammatory, anticarcinogenic and antithrombotic activity. Unlike bromelain, which has already gained FDA approval in topical product NexoBrid, the nisin is only approved as a food additive despite its effectiveness against drug-resistant organisms also in biomedical research. Nonetheless, much effort has been devoted to widening the nisin efficiency from Gram-positive bacteria towards Gram-negative bacteria, where biotechnological approaches or combination with other components (antibiotics, inorganic nanoparticles, chelating agents, . . .) have been applied, which paves its way towards use in more demanding clinical set-ups. Further, the production of different variants (from native and gene-modified bacterial species) with a high degree of purity, securing the safeness of final products are evidencing recognized the potential of this bioactive compound.

To the best of our knowledge, the synergistic action of both bioactive components is yet to be explored as an attractive topic. Before going ahead with a cost-demanding clinical translation of bromelain- or nisin-containing materials developed in a lab, much remains to be learned, particularly about different variants and combinations with conventional antibiotics and cancer drugs, their complex mechanism of action on the human body and pathogens, consequences of long-term clinical trials and choosing suitable optimized immobilization method with high immobilization yield and secured activity/efficiency. As said, most data for bromelain and nisin demonstrated an in vitro efficiency, and the extrapolation of in vitro to in vivo outcome is not that straightforward, yet, same present a solid background, important in future translation in a clinic. With all this, it will be possible to offer novel, safe and efficient natural therapeutic solutions to our society without significant risks to developing resistance in pathogenic organisms and cells.

Author Contributions: Conceptualization, S.G. and U.J.; methodology, S.G.; writing—original draft preparation, S.G. and U.J.; writing—review and editing, S.G. and U.J.; funding acquisition, S.G. All authors have read and agreed to the published version of the manuscript.

Funding: This research was funded by Slovenian Research Agency, young researcher program (P2-0118/0795), the Textile Chemistry Programme (P2-0118) and project J2-2487. The APC was funded by Slovenian Research Agency, project J2-2487.

Institutional Review Board Statement: Not applicable.

Informed Consent Statement: Not applicable.

Conflicts of Interest: The authors declare no conflict of interest.

Abbreviations

AMP	antimicrobial peptide
APTES	(3-aminopropyl)-triethoxysilane
Asp	asparagine
BBT	bromelain-based treatment
CDTA	cyclohexane-1,2-diaminoetetraacetic acid
COX-2	prostaglandin-endoperoxide synthase 2
CP	cysteine proteinase
DETA	diethylenetriamine
Dha	dehydroalanine
Dhb	dehydrobutyrine
ECM	extracellular matrix
EDC	1-ethyl-(3-dimethylaminopropyl) carbodiimide
EDTA	ethylenediaminetetraacetic acid
EMA	European Medicines Agency
GA	glutaraldehyde
HEDTA	hydroxyethyl ethylenediamine triacetic acid
IL	interleukin
Lan	lanthionine
LD_{50}	lethal dose
Leu	leucine
K_m	Michaelis–Menten constant
MBC	minimum bactericidal concentration
MeLan	β-methyl lanthionine
MIC	minimum inhibitory concentration
MRSA	methicillin-resistant *Staphylococcus aureus*
MSN	mesoporous silica nanoparticles
NCBI	National Center for Biotechnology Information
NF-κB	Nuclear factor kappa B
NHS	N-hydroxysuccinimide
PC	phosphatidylcholine
PEG	poly(ethylene glycol)
PEHA	pentaethylenehexamine
PET	polyethylene terephthalate
PGE-2	prostaglandin E_2
PGI-2	prostaglandin I_2
pI	isoelectric point
PS	polystyrene
SEM	scanning electron microscopy
SPRA	self-assembly PEGylation retaining activity
TEPA	tetraethylenepentamine
TETA	triethylenetetramine
TNF	tumour necrosis factor
TXA-2	thromboxane A2
V_{max}	maximum reaction velocity
Val	valine

References

1. Mamo, J.; Assefa, F. Antibacterial and Anticancer Property of Bromelain: A Plant Protease Enzyme from Pineapples (*Ananas comosus*). *Curr. Trends Biomed. Eng. Biosci.* **2019**, *19*, 60–68. [CrossRef]
2. Sulthana, R.; Archer, A. Bacteriocin nanoconjugates: Boon to medical and food industry. *J. Appl. Microbiol.* **2021**, *131*, 1056–1071. [CrossRef] [PubMed]
3. Khosa, S.; Frieg, B.; Mulnaes, D.; Kleinschrodt, D.; Hoeppner, A.; Gohlke, H.; Smits, S.H.J. Structural basis of lantibiotic recognition by the nisin resistance protein from Streptococcus agalactiae. *Sci. Rep.* **2016**, *6*, 18679. [CrossRef]

4. Homem, N.C.; Tavares, T.D.; Miranda, C.S.; Antunes, J.C.; Amorim, M.T.P.; Felgueiras, H.P. Functionalization of Crosslinked Sodium Alginate/Gelatin Wet-Spun Porous Fibers with Nisin Z for the Inhibition of *Staphylococcus aureus*-Induced Infections. *Int. J. Mol. Sci.* **2021**, *22*, 1930. [CrossRef] [PubMed]
5. Majidinia, M.; Mirza-Aghazadeh-Attari, M.; Rahimi, M.; Mihanfar, A.; Karimian, A.; Safa, A.; Yousefi, B. Overcoming multidrug resistance in cancer: Recent progress in nanotechnology and new horizons. *IUBMB Life* **2020**, *72*, 855–871. [CrossRef]
6. Pandey, P.; Hansmann, U.H.E.; Wang, F. Altering the Solubility of the Antibiotic Candidate Nisin—A Computational Study. *ACS Omega* **2020**, *5*, 24854–24863. [CrossRef]
7. Shin, J.M.; Gwak, J.W.; Kamarajan, P.; Fenno, J.C.; Rickard, A.H.; Kapila, Y.L. Biomedical Applications of Nisin. *J. Appl. Microbiol.* **2016**, *120*, 1449–1465. [CrossRef] [PubMed]
8. Lewies, A.; Du Plessis, L.H.; Wentzel, J.F. The Cytotoxic, Antimicrobial and Anticancer Properties of the Antimicrobial Peptide Nisin Z Alone and in Combination with Conventional Treatments. In *Cytotoxicity*; IntechOpen: London, UK, 2018.
9. Wang, X.; Liu, F.; Zhang, Y.; Zhu, D.; Saris, P.E.; Xu, H.; Qiao, M. Effective adsorption of nisin on the surface of polystyrene using hydrophobin HGFI. *Int. J. Biol. Macromol.* **2021**, *173*, 399–408. [CrossRef]
10. Murthy, S.S.; Narsaiah, T.B. Cytotoxic Effect of Bromelain on HepG2 Hepatocellular Carcinoma Cell Line. *Appl. Biochem. Biotechnol.* **2021**, *193*, 1873–1897. [CrossRef]
11. Chobotova, K.; Vernallis, A.B.; Majid, F.A.A. Bromelain's activity and potential as an anti-cancer agent: Current evidence and perspectives. *Cancer Lett.* **2010**, *290*, 148–156. [CrossRef] [PubMed]
12. Tochi, B.N.; Wang, Z.; Xu, S.-Y.; Zhang, W. Therapeutic Application of Pineapple Protease (*Bromelain*): A Review. *Pak. J. Nutr.* **2008**, *7*, 513–520. [CrossRef]
13. Ramli, A.N.M.; Manas, N.H.A.; Hamid, A.A.A.; Hamid, H.A.; Illias, R.M. Comparative structural analysis of fruit and stem bromelain from Ananas comosus. *Food Chem.* **2018**, *266*, 183–191. [CrossRef] [PubMed]
14. George, S.; Bhasker, S.; Madhav, H.; Nair, A.; Chinnamma, M. Functional Characterization of Recombinant Bromelain of Ananas comosus Expressed in a Prokaryotic System. *Mol. Biotechnol.* **2013**, *56*, 166–174. [CrossRef] [PubMed]
15. De Lencastre Novaes, L.C.; Jozala, A.F.; Lopes, A.M.; de Carvalho Santos-Ebinuma, V.; Mazzola, P.G.; Pessoa Junior, A. Stability, purification, and applications of bromelain: A review. *Biotechnol. Prog.* **2016**, *32*, 5–13. [CrossRef]
16. Hidayat, Y.; Hermawati, E.; Setiasih, S.; Hudiyono, S.; Saepudin, E. Antibacterial activity test of the partially purified bromelain from pineapple core extract (*Ananas comosus* [L.] Merr) by fractionation using ammonium sulfate acetone. In *AIP Conference Proceedings*; AIP Publishing: Melville, NY, USA, 2018; Volume 2023, p. 020067.
17. Chakraborty, A.J.; Mitra, S.; Tallei, T.E.; Tareq, A.M.; Nainu, F.; Cicia, D.; Dhama, K.; Emran, T.B.; Simal-Gandara, J.; Capasso, R. Bromelain a Potential Bioactive Compound: A Comprehensive Overview from a Pharmacological Perspective. *Life* **2021**, *11*, 317. [CrossRef]
18. Dutta, S.; Bhattacharyya, D. Enzymatic, antimicrobial and toxicity studies of the aqueous extract of Ananas comosus (*pineapple*) crown leaf. *J. Ethnopharmacol.* **2013**, *150*, 451–457. [CrossRef]
19. Abbas, S.; Shanbhag, T.; Kothare, A. Applications of bromelain from pineapple waste towards acne. *Saudi. J. Biol. Sci.* **2021**, *28*, 1001–1009. [CrossRef]
20. Azarkan, M.; Maquoi, E.; Delbrassine, F.; Herman, R.; M'Rabet, N.; Esposito, R.C.; Charlier, P.; Kerff, F. Structures of the free and inhibitors-bound forms of bromelain and ananain from Ananas comosus stem and in vitro study of their cytotoxicity. *Sci. Rep.* **2020**, *10*, 19570. [CrossRef]
21. Harrach, T.; Eckert, K.; Maurer, H.R.; Machleidt, I.; Machleidt, W.; Nuck, R. Isolation and characterization of two forms of an acidic bromelain stem proteinase. *Protein J.* **1998**, *17*, 351–361. [CrossRef] [PubMed]
22. Bala, M.; Ismail, N.A.; Mel, M.; Jami, M.S.; Mohd Salleh, H.; Amid, A. Bromelain Production: Current Trends and Perspective. *Arch. Des Sci.* **2012**, *65*, 369–399.
23. Arshad, Z.I.M.; Amid, A.; Yusof, F.; Jaswir, I.; Ahmad, K.; Loke, S.P. Bromelain: An overview of industrial application and purification strategies. *Appl. Microbiol. Biotechnol.* **2014**, *98*, 7283–7297. [CrossRef]
24. Ataide, J.A.; Gérios, E.F.; Mazzola, P.G.; Souto, E.B. Bromelain-loaded nanoparticles: A comprehensive review of the state of the art. *Adv. Colloid Interface Sci.* **2018**, *254*, 48–55. [CrossRef] [PubMed]
25. Maurer, H.R. Bromelain: Biochemistry, pharmacology and medical use. *Cell. Mol. Life Sci.* **2001**, *58*, 1234–1245. [CrossRef]
26. Khairunnisa, F.A.; Vedder, M.; Evers, L.; Permana, S. Bromelain content of extract from stem of pineapple (*Ananas comosus* (L.) Merr). In *AIP Conference Proceedings*; AIP Publishing: Melville, NY, USA, 2018; Volume 2019.
27. Benefo, E.O.; Ofosu, I.W. Bromelain Activity of Waste Parts of Two Pineapple Varieties. *Sustain. Food Prod.* **2018**, *2*, 21–28. [CrossRef]
28. Manzoor, Z.; Nawaz, A.; Mukhtar, H.; Haq, I. Bromelain: Methods of Extraction, Purification and Therapeutic Applications. *Braz. Arch. Biol. Technol.* **2016**, *59*, 1–16. [CrossRef]
29. Ataide, J.A.; Geraldes, D.C.; Gérios, E.F.; Bissaco, F.M.; Cefali, L.C.; Oliveira-Nascimento, L.; Mazzola, P.G. Freeze-dried chitosan nanoparticles to stabilize and deliver bromelain. *J. Drug Deliv. Sci. Technol.* **2021**, *61*, 102225. [CrossRef]
30. Chermahini, S.H. Pharmaceutical Sciences and Technology Bromelain as an Anti-Inflammatory and Anti-Cancer Compound. *Int. J. Res. Pharm. Sci. Technol.* **2019**, *1*, 53–57. [CrossRef]
31. Benucci, I.; Liburdi, K.; Garzillo, A.M.V.; Esti, M. Bromelain from pineapple stem in alcoholic–acidic buffers for wine application. *Food Chem.* **2011**, *124*, 1349–1353. [CrossRef]

32. Amid, A.; Ismail, N.A.; Yusof, F.; Mohd-Salleh, H. Expression, purification, and characterization of a recombinant stem bromelain from Ananas comosus. *Process. Biochem.* **2011**, *46*, 2232–2239. [CrossRef]
33. Rowan, A.D.; Buttle, D.J. Pineapple cysteine endopeptidases. *Methods Enzymol.* **1994**, *244*, 555–568. [CrossRef] [PubMed]
34. Hale, L.P.; Greer, P.K.; Trinh, C.T.; James, C.L. Proteinase activity and stability of natural bromelain preparations. *Int. Immunopharmacol.* **2005**, *5*, 783–793. [CrossRef]
35. Pillai, K.; Akhter, J.; Chua, T.C.; Morris, D.L. Anticancer Property of Bromelain with Therapeutic Potential in Malignant Peritoneal Mesothelioma. *Cancer Investig.* **2013**, *31*, 241–250. [CrossRef] [PubMed]
36. Ruchita, D.; Soumya, R.; Murthy, N.Y.S. Optimization of Activity of Bromelain. *Asian J. Chem.* **2012**, *24*, 1429–1431.
37. Gautam, S.S.; Mishra, S.K.; Dash, V.; Goyal, A.K.; Rath, G. Comparative Study of Extraction, Purification and Estimation of Bromelain from Stem and Fruit of Pineapple Plant. *Thai J. Pharm. Sci.* **2010**, *34*, 67–76.
38. Soares, P.A.; Vaz, A.F.; Correia, M.T.; Pessoa, A.; Carneiro-Da-Cunha, M.G. Purification of bromelain from pineapple wastes by ethanol precipitation. *Sep. Purif. Technol.* **2012**, *98*, 389–395. [CrossRef]
39. Arefin, P.; Habib, S.; Arefin, A.; Arefin, S. A review of clinical uses of Bromelain and concerned purification methods to obtain its pharmacological effects efficiently. *Int. J. Pharm. Res.* **2020**, *12*, 469–478. [CrossRef]
40. Nor, M.Z.M.; Ramchandran, L.; Duke, M.; Vasiljevic, T. Application of Membrane-Based Technology for Purification of Bromelain. *Int. Food Res. J.* **2017**, *24*, 1685–1696.
41. Vasiljevic, T. *Pineapple*; Elsevier BV: Amsterdam, The Netherlands, 2020; pp. 203–225.
42. Yin, L.; Sun, C.; Han, X.; Xu, L.; Xu, Y.; Qi, Y.; Peng, J. Preparative purification of bromelain (EC 3.4.22.33) from pineapple fruit by high-speed counter-current chromatography using a reverse-micelle solvent system. *Food Chem.* **2011**, *129*, 925–932. [CrossRef]
43. Fouz, N.; Amid, A.; Hashim, Y.Z.H.-Y. Cytokinetic Study of MCF-7 Cells Treated with Commercial and Recombinant Bromelain. *Asian Pac. J. Cancer Prev.* **2013**, *14*, 6709–6714. [CrossRef]
44. Arshad, Z.I.M.; Amid, A.; Othman, M.E.F. Comparison of Different Cell Disruption Methods And Cell Extractant Buffers For Recombinant Bromelain Expressed In E.Coli Bl21-A1. *J. Teknol.* **2015**, *77*, 83–87. [CrossRef]
45. Razali, R.; Budiman, C.; Kamaruzaman, K.A.; Subbiah, V.K. Soluble Expression and Catalytic Properties of Codon-Optimized Recombinant Bromelain from MD2 Pineapple in Escherichia coli. *Protein J.* **2021**, *40*, 406–418. [CrossRef]
46. Wang, W.; Zhang, L.; Guo, N.; Zhang, X.; Zhang, C.; Sun, G.; Xie, J. Functional Properties of a Cysteine Proteinase from Pineapple Fruit with Improved Resistance to Fungal Pathogens in Arabidopsis thaliana. *Molecules* **2014**, *19*, 2374–2389. [CrossRef] [PubMed]
47. Roeva, O.; Pencheva, T.; Tzonkov, S.; Arndt, M.; Hitzmann, B.; Kleist, S.; Miksch, G.; Friehs, K.; Flaschel, E. Multiple model approach to modelling of Escherichia coli fed-batch cultivation extracellular production of bacterial phytase. *Electron. J. Biotechnol.* **2007**, *10*, 592–603. [CrossRef]
48. Mameli, A.; Natoli, V.; Casu, C. Bromelain: An Overview of Applications in Medicine and Dentistry. *Biointerface Res. Appl. Chem.* **2020**, *11*, 8165–8170. [CrossRef]
49. Ali, A.A.; Milala, M.A.; Gulani, I.A. Antimicrobial Effects of Crude Bromelain Extracted from Pineapple Fruit (*Ananas comosus* (Linn.) Merr.). *Adv. Biochem.* **2015**, *3*, 1. [CrossRef]
50. Praveen, N.C.; Rajesh, A.; Madan, M.; Chaurasia, V.R.; Hiremath, N.V.; Sharma, A.M. In vitro Evaluation of Antibacterial Efficacy of Pineapple Extract (*Bromelain*) on Periodontal Pathogens. *J. Int. Oral Heal.* **2014**, *6*, 96–98.
51. Onken, J.E.; Greer, P.K.; Calingaert, B.; Hale, L.P. Bromelain treatment decreases secretion of pro-inflammatory cytokines and chemokines by colon biopsies in vitro. *Clin. Immunol.* **2008**, *126*, 345–352. [CrossRef]
52. Parodi, A.; Haddix, S.; Taghipour, N.; Scaria, S.; Taraballi, F.; Cevenini, A.; Yazdi, I.; Corbo, C.; Palomba, R.; Khaled, S.Z.; et al. Bromelain Surface Modification Increases the Diffusion of Silica Nanoparticles in the Tumor Extracellular Matrix. *ACS Nano* **2014**, *8*, 9874–9883. [CrossRef]
53. Bhatnagar, P.; Patnaik, S.; Srivastava, A.K.; Mudiam, M.K.R.; Shukla, Y.; Panda, A.K.; Pant, A.B.; Kumar, P.; Gupta, K.C. Anti-cancer activity of bromelain nanoparticles by oral administration. *J. Biomed. Nanotechnol.* **2014**, *10*, 3558–3575. [CrossRef]
54. Lee, J.-H.; Lee, J.-T.; Park, H.R.; Kim, J.-B. The potential use of bromelain as a natural oral medicine having anticarcinogenic activities. *Food Sci. Nutr.* **2019**, *7*, 1656–1667. [CrossRef] [PubMed]
55. Tadikonda, A.; Pentapati, K.-C.; Urala, A.; Acharya, S. Anti-plaque and anti-gingivitis effect of Papain, Bromelain, Miswak and Neem containing dentifrice: A randomized controlled trial. *J. Clin. Exp. Dent.* **2017**, *9*, e649–e653. [CrossRef] [PubMed]
56. Amini, N.; Setiasih, S.; Handayani, S.; Hudiyono, S.; Saepudin, E. Potential antibacterial activity of partial purified bromelain from pineapple core extracts using acetone and ammonium sulphate against dental caries-causing bacteria. *AIP Conf. Proc.* **2018**, *2023*, 020071. [CrossRef]
57. Santi, G.D.; Borgognone, A. The use of Epiprotect®, an advanced wound dressing, to heal paediatric patients with burns: A pilot study. *Burn. Open* **2019**, *3*, 103–107. [CrossRef]
58. Aichele, K.; Bubel, M.; Deubel, G.; Pohlemann, T.; Oberringer, M. Bromelain down-regulates myofibroblast differentiation in an in vitro wound healing assay. *Naunyn-Schmiedebergs Arch. fur Exp. Pathol. und Pharmakol.* **2013**, *386*, 853–863. [CrossRef] [PubMed]
59. Hirche, C.; Citterio, A.; Hoeksema, H.; Koller, J.; Lehner, M.; Martinez, J.R.; Monstrey, S.; Murray, A.; Plock, J.A.; Sander, F.; et al. Eschar removal by bromelain based enzymatic debridement (Nexobrid®) in burns: An European consensus. *Burns* **2017**, *43*, 1640–1653. [CrossRef] [PubMed]
60. Krieger, Y.; Rubin, G.; Schulz, A.; Rosenberg, N.; Levi, A.; Singer, A.; Rosenberg, L.; Shoham, Y. Bromelain-based enzymatic debridement and minimal invasive modality (mim) care of deeply burned hands. *Ann. Burn. Fire Disasters* **2017**, *30*, 198–204.

61. Brien, S.; Lewith, G.; Walker, A.; Hicks, S.M.; Middleton, D. Bromelain as a Treatment for Osteoarthritis: A Review of Clinical Studies. *Evid. Based Complement Altern. Med.* **2004**, *1*, 251–257. [CrossRef] [PubMed]
62. Tallei, T.E.; Fatimawali, A.Y.; Idroes, R.; Kusumawaty, D.; Bin Emran, T.; Yesiloglu, T.Z.; Sippl, W.; Mahmud, S.; Alqahtani, T.; Alqahtani, A.M.; et al. An Analysis Based on Molecular Docking and Molecular Dynamics Simulation Study of Bromelain as Anti-SARS-CoV-2 Variants. *Front. Pharmacol.* **2021**, *12*, 717757. [CrossRef]
63. Ajibade, V.A.; Akinruli, F.T.; Ilesanmi, T.M. Antibacterial Screening of Crude Extract of Oven-Dried Pawpaw and Pineapple. *Int. J. Sci. Res. Publ.* **2015**, *5*, 408–411.
64. López-García, B.; Hernández, M.; Segundo, B.S. Bromelain, a Cysteine Protease from Pineapple (Ananas Comosus) Stem, Is an Inhibitor of Fungal Plant Pathogens. *Lett. Appl. Microbiol.* **2012**, *55*, 62–67. [CrossRef] [PubMed]
65. Colletti, A.; Li, S.; Marengo, M.; Adinolfi, S.; Cravotto, G. Recent Advances and Insights into Bromelain Processing, Pharmacokinetics and Therapeutic Uses. *Appl. Sci.* **2021**, *11*, 8428. [CrossRef]
66. Montazeri, A.; Ramezani, M.; Mohammadgholi, A. Investigation the Effect of Encapsulated Bromelain Enzyme in Magnetic Carbon Nanotubes on Colorectal Cancer Cells. *Jundishapur J. Nat. Pharm. Prod.* **2021**, *16*, e108796. [CrossRef]
67. Gajšek, M.; Jančič, U.; Vasić, K.; Knez, Ž.; Leitgeb, M. Enhanced activity of immobilized transglutaminase for cleaner production technologies. *J. Clean. Prod.* **2019**, *240*, 118218. [CrossRef]
68. Wijayanti, L.; Setiasih, S.; Hudiyono, S. Encapsulation of bromelain in alginate-carboxymethyl cellulose microspheres as an antiplatelet agent. *J. Physics: Conf. Ser.* **2021**, *1943*, 012165. [CrossRef]
69. Bernal, C.; Rodríguez, K.; Martínez, R. Integrating enzyme immobilization and protein engineering: An alternative path for the development of novel and improved industrial biocatalysts. *Biotechnol. Adv.* **2018**, *36*, 1470–1480. [CrossRef] [PubMed]
70. Holyavka, M.; Faizullin, D.; Koroleva, V.; Olshannikova, S.; Zakhartchenko, N.; Zuev, Y.; Kondratyev, M.; Zakharova, E.; Artyukhov, V. Novel biotechnological formulations of cysteine proteases, immobilized on chitosan. Structure, stability and activity. *Int. J. Biol. MacroMolecules* **2021**, *180*, 161–176. [CrossRef] [PubMed]
71. Bahrami, A.; Delshadi, R.; Jafari, S.M.; Williams, L. Nanoencapsulated nisin: An engineered natural antimicrobial system for the food industry. *Trends Food Sci. Technol.* **2019**, *94*, 20–31. [CrossRef]
72. Baker, P.J.; Patwardhan, S.V.; Numata, K. Synthesis of Homopolypeptides by Aminolysis Mediated by Proteases Encapsulated in Silica Nanospheres. *Macro. Mol. Biosci.* **2014**, *14*, 1619–1626. [CrossRef]
73. Putranto, M.A.; Budianto, E.; Hudoyon, S. Encapsulation and dissolution study of bromelain in chitosan-methyl cellulose semi-IPN hydrogel. In *AIP Conference Proceedings*; AIP Publishing: Melville, NY, USA, 2018; Volume 2049, p. 020033.
74. Herfena, N.; Setiasih, S.; Handayani, S.; Hudiyono, S. Evaluation of in-vitro dissolution profiles of partially purified bromelain from pineapple cores (*Ananas comosus* [L.] *Merr*) loaded in glutaraldehyde-crosslinked chitosan microspheres. In Proceedings of the 8th International Conference of The Indonesian Chemical Society (Icics), Bogor, Indonesia, 6–7 August 2019.
75. Bhatnagar, P.; Gupta, K.C. Oral Administration of Eudragit Coated Bromelain Encapsulated PLGA Nanoparticles for Effective Delivery of Bromelain for Chemotherapy in vivo. In Proceedings of the 2013 29th Southern Biomedical Engineering Conference, Miami, FL, USA, 3–5 May 2013; pp. 47–48.
76. Bernela, M.; Ahuja, M.; Thakur, R. Enhancement of anti-inflammatory activity of bromelain by its encapsulation in katira gum nanoparticles. *Carbohydr. Polym.* **2016**, *143*, 18–24. [CrossRef] [PubMed]
77. Esti, M.; Benucci, I.; Liburdi, K.; Garzillo, A.M.V. Immobilized pineapple stem bromelain activity in a wine-like medium: Effect of inhibitors. *Food Bioprod. Process.* **2015**, *93*, 84–89. [CrossRef]
78. Ataide, J.A.; De Carvalho, N.M.; Rebelo, M.D.A.; Chaud, M.V.; Grotto, D.; Gerenutti, M.; Rai, M.; Mazzola, P.; Jozala, A.F. Bacterial Nanocellulose Loaded with Bromelain: Assessment of Antimicrobial, Antioxidant and Physical-Chemical Properties. *Sci. Rep.* **2017**, *7*, 18031. [CrossRef]
79. Costa, S.A.; Cerón, A.A.; Petreca, B.; Costa, S.M. Fibers of cellulose sugarcane bagasse with bromelain enzyme immobilized to application in dressing. *SN Appl. Sci.* **2020**, *2*, 285. [CrossRef]
80. Colmenares, J.M.G.; Cuellar, J.C.R. Immobilization of bromelain on cobalt-iron magnetic nanoparticles ($CoFe_2O_4$) for casein hydrolysis. *Rev. Colomb. De Química* **2020**, *49*, 3–10 [CrossRef]
81. Benucci, I.; Liburdi, K.; Cacciotti, I.; Lombardelli, C.; Zappino, M.; Nanni, F.; Esti, M. Chitosan/clay nanocomposite films as supports for enzyme immobilization: An innovative green approach for winemaking applications. *Food Hydrocoll.* **2018**, *74*, 124–131. [CrossRef]
82. Holyavka, M.; Pankova, S.; Koroleva, V.; Vyshkvorkina, Y.; Lukin, A.; Kondratyev, M.; Artyukhov, V. Influence of UV radiation on molecular structure and catalytic activity of free and immobilized bromelain, ficin and papain. *J. Photochem. Photobiol. B: Biol.* **2019**, *201*, 111681. [CrossRef]
83. Li, X.; Yang, Z.; Peng, Y. The interaction of silver nanoparticles with papain and bromelain. *New J. Chem.* **2018**, *42*, 4940–4950. [CrossRef]
84. Song, M.-M.; Nie, H.-L.; Zhou, Y.-T.; Zhu, L.-M.; Bao, J.-Y. Affinity Adsorption of Bromelain on Reactive Red 120 Immobilized Magnetic Composite Particles. *Sep. Sci. Technol.* **2011**, *46*, 473–482. [CrossRef]
85. Nwagu, T.N.; Ugwuodo, C.J. Stabilizing bromelain for therapeutic applications by adsorption immobilization on spores of probiotic Bacillus. *Int. J. Biol. Macro. Mol.* **2019**, *127*, 406–414. [CrossRef]

86. Croisfelt, F.M.; Ataide, J.A.; Tundisi, L.L.; Cefali, L.C.; Rebelo, M.D.A.; Sánchez, J.L.D.; da Costa, T.G.; Lima, R.; Jozala, A.F.; Chaud, M.V.; et al. Characterization of PNIPAAm-co-AAm hydrogels for modified release of bromelain. *Eur. Polym. J.* **2018**, *105*, 48–54. [CrossRef]
87. Ataide, J.A.; Cefali, L.C.; Rebelo, M.D.; Spir, L.G.; Tambourgi, E.B.; Jozala, A.F.; Chaud, M.V.; Silveira, E.; Gu, X.; Mazzola, P.G. Bromelain Loading and Release from a Hydrogel Formulated Using Alginate and Arabic Gum. *Planta Medica* **2017**, *83*, 870–876. [CrossRef]
88. Sharma, M.; Sharma, R. Implications of designing a bromelain loaded enteric nanoformulation on its stability and anti-inflammatory potential upon oral administration. *RSC Adv.* **2018**, *8*, 2541–2551. [CrossRef]
89. Sharma, M.; Chaudhary, D. Exploration of bromelain laden nanostructured lipid carriers: An oral platform for bromelain delivery in rheumatoid arthritis management. *Int. J. Pharm.* **2021**, *594*, 120176. [CrossRef] [PubMed]
90. Sullivan, G.; Calkins, C. Application of exogenous enzymes to beef muscle of high and low-connective tissue. *Meat Sci.* **2010**, *85*, 730–734. [CrossRef]
91. Chaurasiya, R.S.; Sakhare, P.Z.; Bhaskar, N.; Hebbar, H.U. Efficacy of reverse micellar extracted fruit bromelain in meat tenderization. *J. Food Sci. Technol.* **2014**, *52*, 3870–3880. [CrossRef] [PubMed]
92. Jun-Hui, X.; Hui-Juan, C.; Bin, Z.; Hui, Y. The mechanistic effect of bromelain and papain on tenderization in jumbo squid (Dosidicus gigas) muscle. *Food Res. Int.* **2020**, *131*, 108991. [CrossRef]
93. Tanabe, S.; Arai, S.; Watanabe, M. Modification of Wheat Flour with Bromelain and Baking Hypoallergenic Bread with Added Ingredients. *Biosci. Biotechnol. Biochem.* **1996**, *60*, 1269–1272. [CrossRef] [PubMed]
94. Li-Chan, E.C.Y.; Hunag, S.-L.; Jao, C.-L.; Ho, K.-P.; Hsu, K.-C. Peptides Derived from Atlantic Salmon Skin Gelatin as Dipeptidyl-peptidase IV Inhibitors. *J. Agric. Food Chem.* **2012**, *60*, 973–978. [CrossRef]
95. Choi, W.M.; Lam, C.L.; Mo, W.Y.; Wong, M.H. Upgrading food wastes by means of bromelain and papain to enhance growth and immunity of grass carp (*Ctenopharyngodon idella*). *Environ. Sci. Pollut. Res.* **2015**, *23*, 7186–7194. [CrossRef]
96. Italiano, G.; Raimondo, M.; Giannetti, G.; Gargiulo, A. Benefits of a Food Supplement Containing Boswellia serrata and Bromelain for Improving the Quality of Life in Patients with Osteoarthritis: A Pilot Study. *J. Altern. Complement. Med.* **2020**, *26*, 123–129. [CrossRef]
97. Mo, W.Y.; Man, Y.B.; Wong, M.H. Soybean dreg pre-digested by enzymes can effectively replace part of the fishmeal included in feed pellets for rearing gold-lined seabream. *Sci. Total. Environ.* **2020**, *704*, 135266. [CrossRef]
98. Sarkar, S.; Ahmed, M.; Mohammad, H.; Science, D.; Mozumder, R.; Saeid, A. Isolation and Characterization of Bromelain Enzyme from Pineapple and Its Utilization as Anti-Browning Agent. *Process Eng. J.* **2017**, *1*, 52–58.
99. dos Anjos, M.M.; da Silva, A.A.; de Pascoli, I.C.; Mikcha, J.M.G.; Machinski, M.; Peralta, R.M.; Filho, B.A.A. Antibacterial activity of papain and bromelain on Alicyclobacillus spp. *Int. J. Food Microbiol.* **2016**, *216*, 121–126. [CrossRef] [PubMed]
100. Chen, X.; Wang, X.; Wang, S.; Zhang, X.-H.; Yu, J.; Wang, C. Mussel-inspired polydopamine-assisted bromelain immobilization onto electrospun fibrous membrane for potential application as wound dressing. *Mater. Sci. Eng. C* **2020**, *110*, 110624. [CrossRef] [PubMed]
101. Rosenberg, L.; Krieger, Y.; Bogdanov-Berezovski, A.; Silberstein, E.; Shoham, Y.; Singer, A.J. A novel rapid and selective enzymatic debridement agent for burn wound management: A multi-center RCT. *Burns* **2014**, *40*, 466–474. [CrossRef]
102. Bayat, S.; Zabihi, A.R.; Farzad, S.A.; Movaffagh, J.; Hashemi, E.; Arabzadeh, S.; Hahsemi, M. Evaluation of Debridement Effects of Bromelain-Loaded Sodium Alginate Nanoparticles Incorporated into Chitosan Hydrogel in Animal Models. *Iran. J. Basic Med. Sci.* **2021**, *24*, 1404–1412. [CrossRef]
103. Hu, W.; Wang, A.-M.; Wu, S.-Y.; Zhang, B.; Liu, S.; Gou, Y.-B.; Wang, J.-M. Debriding Effect of Bromelain on Firearm Wounds in Pigs. *J. Trauma: Inj. Infect. Crit. Care* **2011**, *71*, 966–972. [CrossRef]
104. Palao, J.A.-S.R. Use of a selective enzymatic debridement agent (Nexobrid®) for wound management: Learning curve. *World J. Dermatol.* **2017**, *6*, 32. [CrossRef]
105. NexoBrid: EPAR—Product Information. Available online: https://www.ema.europa.eu/en/documents/product-information/nexobrid-epar-product-information_en.pdf (accessed on 14 December 2021).
106. Liu, S.; Zhao, H.; Wang, Y.; Zhao, H.; Ma, C. Oral Bromelain for the Control of Facial Swelling, Trismus, and Pain After Mandibular Third Molar Surgery: A Systematic Review and Meta-Analysis. *J. Oral Maxillofac. Surg.* **2019**, *77*, 1566–1574. [CrossRef]
107. Shoham, Y.; Shapira, E.; Haik, J.; Harats, M.; Egozi, D.; Robinson, D.; Kogan, L.; Elkhatib, R.; Telek, G.; Shalom, A. Bromelain-based enzymatic debridement of chronic wounds: Results of a multicentre randomized controlled trial. *Wound Repair Regen.* **2021**, *19*, 899–907. [CrossRef]
108. Shoham, Y.; Krieger, Y.; Tamir, E.; Silberstein, E.; Bogdanov-Berezovsky, A.; Haik, J.; Rosenberg, L. Bromelain-based enzymatic debridement of chronic wounds: A preliminary report. *Int. Wound J.* **2018**, *15*, 769–775. [CrossRef]
109. Zharfan, R.S.; Purwono, P.B.; Mustika, A. Antimicrobial activity of pineapple (*Ananas comosus* L. Merr) extract against multidrug-resistant of pseudomonas aeruginosa: An In Vitro study. *Indones. J. Trop. Infect. Dis.* **2017**, *6*, 118–123. [CrossRef]
110. Vasconcelos, D.F.P.; Da Silva, F.R.P.; Vasconcelos, A.C.C.G.; Alves, E.H.P.; Junior, P.V.D.O.; De Oliveira, J.S. Bromelain: A potential strategy for the adjuvant treatment of periodontitis. *Dent. Hypotheses* **2016**, *7*, 88. [CrossRef]
111. Alves, E.H.P.; Carvalho, A.D.S.; Silva, F.R.P.; França, L.F.C.; Di Lenardo, D.; Vasconcelos, A.C.C.G.; Nascimento, H.M.S.; Lopes, V.L.R.; Oliveira, J.S.; Vasconcelos, D.F.P. Bromelain reduces the non-alcoholic fatty liver disease and periodontal damages caused by ligature-induced periodontitis. *Oral Dis.* **2020**, *26*, 1793–1802. [CrossRef]

112. Ordesi, P.; Pisoni, L.; Nannei, P.; Macchi, M.; Borloni, R.; Siervo, S. Therapeutic efficacy of bromelain in impacted third molar surgery: A randomized controlled clinical study. *Quintessence Int.* **2014**, *45*, 679–684. [CrossRef]
113. Raeisi, F.; Raeisi, E.; Heidarian, E.; Shahbazi-Gahroui, D.; Lemoigne, Y. Bromelain Inhibitory Effect on Colony Formation: An In Vitro Study on Human AGS, PC3, and MCF7 Cancer Cells. *J. Med. Signals Sens.* **2019**, *9*, 267–273. [CrossRef] [PubMed]
114. Dhandayuthapani, S.; Perez, H.D.; Paroulek, A.; Chinnakkannu, P.; Kandalam, U.; Jaffe, M.; Rathinavelu, A. Bromelain-Induced Apoptosis in GI-101A Breast Cancer Cells. *J. Med. Food* **2012**, *15*, 344–349. [CrossRef] [PubMed]
115. Shahbazi-Gahrouei, D.; Raeisi, E.; Raeisi, F.; Heidarian, E. Evaluation of the radiosensitizing potency of bromelain for radiation therapy of 4T1 breast cancer cells. *J. Med Signals Sens.* **2019**, *9*, 68–74. [CrossRef]
116. Bhui, K.; Tyagi, S.; Srivastava, A.K.; Singh, M.; Roy, P.; Singh, R.; Shukla, Y. Bromelain inhibits nuclear factor kappa-B translocation, driving human epidermoid carcinoma A431 and melanoma A375 cells through G2/M arrest to apoptosis. *Mol. Carcinog.* **2011**, *51*, 231–243. [CrossRef]
117. Morris, D.L.; Ehteda, A.; Moghaddam, S.M.; Akhter, J.; Pillai, K. Cytotoxic effects of bromelain in human gastrointestinal carcinoma cell lines (MKN45, KATO-III, HT29-5F12, and HT29-5M21). *Onco. Targets Ther.* **2013**, *6*, 403–409. [CrossRef] [PubMed]
118. Romano, B.; Fasolino, I.; Pagano, E.; Capasso, R.; Pace, S.; De Rosa, G.; Milic, N.; Orlando, P.; Izzo, A.A.; Borrelli, F. The chemopreventive action of bromelain, from pineapple stem (*Ananas comosus* L.), on colon carcinogenesis is related to antiproliferative and proapoptotic effects. *Mol. Nutr. Food Res.* **2014**, *58*, 457–465. [CrossRef]
119. Gani, M.B.A.; Nasiri, R.; Almaki, J.H.; Majid, F.A.A.; Marvibaigi, M.; Amini, N.; Chermahini, S.H.; Mashudin, M. In Vitro Antiproliferative Activity of Fresh Pineapple Juices on Ovarian and Colon Cancer Cell Lines. *Int. J. Pept. Res. Ther.* **2015**, *21*, 353–364. [CrossRef]
120. Majumder, D.; Debnath, R.; Nath, P.; Kumar, K.V.L.; Debnath, M.; Tribedi, P.; Maiti, D. Bromelain and *Olea europaea* L. leaf extract mediated alleviation of benzo(a)pyrene induced lung cancer through Nrf2 and NFκB pathway. *Environ. Sci. Pollut. Res.* **2021**, *28*, 47306–47326. [CrossRef]
121. Higashi, T.; Kogo, T.; Sato, N.; Hirotsu, T.; Misumi, S.; Nakamura, H.; Iohara, D.; Onodera, R.; Motoyama, K.; Arima, H. Efficient Anticancer Drug Delivery for Pancreatic Cancer Treatment Utilizing Supramolecular Polyethylene-Glycosylated Bromelain. *ACS Appl. Bio Mater.* **2020**, *3*, 3005–3014. [CrossRef]
122. Mohamad, N.E.; Abu, N.; Yeap, S.K.; Alitheen, N.B. Bromelain Enhances the Anti-tumor Effects of Cisplatin on 4T1 Breast Tumor Model In Vivo. *Integr. Cancer Ther.* **2019**, *18*, 1534735419880258. [CrossRef] [PubMed]
123. Raeisi, E.; Aazami, M.H.; Aghamiri, S.M.R.; Satari, A.; Hosseinzadeh, S.; Lemoigne, Y.; Heidarian, E. Bromelain-based chemoherbal combination effect on human cancer cells: In-vitro study on AGS and MCF7 proliferation and apoptosis. *Curr. Issues Pharm. Med. Sci.* **2020**, *33*, 155–161. [CrossRef]
124. Taşkın, A.; Tarakçıoğlu, M.; Ulusal, H.; Örkmez, M.; Taysi, S. Idarubicin-bromelain combination sensitizes cancer cells to conventional chemotherapy. *Iran. J. Basic Med. Sci.* **2019**, *22*, 1172–1178. [CrossRef] [PubMed]
125. Walker, J.A.; Cerny, F.J.; Cotter, J.R.; Burton, H.W. Attenuation of contraction-induced skeletal muscle injury by bromelain. *Med. Sci. Sports Exerc.* **1992**, *24*, 20–25. [CrossRef]
126. Kasemsuk, T.; Saengpetch, N.; Sibmooh, N.; Unchern, S. Improved WOMAC score following 16-week treatment with bromelain for knee osteoarthritis. *Clin. Rheumatol.* **2016**, *35*, 2531–2540. [CrossRef] [PubMed]
127. Thapa, R.K.; Diep, D.B.; Tønnesen, H.H. Topical antimicrobial peptide formulations for wound healing: Current developments and future prospects. *Acta Biomater.* **2020**, *103*, 52–67. [CrossRef]
128. Jenssen, H.; Hamill, P.; Hancock, R.E.W. Peptide Antimicrobial Agents. *Clin. Microbiol. Rev.* **2006**, *19*, 491–511. [CrossRef] [PubMed]
129. Wang, G. APD: The Antimicrobial Peptide Database. *Nucleic Acids Res.* **2004**, *32*, D590–D592. [CrossRef]
130. Martin, E.; Ganz, T.; Lehrer, R.I. Defensins and other endogenous peptide antibiotics of vertebrates. *J. Leukoc. Biol.* **1995**, *58*, 128–136. [CrossRef] [PubMed]
131. Tong, Z.; Ni, L.; Ling, J. Antibacterial peptide nisin: A potential role in the inhibition of oral pathogenic bacteria. *Peptides* **2014**, *60*, 32–40. [CrossRef]
132. Field, D.; Cotter, P.; Hill, C.; Ross, R. Bioengineering Lantibiotics for Therapeutic Success. *Front. Microbiol.* **2015**, *6*, 1363. [CrossRef] [PubMed]
133. Wang, Y.; Chang, R.Y.K.; Britton, W.J.; Chan, H.-K. Advances in the development of antimicrobial peptides and proteins for inhaled therapy. *Adv. Drug Deliv. Rev.* **2021**, *180*, 114066. [CrossRef] [PubMed]
134. Makhlynets, O.V.; Caputo, G.A. Characteristics and therapeutic applications of antimicrobial peptides. *Biophys. Rev.* **2021**, *2*, 011301. [CrossRef]
135. Reiners, J.; Lagedroste, M.; Gottstein, J.; Adeniyi, E.T.; Kalscheuer, R.; Poschmann, G.; Stühler, K.; Smits, S.H.J.; Schmitt, L. Insights in the Antimicrobial Potential of the Natural Nisin Variant Nisin H. *Front. Microbiol.* **2020**, *11*, 573614. [CrossRef] [PubMed]
136. Bin Hafeez, A.; Jiang, X.; Bergen, P.J.; Zhu, Y. Antimicrobial Peptides: An Update on Classifications and Databases. *Int. J. Mol. Sci.* **2021**, *22*, 11691. [CrossRef] [PubMed]
137. Dos Santos, C.A.; Dos Santos, G.R.; Soeiro, V.S.; Dos Santos, J.R.; Rebelo, M.D.A.; Chaud, M.; Gerenutti, M.; Grotto, D.; Pandit, R.; Rai, M.; et al. Bacterial nanocellulose membranes combined with nisin: A strategy to prevent microbial growth. *Cellulose* **2018**, *25*, 6681–6689. [CrossRef]

138. Aveyard, J.; Bradley, J.W.; McKay, K.; McBride, F.; Donaghy, D.; Raval, R.; D'Sa, R.A. Linker-free covalent immobilization of nisin using atmospheric pressure plasma induced grafting. *J. Mater. Chem. B* **2017**, *5*, 2500–2510. [CrossRef] [PubMed]
139. Cooper, L.E.; Li, B.; van der Donk, W.A. Biosynthesis and Mode of Action of Lantibiotics. *Compr. Nat. Prod. II* **2010**, *5*, 217–256. [CrossRef]
140. Shin, J.M.; Ateia, I.; Paulus, J.R.; Liu, H.; Fenno, J.C.; Rickard, A.H.; Kapila, Y.L. Antimicrobial nisin acts against saliva derived multi-species biofilms without cytotoxicity to human oral cells. *Front. Microbiol.* **2015**, *6*, 617. [CrossRef] [PubMed]
141. Caballero, B. (Ed.) *Encyclopedia of Food Sciences and Nutrition*, 2nd ed.; Academic Press: Cambridge, MA, USA, 2003.
142. McAuliffe, O.; Ross, R.P.; Hill, C. Lantibiotics: Structure, Biosynthesis and Mode of Action. *FEMS Microbiol. Rev.* **2001**, *25*, 285–308. [CrossRef] [PubMed]
143. Buchman, G.W.; Banerjee, S.; Hansen, J.N. Structure, Expression, and Evolution of a Gene Encoding the Precursor of Nisin, a Small Protein Antibiotic. *J. Biol. Chem.* **1988**, *263*, 16260–16266. [CrossRef]
144. Li, Q.; Montalban-Lopez, M.; Kuipers, O.P. Increasing the Antimicrobial Activity of Nisin-Based Lantibiotics against Gram-Negative Pathogens. *Appl. Environ. Microbiol.* **2018**, *84*, e00052-18. [CrossRef] [PubMed]
145. Mitchell, S.A.; Truscott, F.; Dickman, R.; Ward, J.; Tabor, A.B. Simplified lipid II-binding antimicrobial peptides: Design, synthesis and antimicrobial activity of bioconjugates of nisin rings A and B with pore-forming peptides. *Bioorganic Med. Chem.* **2018**, *26*, 5691–5700. [CrossRef] [PubMed]
146. Arnison, P.G.; Bibb, M.J.; Bierbaum, G.; Bowers, A.A.; Bugni, T.S.; Bulaj, G.; Camarero, J.A.; Campopiano, D.; Challis, G.; Clardy, J.; et al. Ribosomally synthesized and post-translationally modified peptide natural products: Overview and recommendations for a universal nomenclature. *Nat. Prod. Rep.* **2012**, *30*, 108–160. [CrossRef] [PubMed]
147. O'Sullivan, J.N.; O'Connor, P.M.; Rea, M.C.; O'Sullivan, O.; Walsh, C.J.; Healy, B.; Mathur, H.; Field, D.; Hill, C.; Ross, R.P. Nisin J, a Novel Natural Nisin Variant, Is Produced by Staphylococcus capitis Sourced from the Human Skin Microbiota. *J. Bacteriol.* **2020**, *202*, e00639-19. [CrossRef]
148. Salmieri, S.; Islam, F.; Khan, R.A.; Hossain, F.M.; Ibrahim, H.M.M.; Miao, C.; Hamad, W.Y.; Lacroix, M. Antimicrobial nanocomposite films made of poly(lactic acid)-cellulose nanocrystals (PLA-CNC) in food applications: Part A—effect of nisin release on the inactivation of Listeria monocytogenes in ham. *Cellulose* **2014**, *21*, 1837–1850. [CrossRef]
149. Gharsallaoui, A.; Oulahal, N.; Joly, C.; Degraeve, P. Nisin as a Food Preservative: Part 1: Physicochemical Properties, Antimicrobial Activity, and Main Uses. *Crit. Rev. Food Sci. Nutr.* **2016**, *56*, 1262–1274. [CrossRef]
150. Saini, S.; Sillard, C.; Belgacem, M.N.; Bras, J. Nisin anchored cellulose nanofibers for long term antimicrobial active food packaging. *RSC Adv.* **2016**, *6*, 12422–12430. [CrossRef]
151. Gedarawatte, S.T.; Ravensdale, J.T.; Al-Salami, H.; Dykes, G.A.; Coorey, R. Antimicrobial efficacy of nisin-loaded bacterial cellulose nanocrystals against selected meat spoilage lactic acid bacteria. *Carbohydr. Polym.* **2021**, *251*, 117096. [CrossRef] [PubMed]
152. Nguyen, V.; Gidley, M.; Dykes, G. Potential of a nisin-containing bacterial cellulose film to inhibit Listeria monocytogenes on processed meats. *Food Microbiol.* **2008**, *25*, 471–478. [CrossRef] [PubMed]
153. Gao, G.; Fan, H.; Zhang, Y.; Cao, Y.; Li, T.; Qiao, W.; Wu, M.; Ma, T.; Li, G. Production of nisin-containing bacterial cellulose nanomaterials with antimicrobial properties through co-culturing Enterobacter sp. FY-07 and Lactococcus lactis N8. *Carbohydr. Polym.* **2021**, *251*, 117131. [CrossRef] [PubMed]
154. Liu, W.; Hansen, J.N. Some chemical and physical properties of nisin, a small-protein antibiotic produced by Lactococcus lactis. *Appl. Environ. Microbiol.* **1990**, *56*, 2551–2558. [CrossRef] [PubMed]
155. Garcia-Gutierrez, E.; O'Connor, P.M.; Saalbach, G.; Walsh, C.; Hegarty, J.W.; Guinane, C.M.; Mayer, M.; Narbad, A.; Cotter, P. First evidence of production of the lantibiotic nisin P. *Sci. Rep.* **2020**, *10*, 3738. [CrossRef]
156. Field, D.; Begley, M.; O'Connor, P.M.; Daly, K.M.; Hugenholtz, F.; Cotter, P.D.; Hill, C.; Ross, R. Bioengineered Nisin A Derivatives with Enhanced Activity against Both Gram Positive and Gram Negative Pathogens. *PLoS ONE* **2012**, *7*, e46884. [CrossRef] [PubMed]
157. Mouritzen, M.V.; Andrea, A.; Qvist, K.; Poulsen, S.S.; Jenssen, H. Immunomodulatory potential of Nisin A with application in wound healing. *Wound Repair Regen.* **2019**, *27*, 650–660. [CrossRef]
158. Punyauppa-path, S.; Phumkhachorn, P. Nisin: Production and Mechanism of Antimicrobial Action. *Int. J. Curr. Res. Rev.* **2015**, *7*, 47–53.
159. Joo, N.E.; Ritchie, K.; Kamarajan, P.; Miao, D.; Kapila, Y.L. Nisin, an apoptogenic bacteriocin and food preservative, attenuates HNSCC tumorigenesis via CHAC 1. *Cancer Med.* **2012**, *1*, 295–305. [CrossRef]
160. Wang, P.; Wang, H.; Zhao, X.; Li, L.; Chen, M.; Cheng, J.; Liu, J.; Li, X. Antibacterial activity and cytotoxicity of novel silkworm-like nisin@PEGylated MoS_2. *Colloids Surf. B Biointerfaces* **2019**, *183*, 110491. [CrossRef]
161. Vukomanović, M.; Žunič, V.; Kunej, Š.; Jančar, B.; Jeverica, S.; Podlipec, R.; Suvorov, D. Nano-engineering the Antimicrobial Spectrum of Lantibiotics: Activity of Nisin against Gram Negative Bacteria. *Sci. Rep.* **2017**, *7*, 4324. [CrossRef]
162. Kuwano, K.; Tanaka, N.; Shimizu, T.; Nagatoshi, K.; Nou, S.; Sonomoto, K. Dual antibacterial mechanisms of nisin Z against Gram-positive and Gram-negative bacteria. *Int. J. Antimicrob. Agents* **2005**, *26*, 396–402. [CrossRef] [PubMed]
163. Naghmouchi, K.; Drider, D.; Baah, J.; Teather, R. Nisin A and Polymyxin B as Synergistic Inhibitors of Gram-positive and Gram-negative Bacteria. *Probiotics Antimicrob. Proteins* **2010**, *2*, 98–103. [CrossRef]
164. Pinilla, C.M.B.; Brandelli, A. Antimicrobial activity of nanoliposomes co-encapsulating nisin and garlic extract against Gram-positive and Gram-negative bacteria in milk. *Innov. Food Sci. Emerg. Technol.* **2016**, *36*, 287–293. [CrossRef]

165. Qian, J.; Chen, Y.; Wang, Q.; Zhao, X.; Yang, H.; Gong, F.; Guo, H. Preparation and antimicrobial activity of pectin-chitosan embedding nisin microcapsules. *Eur. Polym. J.* **2021**, *157*, 110676. [CrossRef]
166. Soto, K.M.; Iturriaga, M.H.; Loarca-Piña, G.; Luna-Barcenas, G.; Gómez-Aldapa, C.A.; Mendoza, S. Stable nisin food-grade electrospun fibers. *J. Food Sci. Technol.* **2016**, *53*, 3787–3794. [CrossRef]
167. Lopes, N.A.; Pinilla, C.M.B.; Brandelli, A. Antimicrobial activity of lysozyme-nisin co-encapsulated in liposomes coated with polysaccharides. *Food Hydrocoll.* **2019**, *93*, 1–9. [CrossRef]
168. Brum, L.F.W.; dos Santos, C.; Santos, J.H.Z.; Brandelli, A. Structured silica materials as innovative delivery systems for the bacteriocin nisin. *Food Chem.* **2022**, *366*, 130599. [CrossRef] [PubMed]
169. Dill, J.K.; Auxier, J.A.; Schilke, K.F.; McGuire, J. Quantifying nisin adsorption behavior at pendant PEO layers. *J. Colloid Interface Sci.* **2013**, *395*, 300–305. [CrossRef] [PubMed]
170. Malheiros, P.D.S.; Daroit, D.J.; da Silveira, N.P.; Brandelli, A. Effect of nanovesicle-encapsulated nisin on growth of Listeria monocytogenes in milk. *Food Microbiol.* **2010**, *27*, 175–178. [CrossRef] [PubMed]
171. Alishahi, A. Antibacterial Effect of Chitosan Nanoparticle Loaded with Nisin for the Prolonged Effect. *J. Food Saf.* **2014**, *34*, 111–118. [CrossRef]
172. Maresca, D.; De Prisco, A.; La Storia, A.; Cirillo, T.; Esposito, F.; Mauriello, G. Microencapsulation of nisin in alginate beads by vibrating technology: Preliminary investigation. *LWT* **2016**, *66*, 436–443. [CrossRef]
173. Hassan, H.; Gomaa, A.; Subirade, M.; Kheadr, E.; St-Gelais, D.; Fliss, I. Novel design for alginate/resistant starch microcapsules controlling nisin release. *Int. J. Biol. Macromol.* **2020**, *153*, 1186–1192. [CrossRef] [PubMed]
174. Bekhit, M.; Sánchez-González, L.; Ben Messaoud, G.; Desobry, S. Encapsulation of Lactococcus lactis subsp. lactis on alginate/pectin composite microbeads: Effect of matrix composition on bacterial survival and nisin release. *J. Food Eng.* **2016**, *180*, 1–9. [CrossRef]
175. Chandrasekar, V.; Coupland, J.N.; Anantheswaran, R.C. Characterization of nisin containing chitosan-alginate microparticles. *Food Hydrocoll.* **2017**, *69*, 301–307. [CrossRef]
176. Qi, X.; Poernomo, G.; Wang, K.; Chen, Y.; Chan-Park, M.B.; Xu, R.; Chang, M.W. Covalent immobilization of nisin on multi-walled carbon nanotubes: Superior antimicrobial and anti-biofilm properties. *Nanoscale* **2011**, *3*, 1874–1880. [CrossRef]
177. Hrabalikova, M.; Holcapkova, P.; Suly, P.; Sedlarik, V. Immobilization of bacteriocin nisin into a poly(vinyl alcohol) polymer matrix crosslinked with nontoxic dicarboxylic acid. *J. Appl. Polym. Sci.* **2016**, *133*, 1–10. [CrossRef]
178. Wang, H.; Guo, L.; Liu, L.; Han, B.; Niu, X. Composite chitosan films prepared using nisin and Perilla frutescense essential oil and their use to extend strawberry shelf life. *Food Biosci.* **2021**, *41*, 101037. [CrossRef]
179. Wu, C.; Wu, T.; Fang, Z.; Zheng, J.; Xu, S.; Chen, S.; Hu, Y.; Ye, X. Formation, characterization and release kinetics of chitosan/γ-PGA encapsulated nisin nanoparticles. *RSC Adv.* **2016**, *6*, 46686–46695. [CrossRef]
180. Da Silva, I.M.; Boelter, J.F.; Da Silveira, N.P.; Brandelli, A. Phosphatidylcholine nanovesicles coated with chitosan or chondroitin sulfate as novel devices for bacteriocin delivery. *J. Nanoparticle Res.* **2014**, *16*, 2479. [CrossRef]
181. Boelter, J.F.; Brandelli, A. Innovative bionanocomposite films of edible proteins containing liposome-encapsulated nisin and halloysite nanoclay. *Colloids Surf. B Biointerfaces* **2016**, *145*, 740–747. [CrossRef]
182. Karam, L.; Jama, C.; Nuns, N.; Mamede, A.-S.; Dhulster, P.; Chihib, N.-E. Nisin adsorption on hydrophilic and hydrophobic surfaces: Evidence of its interactions and antibacterial activity. *J. Pept. Sci.* **2013**, *19*, 377–385. [CrossRef] [PubMed]
183. Ibarguren, C.; Audisio, M.C.; Sham, E.L.; Müller, F.A.; Torres, E.M.F. Adsorption of Nisin on Montmorillonite: A Concentration Strategy. *J. Food Process. Preserv.* **2016**, *41*, e12788. [CrossRef]
184. Bouaziz, Z.; Djebbi, M.A.; Soussan, L.; Janot, J.-M.; Amara, A.B.H.; Balme, S. Adsorption of nisin into layered double hydroxide nanohybrids and in-vitro controlled release. *Mater. Sci. Eng. C* **2017**, *76*, 673–683. [CrossRef]
185. Auxier, J.A.; Schilke, K.F.; McGuire, J. Activity Retention after Nisin Entrapment in a Polyethylene Oxide Brush Layer. *J. Food Prot.* **2014**, *77*, 1624–1629. [CrossRef] [PubMed]
186. Behary, N.; Kerkeni, A.; Perwuelz, A.; Chihib, N.-E.; Dhulster, P. Bioactivation of PET woven fabrics using alginate biopolymer and the bacteriocin nisin. *Text. Res. J.* **2013**, *83*, 1120–1129. [CrossRef]
187. Nostro, A.; Scaffaro, R.; Ginestra, G.; D'Arrigo, M.; Botta, L.; Marino, A.; Bisignano, G. Control of biofilm formation by poly-ethylene-co-vinyl acetate films incorporating nisin. *Appl. Microbiol. Biotechnol.* **2010**, *87*, 729–737. [CrossRef] [PubMed]
188. Cunha, E.; Freitas, F.B.; Braz, B.S.; Da Silva, J.M.; Tavares, L.; Veiga, A.S.; Oliveira, M. Polyphasic Validation of a Nisin-Biogel to Control Canine Periodontal Disease. *Antibiotics* **2020**, *9*, 180. [CrossRef] [PubMed]
189. Santos, G.R.; Soeiro, V.S.; Ataide, J.A.; Lopes, A.M.; Mazzola, P.G.; Grotto, D.; Jozala, A.F. Nisin-Loaded Bacterial Cellulose: Evaluation of Its Antimicrobial Activity Stability Gabriela. *Osteoarthr. Cartil.* **2020**, *28*, 1–43. [CrossRef]
190. de Arauz, L.J.; Jozala, A.F.; Mazzola, P.G.; Penna, T.C.V. Nisin biotechnological production and application: A review. *Trends Food Sci. Technol.* **2009**, *20*, 146–154. [CrossRef]
191. Jia, W.; Wu, X.; Li, R.; Liu, S.; Shi, L. Effect of nisin and potassium sorbate additions on lipids and nutritional quality of Tan sheep meat. *Food Chem.* **2021**, *365*, 130535. [CrossRef]
192. Malvano, F.; Pilloton, R.; Albanese, D. A novel impedimetric biosensor based on the antimicrobial activity of the peptide nisin for the detection of Salmonella spp. *Food Chem.* **2020**, *325*, 126868. [CrossRef]
193. Cao, L.; Wu, J.; Xie, F.; Hu, S.; Mo, Y. Efficacy of Nisin in Treatment of Clinical Mastitis in Lactating Dairy Cows. *J. Dairy Sci.* **2007**, *90*, 3980–3985. [CrossRef] [PubMed]

194. Broadbent, J.; Chou, Y.; Gillies, K.; Kondo, J. Nisin Inhibits Several Gram-Positive, Mastitis-Causing Pathogens. *J. Dairy Sci.* **1989**, *72*, 3342–3345. [CrossRef]
195. Castelani, L.; Arcaro, J.; Braga, J.; Bosso, A.; Moura, Q.; Esposito, F.; Sauter, I.; Cortez, M.; Lincopan, N. Short communication: Activity of nisin, lipid bilayer fragments and cationic nisin-lipid nanoparticles against multidrug-resistant Staphylococcus spp. isolated from bovine mastitis. *J. Dairy Sci.* **2019**, *102*, 678–683. [CrossRef] [PubMed]
196. Fernández, L.; Delgado, S.; Herrero, H.; Maldonado, A.; Rodríguez, J.M. The Bacteriocin Nisin, an Effective Agent for the Treatment of Staphylococcal Mastitis During Lactation. *J. Hum. Lact.* **2008**, *24*, 311–316. [CrossRef]
197. Salgado-Ruiz, T.B.; Rodríguez, A.; Gutiérrez, D.; Martínez, B.; García, P.; Espinoza-Ortega, A.; Campos, A.R.M.; Lagunas-Bernabe, S.; Vicente, F.; Arriaga-Jordán, C.M. Molecular characterization and antimicrobial susceptibility of Staphylococcus aureus from small-scale dairy systems in the highlands of Central México. *Dairy Sci. Technol.* **2015**, *95*, 181–196. [CrossRef]
198. Mukherjee, R.; Jadhav, R.K.; De, U.K. Expression of L Selectin Molecule on Peripheral Leukocyte in Response to Nisin Treatment during Acute Bovine Mastitis. *Vet. Arch.* **2010**, *80*, 355–364.
199. De Kwaadsteniet, M.; Doeschate, K.; Dicks, L. Nisin F in the treatment of respiratory tract infections caused byStaphylococcus aureus. *Lett. Appl. Microbiol.* **2009**, *48*, 65–70. [CrossRef]
200. Valenta, C.; Bernkop-Schnürch, A.; Rigler, H.P. The Antistaphylococcal Effect of Nisin in a Suitable Vehicle: A Potential Therapy for Atopic Dermatitis in Man. *J. Pharm. Pharmacol.* **2011**, *48*, 988–991. [CrossRef]
201. Döşler, S.; Gerçeker, A.A. In vitro Activities of Nisin Alone or in Combination with Vancomycin and Ciprofloxacin against Methicillin-Resistant and Methicillin-Susceptible Staphylococcus aureus Strains. *Chemotherapy* **2011**, *57*, 511–516. [CrossRef]
202. Severina, E.; Severin, A.; Tomasz, A. Antibacterial efficacy of nisin against multidrug-resistant Gram- positive pathogens. *J. Antimicrob. Chemother.* **1998**, *41*, 341–347. [CrossRef]
203. Ellis, J.-C.; Ross, R.; Hill, C. Nisin Z and lacticin 3147 improve efficacy of antibiotics against clinically significant bacteria. *Futur. Microbiol.* **2019**, *14*, 1573–1587. [CrossRef]
204. Webber, J.L.; Namivandi-Zangeneh, R.; Drozdek, S.; Wilk, K.A.; Boyer, C.; Wong, E.H.H.; Bradshaw-Hajek, B.H.; Krasowska, M.; Beattie, D.A. Incorporation and antimicrobial activity of nisin Z within carrageenan/chitosan multilayers. *Sci. Rep.* **2021**, *11*, 1690. [CrossRef] [PubMed]
205. Thomas, V.M.; Brown, R.M.; Ashcraft, D.S.; Pankey, G.A. Synergistic effect between nisin and polymyxin B against pandrug-resistant and extensively drug-resistant Acinetobacter baumannii. *Int. J. Antimicrob. Agents* **2019**, *53*, 663–668. [CrossRef] [PubMed]
206. Tong, Z.; Dong, L.; Zhou, L.; Tao, R.; Ni, L. Nisin inhibits dental caries-associated microorganism in vitro. *Peptides* **2010**, *31*, 2003–2008. [CrossRef] [PubMed]
207. Radaic, A.; Ye, C.; Parks, B.; Gao, L.; Kuraji, R.; Malone, E.; Kamarajan, P.; Zhan, L.; Kapila, Y.L. Modulation of pathogenic oral biofilms towards health with nisin probiotic. *J. Oral Microbiol.* **2020**, *12*, 1809302. [CrossRef]
208. Cunha, E.; Valente, S.; Nascimento, M.; Pereira, M.; Tavares, L.; Dias, R.; Oliveira, M. Influence of the dental topical application of a nisin-biogel in the oral microbiome of dogs: A pilot study. *PeerJ* **2021**, *9*, e11626. [CrossRef]
209. Preet, S.; Bharati, S.; Panjeta, A.; Tewari, R.; Rishi, P. Effect of nisin and doxorubicin on DMBA-induced skin carcinogenesis—A possible adjunct therapy. *Tumor Biol.* **2015**, *36*, 8301–8308. [CrossRef]
210. Rana, K.; Sharma, R.; Preet, S. Augmented therapeutic efficacy of 5-fluorouracil in conjunction with lantibiotic nisin against skin cancer. *Biochem. Biophys. Res. Commun.* **2019**, *520*, 551–559. [CrossRef] [PubMed]
211. Hosseini, S.S.; Goudarzi, H.; Ghalavand, Z.; Hajikhani, B.; Rafeieiatani, Z.; Hakemi-Vala, M. Anti-proliferative effects of cell wall, cytoplasmic extract of Lactococcus lactis and nisin through down-regulation of cyclin D1 on SW480 colorectal cancer cell line. *Iran. J. Microbiol.* **2020**, *12*, 424–430. [CrossRef]
212. Tavakoli, S.; Gholami, M.; Ghorban, K.; Nojoumi, F.; Faghihloo, E.; Dadmanesh, M.; Rouzbahani, N.H. Transcriptional regulation of T-bet, GATA3, RORT, HERV-K env, Syncytin-1, microRNA-9, 192 and 205 induced by nisin in colorectal cancer cell lines (SW480, HCT116) and human peripheral blood mononuclear cell. *Gene Rep.* **2021**, *23*, 101025. [CrossRef]
213. Wu, Z.; Shi, L.; Yu, X.; Zhang, S.; Chen, G. Co-Immobilization of Tri-Enzymes for the Conversion of Hydroxymethylfurfural to 2,5-Diformylfuran. *Molecules* **2019**, *24*, 3648. [CrossRef]
214. Baronia, A.K.; Ahmed, A. Current concepts in combination antibiotic therapy for critically ill patients. *Indian J. Crit. Care Med.* **2014**, *18*, 310–314. [CrossRef] [PubMed]
215. Giacometti, A.; Cirioni, O.; Barchiesi, F.; Scalise, G. In-vitro activity and killing effect of polycationic peptides on methicillin-resistant Staphylococcus aureus and interactions with clinically used antibiotics. *Diagn. Microbiol. Infect. Dis.* **2000**, *38*, 115–118. [CrossRef]
216. Brumfitt, W.; Salton, M.R.J.; Hamilton-Miller, J.M.T. Nisin, alone and combined with peptidoglycan-modulating antibiotics: Activity against methicillin-resistant Staphylococcus aureus and vancomycin-resistant enterococci. *J. Antimicrob. Chemother.* **2002**, *50*, 731–734. [CrossRef]
217. Naghmouchi, K.; Le Lay, C.; Baah, J.; Drider, D. Antibiotic and antimicrobial peptide combinations: Synergistic inhibition of Pseudomonas fluorescens and antibiotic-resistant variants. *Res. Microbiol.* **2012**, *163*, 101–108. [CrossRef]
218. Field, D.; O'Connor, R.; Cotter, P.D.; Ross, R.P.; Hill, C. In Vitro Activities of Nisin and Nisin Derivatives Alone and In Combination with Antibiotics against Staphylococcus Biofilms. *Front. Microbiol.* **2016**, *7*, 508. [CrossRef]

219. Alves, D.; Magalhães, A.; Grzywacz, D.; Neubauer, D.; Kamysz, W.; Pereira, M.O. Co-immobilization of Palm and DNase I for the development of an effective anti-infective coating for catheter surfaces. *Acta Biomater.* **2016**, *44*, 313–322. [CrossRef]
220. ClinicalTrials.gov. Available online: https://clinicaltrials.gov/ct2/results?cond=&term=bromelain&cntry=&state=&city=&dist= (accessed on 14 December 2021).

MDPI
St. Alban-Anlage 66
4052 Basel
Switzerland
Tel. +41 61 683 77 34
Fax +41 61 302 89 18
www.mdpi.com

Pharmaceutics Editorial Office
E-mail: pharmaceutics@mdpi.com
www.mdpi.com/journal/pharmaceutics

www.ingramcontent.com/pod-product-compliance
Lightning Source LLC
LaVergne TN
LVHW070404100526
838202LV00014B/1386